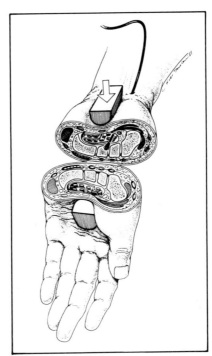

NERVE COMPRESSION SYNDROMES

Diagnosis and Treatment

Robert M. Szabo, MD

SLACK International Book Distributors

In the Europe, the Middle East and Africa.
John Wiley & Sons Limited
Baffins Lane
Chichester, West Sussex PO19 1UD
England

In Canada:
McAinsh and Company
2760 Old Leslie Street
Willowdale, Ontario M2K 2X5

In Australia and New Zealand:
MacLennan & Petty Pty Limited
P.O. Box 425
Artarmon, N.S.W. 2064
Australia

In Japan:
Central Foreign Books Limited
1-13 Jimbocho-Kanda
Tokyo, Japan

In Asia and India:
PG Publishing Pte Limited.
36 West Coast Road, #02-02
Singapore 0512

Printed in the United States of America

Library of Congress Catalog Card Number: 86-42556

ISBN: 0943432-79-0

Published by: SLACK Incorporated
6900 Grove Rd.
Thorofare, NJ 08086

Last digit is print number: 10   9   8   7   6   5   4   3   2   1

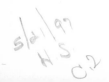

In Memoriam

This work is dedicated to the memory of my father, Gustav Szabo, M.D., and mother, Jette Szabo, to whom I owe everything.

Contents

Preface

Several studies over the past decade have distinguished nerve compression from nerve repair and regeneration as two different biological processes. Excellent textbooks are available which merge these two aspects of nerve behavior into one volume; however, more pages are devoted to the diagnosis and assessment of functional recovery, anatomic studies of internal topography, and techniques of nerve suture than to the clinical and biological problems of nerve compression. Hence, the reason for this book's existence. The first part of the volume indicates the history, pathophysiology and electrodiagnosis of nerve compression lesions. The remainder is devoted to specific clinical syndromes found both in the upper and lower extremities including the spinal column.

The contributors to this volume are some of the outstanding surgeons from throughout the world and leaders in investigation of problems related to nerve compression. Their previous work has, in a large part, been responsible for my interest and pursuit of this field. My thanks to the authors for their cooperation and their efforts, without which this book would not exist.

Special words of thanks go to Richard H. Gelberman, M.D., who has been my inspiration, and to my wife, Mary, for her understanding and support.

Acknowledgements

I would like to thank my secretary, Peggy Gunderson, for the many hours of work in helping me put together this book, and Michael Madison, M.D., Ph.D., for his help and guidance in the editing process.

Contributors

ROBERT M. SZABO, M.D., *Editor*
Associate Professor
Chief, Hand & Upper Extremity
  Service
Dept. of Orthopaedic Surgery
University of California, Davis
2230 Stockton Blvd.
Sacramento, CA 95817

MICHAEL J. BOTTE, M.D.
Assistant Professor
University of California, San Diego
Medical Center
Division of Orthopaedics & Rehab.
225 Dickinson Street
San Diego, CA 92103

TIMOTHY J. BRAY, M.D.
Assistant Clinical Professor
University of California, Davis
Reno Orthopedic Clinic
555 North Arlington Avenue
Reno, NV 89520

LARRY K. CHIDGEY, M.D.
Assistant Professor
Department of Orthopaedics
University of Florida
Box J-246, JHM Health Center
Gainesville, FL 32610

LARS B. DAHLIN, M.D., Ph.D.
Assistant Professor
Laboratory for Experimental
Biology
Department of Anatomy
University of Goteborg
Box 33031, S-400 33 Goteborg,
Sweden

STEVEN R. GARFIN, M.D.
Associate Professor
University of California, San Diego
Medical Center
Division of Orthopedics and Rehab.
225 Dickinson Street
San Diego, CA 92103

RICHARD GELBERMAN, M.D.
Professor of Orthopaedics
Chief of Upper Extremity service
Harvard University
Massachussetts General Hospital
AAC-427
Boston, MA 02114

ALAN R. HARGENS, Ph.D.
Professor of Surgery
University of California, San Diego
Chief of Space Physiology Branch
239-17, NASA-AIMS Research Center
Moffett Field, CA 94035

PATRICIA HOWSON, M.D.,
  C.M., F.R.C.S.(C)
Hand Fellow
Duke University Medical Center
P.O. Box 3000
Durham, NC 27710

RICHARD K. JOHNSON, M.D.
Professor of Anatomy
Stanford University and
San Jose State, San Jose
15215 National Avenue
Los Gatos, CA

L. ANDREW KOMAN, M.D.
Associate Professor
Section of Orthopaedics
Bowman Gray School of Medicine
300 South Hawthorne
Winston-Salem, N.C. 27103

ROSS K. LEIGHTON, B.SC., M.D.
100 Arden Street, Suite 407
Moncton, N.B., E1C 4B7
Canada

JAMES S. LIEBERMAN, M.D.
Professor and Chairman
Department of PM&R
4301 "X" Street, Room 202
Sacramento, CA 95817

PAUL R. LIPSCOMB, M.D.
Professor Emeritus
Department of Orthopaedic Surgery
University of Calif., Davis
TB 150
Davis, CA 95616

GORAN LUNDBORG, M.D.,
  Ph.D.
Professor
Department of Hand Surgery
University of Lund
Malmoł General Hospital
21401 Malmo
Sweden

ROGER MANN, M.D.
237 Estudillo Avenue
San Leandro, CA 94577

ALGIAMANTAS NARAKAS, M.D.
Associate Professor
Lausanne Medical School
Surgeon in Chief
Clinique Longeraie
9 Av de la Gare
1003 Lausanne,
Switzerland

JAMES NUNLEY, II, M.D.,
  F.A.C.S.
Assistant Professor
Department of Surgery
Duke University Medical Center
P.O. Box 2919
Durham, NC 27710

GEORGE E. OMER, M.D., M.S.,
  F.A.C.S.
Professor and Chairman
Department of Orthopaedics & Rehab.
University of New Mexico
Medical School
Albuquerque, NM 87131

CLAYTON A. PEIMER, M.D.
Associate Professor
Chief, Hand Surgery
University of Buffalo S.U.N.Y.
462 Grider Street
Buffalo, NY 14215

PAUL F. PLATTNER, M.D.
3300 Webster Street, #1200
Oakland, CA 94609

BJORN RYDEVIK, M.D., Ph.D.
Department of Orthopaedics
University of Goteborg
Sahlgren Hospital
S-413 45, Goteborg
Sweden

MORTON SPINNER, M.D.
Clinical Professor of
  Orthopaedic Surgery
Albert Einstein College of Medicine
557 Central Avenue
Cedarhurst, NY 11516

ROBERT G. TAYLOR, M.D.
*Deceased
Professor
Dept. of P.M.&R.
University of California, Davis
Medical Center
4301 "X" Street, Room 201
Sacramento, CA 95817

E. BRUCE TOBY, M.D.
Instructor, Orthopaedics
Wake Forest University
Medical Center
300 S. Hawthorne Road
Winston-Salem, NC 27103

FRANKLIN C. WAGNER, JR.,
M.D.
Professor and Chairman
Department of Neurology
University of California, Davis
Medical Center
4301 "X" Street, Room 255
Sacramento, CA 95817

DALE R. WHEELER, M.D.
Assistant Professor
Department of Orthopaedic Surgery
School of Medicine
State Univ. of New York
Buffalo, NY 14209

CHAPTER 1

Historical Perspective On Nerve Compression Syndromes

Paul R. Lipscomb, M.D.

Theoretically, any nerve root, plexus, or peripheral nerve may be subjected to continuous or intermittent pressure. Certain nerves, however, course through specific anatomic regions in which they are easily compressed. The historical aspects of the more common nerve compression syndromes will be discussed briefly in accord with the order of subsequent chapters.

Electrodiagnostic tests are most helpful in identifying and localizing the site of nerve compression. This test is accomplished by determination of the amplitude and evoked action potentials using electromyography and the comparison of nerve conduction velocity to electrical stimuli with a table of normal values. Dawson and Scott,[1] in 1949, first reported the recording of nerve action potentials through the skin in man. Others followed with descriptions of techniques and comparative studies.[2-6]

Upper Extremity

Carpal Tunnel Syndrome

In 1836, Gensoul[7] reported compression of the median nerve associated with a fracture of the radius in a girl who succumbed to tetanus. Postmortem examination revealed that the median nerve was caught between the ends of the fractured radius.

Paget[8] discussed a case of Hilton in 1854, in which the median nerve was compressed by excessive callus after a fracture of the distal radius.

In 1913, Marie and Foix[9] performed an autopsy on a patient with marked atrophy of the thenar muscles but with no history of injury. Neuromas were noted in both median nerves just proximal to the transverse carpal ligament. They were the first physicians to recommend decompression of the median nerve by sectioning the transverse carpal ligament to prevent paralysis of the thenar muscles.

The most common of all nerve compressions, the carpal tunnel syndrome, was not recognized clinically in most patients with this condition until after 1950. This was true even at the Mayo Clinic where Moersch,[10] a neurologist, in 1938 recommended section of the transverse carpal ligament in a patient with bilateral median nerve neuritis. Also, Woltman,[11] another neurologist at the Mayo Clinic, in 1941 described cases that were associated with acromegaly. Cannon and Love,[12] neurosurgeons at the same institution, in 1946 reported 38 cases of tardy median nerve palsy, but only nine of these patients were treated by sectioning of the transverse carpal ligament.

Earlier in this century, in 1905, deRouville,[13] described a pseudoneuroma in a patient who developed paralysis of the median nerve some time after a radial fracture. Following this, Blecher[14] in 1908, Kircheim[15] in 1910, Lewis and Miller[16] in 1922, Abbott and Saunders[17] in 1933, Zachary[18] in 1945, and others added information about the frequency of the carpal tunnel syndrome in association with Colles' fractures, other fractures of the distal radius, and carpal injuries. In 1949, Watson-Jones[19] reported that Léri's pleonosteosis could cause carpal tunnel syndrome.

Phalen[20] in 1949 gave a paper at the annual meeting of the American Society for Surgery of the Hand, which was published one year later entitled, "Neuropathy of the Median Nerve Due to Compression Beneath the Transverse Carpal Ligament." He stated in summary, "The authors are confident that this condition is not a rarity, as one might assume from the paucity of previous reports in the literature." In 1954, Phalen[21] described and demonstrated the wrist flexion test that now is known as Phalen's sign at the meeting of the American Society for Surgery of the Hand. It was my good fortune to hear Phalen's papers and soon I too was recognizing the condition and spreading the word to colleagues at the Mayo Clinic. Yamaguchi (a resident), Soule (a pathologist), and I[22] reported in 1963 at the American Society for Surgery of the Hand meeting a clinicopathologic study of 1215 patients with carpal tunnel syndrome seen at the Mayo Clinic from 1930 to 1960. Of the 1215 patients, 756 were observed or treated nonsurgically and 459 were treated surgically. In 1966, Phalen[23] reviewed his experience in the diagnosis and treatment of 654 hands with carpal tunnel syndrome.

There have been other reports through the years of lesions of the median nerve that were due to what is now known as the carpal tunnel syndrome. Only a few are listed.[24-29]

Ulnar Nerve Compression at the Wrist

Entrapment of the ulnar nerve at the wrist is proximal to or within the canal, or "loge" described by Guyon[30] in 1861. Hunt,[31] in 1908, provided the classic description of ulnar nerve compression. Occupational factors predisposing to the syndrome were first discussed by Worster-Drought[32] in

1929, tumorous conditions or ganglia by Seddon[33] in 1952, and fractures of the carpal and metacarpal bones by Howard[34] in 1961. Bacorn and Kurtze,[35] in 1953, reported a study of 2000 Colles' fractures and commented that in one case there was a traumatic neuritis of the ulnar nerve. Zoega,[36] in 1966, reported three cases of fracture of the lower end of the radius with ulnar nerve palsy. A case report of anomalous muscles as a cause for ulnar tunnel syndrome was reported by Salgebac[37] in 1977. Kaplan[38] first discussed variation of the ulnar nerve at the wrist in 1963.

Median Nerve Forearm Compression Syndromes

The most proximal entrapment neuropathy of the median nerve is due to compression in the distal third of the humerus beneath a supracondylar process and the ligament of Struthers.[39] Solieri[40] in 1929 reported a nineteen-year-old man who had severe paresthesia and hyperesthesia in the median nerve distribution of the hand and fingers caused by the presence of a supracondyloid process. Mandruzzato[41] reported two cases in 1938 and Barnard and McCoy[42] one in 1946. All were relieved by decompression of the median nerve and resection of the process. Other cases have been reported since.

The next potential site of compression of the median nerve is at the level of the elbow where the lacertus fibrosis courses across the nerve. The third site is within the pronator muscle as the result of hypertrophy of the muscle or by the aponeurotic fascia between the superficial and deep heads of this muscle. The fourth area of potential compression in the pronator syndrome is at the arch of the flexor digitorum superficialis muscle where the median nerve passes beneath the muscle to lie deep to and within the muscle fascia of the flexor digitorum superficialis. Seyffarth[43] in 1951 published a paper describing primary abnormalities in the pronator teres muscle as cause of the pronator syndrome.

Cubital Tunnel Syndrome

Panas[44] in 1878 described for the first time the condition that is now known as *tardy ulnar palsy*. Entrapment of the ulnar nerve as it passes behind the medial epicondyle of the humerus may be associated with recurrent dislocation of the nerve, which was discussed by Collinet[45] in 1896 and then by Cobb[46] and Momberg,[47] both in 1903. Platt[48] in 1926 wrote on the pathogenesis and treatment of traumatic neuritis of the ulnar nerve in the postcondylar groove. There have been other publications discussing entrapment, not only at the level of the medial epicondyle, but also by the aponeurosis between the heads of the flexor carpi ulnaris and in the muscle itself.[49-52]

Radial Tunnel Syndrome

Compression neuropathies of the radial nerve along its course in the arm above the elbow occur at the site of the lateral intermuscular septum and are comparatively infrequent. The most common entrapment neuropathy of the radial nerve, the radial tunnel syndrome, occurs in its course from the level of the radial head to the supinator muscle and was first described as the radial tunnel syndrome by Roles and Maudsley[53] in 1972. After this report and that by Lister, Belsole and Kleinert[54] in 1979, many cases of "intractable tennis elbow" have been relieved by decompression of the radial nerve and its divisions (the superficial branch and the posterior interosseous nerve) in the radial tunnel, which includes the arcade of Frohse.[55]

A compression neuropathy of the superficial branch of the radial nerve distal to its exit from the radial tunnel and along its course in the forearm and wrist is relatively uncommon and was described by Wartenberg[56] in 1932.

Lateral Antebrachial Nerve Compression

Entrapment of the peripheral sensory portion (the lateral antebrachial nerve) of the musculocutaneous nerve at the elbow was first described by Bassett and Nunley[57] in 1982. Four of 11 patients responded to nonoperative management and seven to surgical decompression.

Thoracic Outlet Syndrome

Compression neuropathies of the brachial plexus are usually included in the term **thoracic outlet syndrome** which is used to designate a spectrum of signs and symptoms resulting from the neurovascular structures in the interval between the intervertebral foramina and the axilla.[58]

Coute[59] in 1861, described the removal of an "exostosis" which was thought to arise from the transverse process of the seventh cervical vertebra, which was surrounded by blood vessels and nerves.[60] It is probable that the "exostosis" was a cervical rib that was causing what we now designate the thoracic outlet syndrome. In 1907, Keen[61] published a paper entitled, "The Symptomatology, Diagnosis and Surgical Treatment of Cervical Ribs." In 1935, Ochsner, Gage, and DeBakey[62] first wrote on the scalenus anticus syndrome, and in 1947 Adson[63] published a paper entitled, "Surgical Treatment for Symptoms Produced by Cervical Ribs and the Scalenus Anticus Muscle." Bonney[64] in 1965 published a paper, "The Scalenus Medius Band: A Contribution to the Study of the Thoracic Outlet Syndrome," and made it clear that the 13 cases he discussed were due to compression of the lower trunk of the brachial plexus and were distinct from the vascular syndrome in which symptoms are produced by direct affection of the subclavian artery.

Neurovascular structures passing from the thorax may also be compressed by the pectoralis minor at its attachment to the coracoid.[65]

Nerve Compression in the Spinal Column

Anterior displacement of a vertebral body on the adjacent caudal segment of the spine was described in 1855 by Rokitansky[66] and the term, "spondylolisthesis" (slipped vertebra) was coined by Neugeberger.[67] Killian[68] in 1854, pointed out its clinical significance as a barrier to normal delivery in the obstetrical patient. Since that time the literature on the subject has become extensive.[69]

In 1934, Mixter and Barr[70] first described the syndrome of the ruptured intervertebral disc in the lumbar spine.

Semmes and Murphy[71] in 1943 reported four cases of unilateral rupture of the sixth cervical intervertebral disc with compression of the seventh cervical root and symptoms simulating coronary disease.

The first description of spinal stenosis relieved by laminectomy was by Sachs and Fraenkel[72] in 1900. Bailly and Casamajor[73] in 1911 and Elsberg[74] in 1913 described similar pathologic findings and relief following surgery. The syndrome was not widely diagnosed until Verbiest[75] in 1954 described the classic findings in middle-aged and older adults.

Ruptures of thoracic discs, which are infrequent, have been discussed by Young,[76] Love and Kiefer,[77] Arseni and Nash,[78] and Simmons.[79]

Spine and Pelvis

Lumbosacral and Sciatic Nerve Compression Syndromes

Tumors within the pelvis, compressing the lumbosacral segments of the sciatic nerve, are difficult to differentiate from a sciatic neuritis or a sciatica of intraspinal origin.[80] Also, it has long been known that sciatic palsy is frequently associated with fractures of the pelvis, dislocations of the hip, and space-occupying lesions in the buttock and thigh along the course of the sciatic nerve.

Casagrande and Danahy[81] in 1971 described a case of delayed sciatic nerve entrapment following the use of self-curing acrylic seven months after a total hip replacement. Dorr, Conaty, and Harvey[82] in 1974 reported a case of a false aneurysm of the femoral artery following a total hip surgery that caused sciatic palsy nine months following the operation. Apparently a spur of methyl methacrylate caused a late perforation of the artery.

Kaufman and Bok[83] in 1972 reported the case of a patient with a sickle cell trait who developed a large mass in the buttock that produced a partial sciatic nerve palsy. At surgery the mass was associated with necrosis of the gluteus minimus and piriformis muscles and compression of the sciatic nerve.

Miller and associates[84] in 1974 reported the case of a patient with sciatic palsy occurring eight weeks after a pelvic fracture caused by an aneurysm of the gluteal artery. This was excised one week later and the foot drop cleared.

Meralgia Paresthetica

The lateral femoral cutaneous nerve is formed from the roots of L2 and L3. It exits the pelvis under the inguinal ligament, deep and just medial to the anterior superior iliac spine. Compression there or as it passes over the sartorious muscle causes the syndrome which was reported by Bernhardt[85] in 1895. Musser and Sailer,[86] in 1940, reported ten cases. Cohen,[87] in 1946 reported a case due to an abnormal fibrous band, which on microscopic study proved to be caused by trichinosis. Edelson,[88] in 1975 reported that 51 percent of adult cadavers had a significant enlargement—pseudoganglion—in the lateral femoral cutaneous nerve where it passed under the inguinal ligament to turn sharply downward into the thigh.

Obturator Nerve

The obturator nerve is formed by union of the anterior divisions of the L2, L3, and L4 roots. It decends through the pelvis posterior to the common iliac vessels and exits through the obturator foramen. I recall two patients before the antibiotic era who had osteomyelitis involving the pubis and ischium and associated adduction contracture of the extremity with scarring and compression of the obturator nerve in the foramen. Both were cured by resection of the decending ramus of the pubis, the ascending ramus of the ischium, and the obturator nerve.

Femoral Nerve

The femoral nerve is formed by union of the posterior divisions of L2, L3, and L4 roots. It is lateral to the femoral artery as it enters the thigh. Femoral compression neuropathies have been reported in hemorrhagic disorders and following arterial punctures in anticoagulated patients.[89-91] Compression of the femoral nerve in the thigh is relatively uncommon but may result from pressure due to lipomas, other larger tumors, and cysts.

Pudendal Nerve

Aboulker and associates[92] in 1974 reported three cases of pudendal nerve neurapraxia as a complication of traction on the fracture table. Since then, there have been similar reports by Schulak and associates,[93] Hoffman and associates[94] and Lindenbaum and associates.[95] It was agreed that pressure on the perineal nerve as a result of positioning against the perineal post was an etiologic factor. It was also agreed that pudendal nerve neurapraxia can frequently be a preventable complication of operative treatment of hip and femoral shaft fractures.

Lower Extremity

Common Peroneal Nerve

Compression neuropathies of the peroneal nerve are relatively uncommon when compared with traction injuries associated with fractures, ligamentous injuries, and dislocations of the knee. Because of its superficial position, pressure on the peroneal nerve by external hard objects makes it more susceptible to neurapraxia than the tibial nerve. Cross-leg palsy is not uncommon. In the past, pressure from improperly molded plaster casts was responsible for a number of palsies of the common peroneal nerve. Also, years ago I occasionally saw a patient with peroneal palsy due to pressure from huge popliteal cysts.

Sultan,[96] in 1921 was the first to report compression of the peroneal nerve by a ganglion. Wadstein,[97] in 1931 thought the ganglia arose in the sheaths of the peroneal nerve in the two cases he discussed. Likewise, Ellis,[98] in 1936 reported two cases of ganglia in the sheath of peroneal nerves. Similar reports followed from Ferguson[99] in 1937, Clark[100] and Parkes[101], both in 1961.

Brooks,[102] in 1952 described 13 cases of nerve compression due to ganglion. In three of these, the ganglion definitely arose from the superior tibiofibular joint. He suggested that ganglia of nerve sheaths and simple ganglia were anatomic variants of the same entity.

Barber, Bianco, Soule, and MacCarty[103] of the Mayo Clinic in a 1962 report, "Benign Extraneural Soft-tissue Tumors of the Extremities Causing Compression of Nerves," noted that in 32 cases there were five ganglion cysts involving peroneal nerves, three the ulnar nerve and one the median nerve. Three years later, Stack, Bianco, and MacCarty[104] added four cases involving the peroneal nerve to the Mayo Clinic series when they reported on nine patients who had been treated for involvement of the common peroneal nerve by a ganglion cyst since 1934.

Maudsley[105] in 1967 described nine patients with pain down the lateral side of the leg due to a tight crescentic band that constricted the peroneal nerve at the origin of the peroneus longus. He called this the **fibular tunnel syndrome**.

Mangieri,[106] in 1973 reported a case of peroneal nerve compression from an enlarged fabella. Excision resulted in cure. Yamahiro[107] of Tokyo reported a similar case in 1967.

Sural Nerve

Pringle, Prothero, and Mukherjee[108] in 1974 reported four cases of sural nerve entrapment at the lateral side of the foot and ankle. Two of the entrapments were associated with a ganglion. One occurred following an injury to the foot; at operation when the sural nerve was exposed on the lateral side of the foot, a thickened band of soft tissue was found across the nerve, compressing it. In the fourth patient no clear abnormality was noted at the time the sural nerve was freed from the surrounding tissues on the lateral side of the foot. Nevertheless, she gained and maintained complete relief of her preoperative symptoms, which had been present for several months.

Tibial Nerve Compression in the Tarsal Tunnel

The tarsal tunnel syndrome was first described in 1932 by Pollock and Davis.[109] In 1960, Kopell and Thompson[110] reviewed the mechanisms by which nerves, including the tibial, are compressed in the lower extremity.

Two isolated cases of the tarsal tunnel syndrome with compression of the tibial nerve or its branches on the medial side of the ankle and foot were described by Keck[111] and Lam[112] in 1962. Additional cases were reported by Kojima[113] in 1963 and McGill[114] in 1964. In 1967 Lam[115] reviewed 10 cases in an excellent article. Edwards and associates[116] in 1969 described the pathogenesis and symptoms of the syndrome. In 1975, at the annual meeting of the Western Orthopedic Association, Mann[117] reported on 20 cases of the tarsal tunnel syndrome.

Janecki and Dovberg[118] in 1977 reported a case of tarsal tunnel syndrome that was due originally to a neurilemoma of the medial plantar nerve. The posterior tibial nerve was found to have bifurcated into the medial and lateral plantar nerves well above the ankle. After removal of the 5 mm diameter tumor, the patient was relieved of symptoms for one year, at which time they recurred. The operative site was reexplored and the medial plantar nerve was decompressed and placed in a bed of adipose tissue. The patient remained asymptomatic when last contacted two years later.

Garcia and associates[119] reported on 56 cases of tarsal tunnel syndrome at the combined meeting of the British and Spanish Orthopaedic Associations in 1978. In this series there was a high frequency of the syndrome following fractures of the os calcis. Wileman[120] in 1979 reported on two cases of tarsal tunnel syndrome and a 50-year survey of the world literature.

Plantar Digital Neuroma (Morton's Toe)

Morton of Philadelphia[121] in 1876 in a classic paper described the symptoms of the typical plantar neuroma but did not recognize the true etiology. It was not until 1940 that Betts[122] of Adelaide, Australia reported a series of 19 patients in each of whom the common plantar digital nerve to the third and fourth toes was exposed through a longitudinal incision in the sole of the foot. In every case what we now call a plantar neuroma was found and excised. In all, the pain was relieved and in none was there trouble from the scar. W.J. Betts[123] stated that his father thought the condition was due to pressure on the nerve by the transverse metatarsal ligament.

McElvenny[124] in 1943 reported a series in which 12 nerve tumors were removed from 11 patients. In five the tumors were studied microscopically and appeared to be either neurofibromata or angioneurofibromata. McElvenny stated that the incision on the sole of the foot was far inferior to the dorsal web-splitting approach.

Watson Jones[125] in 1949 reported that Léri's pleonosteosis could be a cause of Morton's metatarsalgia.

Most authors[126-128] have found the neuroma to be far more frequent in the common digital nerve between the bases of the third and fourth toes. This nerve is formed from the lateral branch of the medial plantar nerve and the communicating branch of the lateral plantar nerve. The latter branch is absent in some individuals.

Baker and Kuhn[129] in 1944 and Winkler and associates[130] in 1948 determined that the etiologic conception of the syndrome is essentially that which was proposed by Betts and that the marked fusiform thickening of the nerve was degenerative in nature, trauma being its most probable cause.

Hauser[131] found the "neuroma" between the second and third metatarsal heads in 52 percent of 100 patients with 116 lesions. This has not been the experience of other authors.

McKeever[132] in 1952 emphasized the superiority of the dorsal web-splitting incision and described the technique, which is done quickly through an incision one inch in length.

As this historical perspective began with discussion of the most common nerve compression syndrome in the upper extremity, the carpal tunnel syndrome, it is appropriate that this chapter ends with the most common nerve compression syndrome in the lower extremity, the plantar neuroma.

References

1. Dawson GD, Scott JW: Recording of nerve action potentials through skin in man. J Neurosurg Psychiatry 12:259, 1949.
2. Buchthal F, Rosenfalck A: Evoked potentials and conduction velocity in human sensory nerves. Brain Res 3:1, 1966.
3. Melvin JL, Harris DH, Johnson EW: Sensory and motor conduction velocities in the ulnar and median nerves. Arch Phys Med Rehabil 47:511, 1966.
4. Goodgold J: Anatomical correlates of clinical electromygraphy. Baltimore: Williams and Wilkins, 1974, p 62.
5. Buchthal F, Rosenfalck A, Trojaborg W: Electrophysiological findings in entrapment of the median nerve at wrist and elbow. J Neurol Neurosurg Psychiatry 37:340, 1974.
6. Goodgold J, Eberstein A: Electrodiagnosis of neuromuscular diseases. Ed 2. Baltimore: Williams and Wilkins, 1978, p 97.
7. Gensoul, quoted by Lobert M: Observation et réflexions sur une complication grave des fractures. Arch Gen Med 41:198, 1836.
8. Paget J: Lectures on surgical pathology. Ed 1. Philadelphia: Lindsay and Blakiston, 1854, p 42.
9. Marie P, Foix C: Atrophie isole de l'éminence thènar d'origine névritiquè: rôle du ligament annulaire antérieur du carpe dans la pathogènie de la lèsion. Rev Neurol 26:647, 1913.
10. Moersch FP: Median thenar neuritis. Proc Staff Meet Mayo Clinic 13:220, 1938.
11. Woltman HW: Neuritis associated with acromegaly. Arch Neurol Psychiatry 45:680, 1941.
12. Cannon BW, Love JG: Tardy median palsy: Median neuritis: Median thenar neuritis amenable to surgery. Surgery 20:210, 1946.
13. deRouville G: Section du nerf radial: suture secondaire et guérison. Bull Soc Chir Paris 32:1046, (Dec) 1905.
14. Blecher S: Die schädigung des nervus medianus als komplikation des typischen radiusbruches. Deutsch Z Chir 93:34, 1908.
15. Kircheim GWT: Ueber verletzungen des N. medianus bei fractura radii an klassicher stelle. Thesis, Friedrich-Wilhelm Universitaet Zee Berlin: G Schade, 1910, 30 p.
16. Lewis D, Miller EM: Peripheral nerve injuries associated with fractures. Trans Amer Surg Assoc 40:489, 1922.
17. Abbott LC, Saunders JB deC: Injuries of the median nerve in fractures of the lower end of the radius. Surg Gynecol Obstet 57:507, 1933.
18. Zachary RB: Thenar palsy due to compression of the median nerve in the carpal tunnel. Surg Gynecol Obstet 81:213, 1945.
19. Watson-Jones R: Léri's pleonosteosis, carpal tunnel compression and Morton's metatarsalgia. J Bone Joint Surg 31B:560, 1949.

20. Phalen GS, Gardner WJ, LaLonde AA: Neurpathy of the median nerve due to compression beneath the transverse carpal ligament. J Bone Joint Surg 32A:109, 1950.

21. Phalen GS: Spontaneous compression of the median nerve at the wrist. Proceedings, Am Soc Surg of the Hand. J Bone Joint Surg 36A:663, 1954.

22. Yamaguchi DM, Lipscomb PR, Soule EH: Carpal tunnel syndrome. Minn Med 48:22, 1965.

23. Phalen GS: The carpal tunnel syndrome: Seventeen years' experience in diagnosis and treatment of 654 hands. J Bone Joint Surg 48A:211, 1966.

24. Hartwell AS: Cystic tumor of median nerve: Operation: Restoration of function. Boston: Med Surg J 144:582, 1901.

25. Cannon BW, Love JG: Tardy median palsy; Median neuritis; Median thenar neuritis amenable to surgery. Surgery 20:210, 1946.

26. Goodman HV, Gilliat RW: The effect of treatment on median nerve conduction in patients with the carpal tunnel syndrome. Ann Phys Med 6:137, 1961.

27. Lynch AC, Lipscomb PR: The carpal tunnel syndrome and Colles' fractures. JAMA 185:363, 1963.

28. Salgebac S: Ulnar tunnel syndrome caused by anomalous muscles. Case report. Scand J Plast Reconstr Surg 11:255, 1977.

29. Eversmann WW: Entrapment and compression neuropathies. *In* Green DP (ed): Operative Hand Surgery. New York: Churchill Livingstone, 1982, pp 957.

30. Guyon F: Note sur une disposition anatomique propre á la face antérieure de la région du poignet et non encores décrite par le docteur. Bull Soc Anat Paris, 2nd series 6:184, 1861.

31. Hunt JR: Occupation neuritis of the deep palmar branch of the ulnar nerve. A well defined clinical type of professional palsy of the hand. J Nerv Ment Dis 35:673, 1908.

32. Worster-Drought C: Pressure neuritis of the deep palmar branch of the ulnar nerve. Br Med J 1:247, 1929.

33. Seddon HJ: Carpal ganglion as a cause of paralysis of the deep branch of the ulnar nerve. J Bone Joint Surg 34B:386, 1952.

34. Howard FM: Ulnar nerve palsy in wrist fractures. J Bone Joint Surg 43A:1197, 1961.

35. Bacorn RW, Kurtze JF: Colles' fracture: A study of two thousand cases from the New York State Workmen's Compensation Board. J Bone Joint Surg 35A:643, 1953.

36. Zoega H: Fracture of the lower end of the radius with ulnar nerve palsy. J Bone Joint Surg 48B:514, 1966.

37. Salgebac S: Ulnar tunnel syndrome caused by anomalous muscles. Case report. Scand J Plast Reconstr Surg 11:255, 1977.

38. Kaplan EB: Variation of the ulnar nerve at the wrist. Bull Hosp Joint Dis 24:85, 1963.

39. Struthers J: Anatomical and physiological observations. Part 1. Edinburgh: Sutherland & Knox, 1854.

40. Solieri S: Neuralgia del nervo mediano da processo sopraepitrocleare. Chir d Org di Movimento 4:171, 1929.

41. Mandruzzato F: Patologia e chiurgia del processo sopraepitrocleare dell'omero. Chi d Org di Movimento 24:123, 1938.

42. Barnard LB, McCoy SM: The supracondyloid process of the humerus. J Bone Joint Surg 28:845, 1946.

43. Seyffarth HJ: Primary myoses in the M. pronator teres as cause of lesion of the N. medianus (the pronator syndrome). Acta Psychiatr Neurol (suppl) 74:251, 1951.

44. Panas J: Sur une cause peu connue de paralysie du nerf cubital. Arch Gén de Méd 2:5, 1878.

45. Collinet P: Luxation congenital du nerf cubital. Bull Soc Anat Paris 79:358, 1896.

46. Cobb F: Recurrent dislocation of the ulnar nerve. Ann Surg 21:652, 1903.

47. Momberg: Die luxation des nervus ulnaris. Arch f Klin Chir 70:215, 1903.

48. Platt H: The pathogenesis and treatment of traumatic neuritis of the ulnar nerve in the postcondylar groove. Br J Surg 13:409, 1926.

49. Davidson AJ, Horwitz MT: Late or tardy ulnar nerve paralysis. J Bone Joint Surg 17:224, 1911.

50. Adson AW: The surgical treatment of progressive ulnar paralysis. Minn Med 1:445, 1918.

51. Gay JR, Love JG: Diagnosis and treatment of tardy paralysis of the ulnar nerve. J Bone Joint Surg 29:1087, 1947.

52. Barber KW Jr, Bianco AJ Jr, Soule EH, MacCarty CS: Benign extraneural soft-tissue tumors of the extremities causing compression of nerves. J Bone Joint Surg 44A:98, 1962.

53. Roles NC, Maudsley RH: Radial tunnel syndrome. Resistant tennis elbow as a nerve entrapment. J Bone Joint Surg 54B:499, 1972.

54. Lister GD, Belsole RB, Kleinert HE: The radial tunnel syndrome. J Hand Surg 4:52, 1979.

55. Frohse F, Frankel M: Die muskeln des menschlichen armes. *In* Bardeleben's Handbuch der Anatomie des Menschlichen. Jena, Fisher, 1908, pp 164.

56. Wartenberg R: Cheiralgia paresthetica (isolierte neuritis des ramus superficialis nervi radialis). Z Ges Neurol Psychiatr 141:145, 1932.

57. Bassett EH, Nunley JA: Compression of the musculocutaneous nerve at the elbow. J Bone Joint Surg 64A:1050, 1982.

58. Leffert RD: Lesions of the brachial plexus including thoracic outlet syndrome. AAOS Instructional Course Lectures, 26:77, St. Louis: C.V. Mosby, 1977.

59. Coute H: Exostosis of the left transverse process of the seventh cervical vertebra surrounded by blood vessels and nerves: Successful removal. Lancet 1:360, 1861.

60. Roos DB, Owen JC: Thoracic outlet syndrome. Arch Surg 93:71, 1966.

61. Keen WW: The symptomatology, diagnosis and surgical treatment of cervical ribs. Am J Med Sci 133:173, 1907.

62. Ochsner A, Gage M, DeBakey M: Scalenus anticus syndrome. Am J Surg 28:669, 1935.

63. Adson AW: Surgical treatment for symptoms produced by cervical ribs and the scalenus anticus muscle. Surg Gynec Obstet 85:687, 1947.

64. Bonney G: The scalenus medius band. A contribution to the study of the thoracic outlet syndrome. J Bone Joint Surg 47B:268, 1965.

65. Wright PE, Simmons JCH: Brachial plexus compression syndrome. *In* Campbell's Operative Orthopaedics, 6th ed. St. Louis: C.V. Mosby Co., 1980, p 1675.

66. Rokitansky C: Lehrbuch der pathologischen anatomie. Wien: Braumüller, 1855. (English translation by WE Swaine, Edward Sievking, Otto Moore and GE Day. Philadelphia: Blanchard and Ler.)

67. Neuberger FL: Entwicklungsgeschichte des spondylolesthetischen beckens und seiner diagnose (mit beruckichtigung von Korperhaltung und Gangspur). Casuistischkritische Monographie. Halle, Max Niemeyer, 1882.

68. Killian HF: De spondylolisthesi gravissimae pelvangustiae caussa nupe detecta. Commentatio anatomica—obstetrica. Bonn: Lit. C. Georgii, 1854.

69. Barr JS: Editorial: Spondylolisthesis. J Bone Joint Surg 37A:878, 1955.

70. Mixter WJ, Barr JS: Rupture of the intervertebral disc with involvement of the spinal canal. N Engl J Med 211:210, 1934.

71. Semmes RE, Murphy F: The syndrome of unilateral rupture of the sixth cervical intervertebral disc, with compression of the seventh cervical root: Report of four cases with symptoms simulating coronary disease. JAMA 121:1209, 1943.

72. Sachs B, Fraenkel J: Progressive and kyphotic rigidity of the spine (spondylorhizomelique). J Nerv Ment Dis 27:1, 1900.

73. Bailly P, Casamajor L: Osteoarthritis of the spine as a cause of compression of the spinal cord and its roots with reports of 5 cases. J Nerv Ment Dis 38:588, 1911.

74. Elsberg CA: Experiences in spinal surgery: Observations upon 60 laminectomies for spinal disease. Surg Gynecol Obstet 16:117, 1913.

75. Verbiest H: A radicular syndrome from developmental narrowing of the lumbar vertebral canal. J Bone Joint Surg 36B:230, 1954.

76. Young JH: Cervical and thoracic intervertebral disc disease. Med J Aust 2:833, 1946.

77. Love JG, Kiefer E Jr: Root pain and paraplegia due to protrusion of thoracic intervertebral discs. J Neurosurg 15:62, 1950.

78. Arseni C, Nash F: Protrusion of thoracic intervertebral discs. Acta Neurochir 11:1, 1963.

79. Simmons JCH: Rupture of intervertebral discs. *In* The Spine, Campbell's Operative Orthopaedics, 6th Ed. St. Louis: C.V. Mosby Co., 1980.

80. Cramer F: Sciatica and the sciatic nerve. *In* Howorth MB, A Textbook of Orthopedics. Published by author, Stanford, Connecticut, 1959, p 982.

81. Casagrande PA, Danahy PR: Delayed sciatic nerve entrapment following the use of self curing acrylic. J Bone Joint Surg 53A:167, 1971.

82. Dorr LD, Conaty RK, Harvey JP: False aneurysm of the femoral artery following total hip surgery. J Bone Joint Surg 56A:1059, 1974.

83. Kaufman G, Bok C: Ischemic necrosis of muscles of the buttock. J Bone Joint Surg 54A:1079.

84. Miller JW, Stuart ME, Tytus JS, et al: Gluteal artery aneurysms. J Bone Joint Surg 56A:620, 1974.

85. Bernhardt M: Ueber isolirt im gebeite des N. cutaneous femoris externus vorkommende parasthesien. Neurol Centralbl 14:242, 1895.

86. Musser JH, Sailer J: Meralgia paresthetica with the report of ten cases. J Nerv Ment Dis 17:16, 1900.

87. Cohen HB: Trichinosis as a cause of meralgia paresthetica. J Bone Joint Surg 28:153, 1946.

88. Edelson EG: Meralgia paresthetica: An anatomical interpretation. Proceedings, J Bone Joint Surg 58A:284, 1976.

89. Kettlecamp DB, Powers SR: Femoral compression neuropathy in hemorrhagic disorders. Arch Surg 98:367, 1969.

90. Spiegel PG, Meltzer JL: Femoral nerve neuropathy secondary to anticoagulation: Report of a case. J Bone Joint Surg 56A:425, 1974.

91. Neviaser RJ, Adams JP, May GI: Complications of arterial puncture in anticoagulated patients. J Bone Joint Surg 58A:218, 1976.

92. Aboulker P, Benassayag E, Steg A: Les traumatismes due perinee par traction sur table orthopedique avec pelvi-support (3 observations). Rev Chir Orthop 60:165, 1974.

93. Schulak DJ, Bear TF, Summers JL: Transient impotence from positioning on the fracture table. J Trauma 20:420, 1980.

94. Hoffman A, Jones RE, Schoenvogel R: Pudendal-nerve neurapraxia as a result of traction on the fracture table: A report of four cases. J Bone Joint Surg 64A:136, 1982.

95. Lindenbaum SD, Fleming LL, Smith DW: Pudendal-nerve palsies associated with closed intramedullary femoral fixation: A report of two cases and a study of the mechanism of injury. J Bone Joint Surg 64A:934, 1982.

96. Sultan C: Ganglion der nervenscheide des nervus peroneus. Zentralbl f Chir 48:963, 1921.

97. Wadstein T: Two cases of ganglia in the sheath of the peroneal nerve. Acta Orthopaedica Scandinavica 2:221, 1931.

98. Ellis VH: Two cases of ganglia in sheath of the peroneal nerve. Br J Surg 24:141, 1936.

99. Ferguson LK: Ganglion of the peroneal nerve. Ann Surg 106:313, 1937.

100. Clark K: Ganglion of the lateral popliteal nerve. J Bone Joint Surg 43B:778, 1961.

101. Parkes A: Intraneural ganglion of the lateral popliteal nerve. J Bone Joint Surg 43B:784, 1961.

102. Brooks DM: Nerve compression by simple ganglia. J Bone Joint Surg 34B:391, 1952.

103. Barber KW Jr, Bianco AJ Jr, Soule EH, et al: Benign extraneural soft tissue tumors of the extremities causing compression of nerves. J Bone Joint Surg 44A:98, 1962.

104. Stack RE, Bianco AJ Jr, MacCarty CS: Compression of the common peroneal nerve by ganglion cysts: Report of nine cases. J Bone Joint Surg 47A:773, 1965.

105. Maudsley RH: Fibular tunnel syndrome. *In* Proceedings, Northwest Metropolitan Club. J Bone Joint Surg 49B:384, 1967.

106. Mangieri JV: Peroneal nerve injury from an enlarged fabella. J Bone Joint Surg 55A:395, 1973.

107. Yamahiro K: Case of fibular nerve paralysis possibly caused by fabella. Orthop Surg (Tokyo) 18:145, 1967.

108. Pringle RM, Prothero K, Mukherjee SK: Entrapment neuropathy of the sural nerve. J Bone Joint Surg 56B:465, 1974.

109. Pollock LJ, Davis L: Peripheral nerve injuries. Am J Surg 18:361, 1932.

110. Kopell HP, Thompson WA: Peripheral entrapment neuropathies of the lower extremity. N Engl J Med 262:56, 1960.

111. Keck C: The tarsal-tunnel syndrome. J Bone Joint Surg 44A:180, 1962.

112. Lam SJS: A tarsal-tunnel syndrome. Lancet 2:1354, 1962.

113. Kojima T: A case of carpal tunnel syndrome associated with tarsal tunnel syndrome. Tohuka J Orthopaedics Traumatol 7:214, 1963.

114. McGill DA: Tarsal tunnel syndrome. Proc R Soc Med 57:1125, 1964.

115. Lam SJS: Tarsal tunnel syndrome. J Bone Joint Surg 49B:87, 1967.

116. Edwards WG, Lincoln CR, Bassett FH III, et al: The tarsal tunnel syndrome. Diagnosis and treatment. JAMA 207:716, 1969.

117. Mann RA: Tarsal tunnel syndrome. *In* Proceedings, the Western Orthopaedic Association. J Bone Joint Surg 58A:283, 1976.

118. Janecki CJ, Dovberg JL: Tarsal-tunnel syndrome caused by neurilemoma of the medial plantar nerve. J Bone Joint Surg 59A:127, 1977.

119. Garcia PG, Garcia-Rubio M, Lopez VC, et al: Tarsal tunnel syndrome: A report of fifty-six cases. Proceedings, British Orthopaedic Assoc. Meeting with Sociedad Espnaolade Cirugia Ortopedica y Traumatologia. J Bone Joint Surg 61B:123, 1979.

120. Wileman WK: Tarsal tunnel syndrome: A fifty year survey and a report of two new cases. Orthop Rev 8:111, 1979.

121. Morton TG: A peculiar and painful affection of the fourth metatarso-phalangeal articulation. Am J Sci 71:37, 1876.

122. Betts LO: Morton's metatarsalgia: Neuritis of the fourth digital nerve. Med J Aust 1:514, 1940.

123. Betts WJ: Plantar neuroma: Etiology: Thoughts of his father. Personal communication, 1986.

124. McElvenny RT: The etiology and surgical treatment of intractable pain about the fourth metatarso-phalangeal joint (Morton's toe). J Bone Joint Surg 25:675, 1943.

125. Watson-Jones R: Leri's pleonosteosis, carpal tunnel compression of the median nerves and Morton's metatarsalgia. J Bone Joint Surg 31B:560, 1949.

126. Bickle WH, Dockerty MB: Plantar neuromas, Morton's toe. Surg Gynecol Obstet 84:111, 1947.

127. Brahms MA: Common foot problems. J Bone Joint Surg 49A:1658, 1967.

128. Nissen KI: Plantar digital neuritis (Morton's Metatarsalgia). J Bone Joint Surg 30B:84, 1948.

129. Baker LD, Kuhn HH: Morton's metatarsalgia. Localized degenerative fibrosis with neuromatous proliferation of the fourth plantar nerve. South Med J. 37:123, 1944.

130. Winkler H, Feltner JB, Kimmelstiel P: Morton's metatarsalgia. J Bone Joint Surg 30A:496,1948.

131. Hauser EDW: Interdigital neuroma of the foot. Surg Gynecol Obstet 133:265, 1971.

132. McKeever DC: Surgical approach for neuroma of plantar digital nerve (Morton's metatarsalgia). J Bone Joint Surg 34A:490, 1952.

CHAPTER 2

Pathophysiology of Nerve Compression

Göran Lundborg, M.D., Ph.D.
Lars B. Dahlin, M.D., Ph.D.

Chronic nerve compression lesions usually represent the product of several types of traumas including traction, friction, and repetitive compression. Nerve trunks pass through several anatomically narrow canals during their course from the intervertebral foramina down the extremities. Nerves are not static structures: with movements of the extremity they normally slide over several millimeters within such tight canals. However, a local edema in the surrounding tissues may easily interfere with this sliding. A stuck nerve is, with movements of the extremity, subjected to stretching forces which could result in further tissue irritation, edema, microbleeding, and scarring. A constricting scar might induce a permanent compression (entrapment) of the nerve trunk.

Anatomic bases for development of these types of lesions can be formed by, for instance, fibro-osseus tunnels (e.g., intervertebral foramina, cubital tunnel, carpal tunnel), or fascia edges and contracting muscles (Frohse's arcade or the superficial part of the supinator muscle, the proximal part of the flexor carpi ulnaris muscle, the flexor digitorum superficialis muscle at elbow or forearm level). Among several factors possibly contributing to development of a compressing or stretching lesion at such locations are an unphysiologic body posture, unphysiologic movements, repetitive muscle contractions, as well as increase in the volume of structures in the space or decrease in the volume of available space.

Understanding of the complex pathophysiology of compression lesions must be based upon knowledge of the structure and physiology of the neuron as well as the nerve trunk. Knowledge of the microanatomy of nerve trunks is essential, since the nerve trunk contains multiple tissue components, each of them responding individually to compression. Nerve compression lesions do not represent a *mechanical* problem only. Early signs and symptoms presented by these patients often result from changes in intraneural microenvironment, microcirculation, and tissue pressure rather than structural damage to nerve fibers.

The Neuron and Microanatomy of the Nerve Trunk

The Neuron

A neuron, consisting of a nerve cell body (perikaryon) and its elongated processes, represents a highly specialized cell type. The cell bodies, situated in the anterior horn of the spinal cord (motor neurons) or in the dorsal root ganglia (sensory neurons), extend processes to peripheral targets. This extension may be for a length corresponding to many thousands of the cell body diameter. The production of a broad spectrum of substances essential for the neuron is concentrated in the cell body, and the distal parts of the axon, including the synapse, are functionally and structurally dependent on connections with the cell body. The requirements for intracellular transport in neurons—*axonal transport*—are consequently very high. By axonal transport a wide range of substances produced in the nerve cell body are transported from the perikaryon down the axon at different rates by anterograde axonal transport. The materials transported include proteins, membraneous vesicles, neurotransmitters, lipids, mitochondria, and RNA. Five main groups of anterograde axonal transport have been defined.[12,15,26,43,60,82] Slow transport (0.1-30 mm/day; group III-V) involves cytoskeletal elements (subunits of microtubules and neurofilaments) and elements of the axoplasmic or microtrabecular matrix (e.g., actin). Fast transport (20 up to 400 mm/day; Group I-II) consists mainly of small vesicular organelles and both membranous and soluble materials.

Axonal transport in neurons is bidirectional. Normally there is also a constant translocation of materials from the axon terminals toward the cell body, termed "retrograde transport".[9,10,11,23,57,58,69] The velocity of retrograde transport (up to 300 mm/day) is less than that of fast transport[10] and a slow component was recently described (3 to 8 mm/day).[36] Part of the materials in the retrograde stream appear to be recycled materials which originally were transported in the anterograde direction. Various extracellular materials can be taken up by the nerve terminals or by the cut end of transected axons and transported to the cell body via retrograde transport. Retrograde transport may involve transfer of information to the cell body about the status of the axon, its terminals, its general environment, and its target tissues. Such information can be carried with substances derived from target tissues or glia cells (Schwann cells) with trophic effects on the cell body.[10,11,56,108,129,130] There are several indications that nerve cell bodies are under trophic influence of their respective target tissues, and that this influence is mediated via the retrograde axonal transport. Typical morphologic changes in the cell body, including changes in cell volume and nuclear volume, eccentricity of the nucleus and dispersion of the Nissl substance (chromatolysis) are seen after transection of an axon,[5,19,42,62,63,95] and similar changes have been seen also following local compression.[24] It

has been suggested that lack of retrograde transported materials may provide a signal for initiation of nerve cell body changes in such situations; addition of agents blocking retrograde axonal transport may also provide "chromatolytic" reactions.[44,105,109]

The interaction between nerve cell bodies and their peripheral targets, mediated via bidirectional axonal transport, is of fundamental importance for our understanding of the pathophysiology of nerve compression lesions. Recognition of the cell body and the axon as being parts of *one cell*, continuous from the spinal cord to the periphery, helps to understand why compression at one level might induce functional changes also at other levels (see the following discussions).

The Nerve Trunk

The peripheral nerve is a composite tissue in which the nerve fibers are closely packed within *fascicles* or funicles. The various components of a nerve trunk have the purpose of maintaining continuity, nutrition, and protection of the fibers. A well-developed intraneural microvascular system forms a base for a continuous energy supply, necessary to maintain impulse conduction as well as axonal transport.

Each fascicle is surrounded by a *perineurium* (Fig. 2-1), a laminated sheath of considerable mechanical strength. The perineurium constitutes a diffusion barrier to various externally applied substances such as

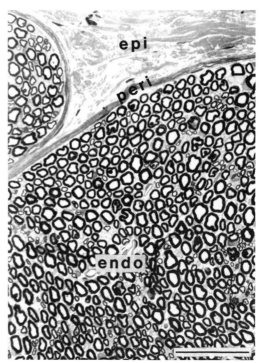

Figure 2-1. Cross section of a rat sciatic nerve showing the different layers of connective tissue of a peripheral nerve. The picture shows part of two fascicles. The nerve fibers are located in endoneurium (endo). Each fascicle is surrounded by a perineurium (peri) and the fascicles are embedded in loose connective tissue, epineurium (epi). Length of bar 50 m.

ferritin,[100,131] horseradish peroxidase (HRP),[55,103,104] and exogenous proteins.[70,74,79,127] The perineurium contributes to chemical isolation of the nerve fibers from the surrounding tissues, thereby creating an intrafascicular ionic environment of its own—a specialized "milieu intérieur". Inside the fascicles the nerve fibers are closely packed in connective tissue—the endoneurium—which consists of fibroblasts and collagen fibrils. The endoneurium of cutaneous nerves seems to consist of more collagen fibrils than that of more deeply placed nerves, which may reflect the extra protection required for the nerve fibers of superficially located nerves.[124]

Fascicles are embedded in an *epineurium* (Fig. 2-1) carrying the main supplying channels of the intraneural vascular system. The epineurium represents a loose and soft connective tissue embedding and protecting the fascicles. The relative amount of epineurium and perineurium varies between nerves, levels, and individuals.[124,125] Nerves usually contain more epineurium where they cross joints, which helps to minimize the effects of compression, friction, and traction caused by joint movements. Superficially the epineurium is condensed to a sheath, delimiting the nerve from surrounding structures to which the nerve is very loosely attached by a conjunctiva-like layer allowing a great deal of motion.

Intraneural Microvascular System

Peripheral nerves are well vascularized structures with well-developed microvascular systems in the epineurium, perineurium, and endoneurium (Fig. 2-2).[1,6,7,13,29,70-73] The vessels in various layers of the nerve are extensively interconnected with each others through numerous anastomoses. Impulse transmission as well as axonal transport require a continuous energy supply provided by the intraneural microvessels, and the microvascular system seems to possess a great reserve capacity to compensate for mobilization or damage to local regional vessels.[70,71] In the epineurium large, longitudinally oriented vessels exhibit a characteristic pattern. Vessels are present in all layers of the epineurium, that is, superficially as well as between the fascicular bundles in the deep layers of the nerve. The epineurial vessels anastomose with a perineurial vascular plexus, exhibiting longitudinally running vessels at various depths between the lamellae of the perineurium. Anastomoses from the perineurial vessels traverse the inner perineurial layer in a characteristic oblique way into the endoneurial space. This oblique passage of the perineurial vessels might constitute a "valve mechanism" at those points where the vessels are especially liable to obliteration if there is an increase in intrafascicular fluid pressure (see later discussion).

Intrafascicularly there is an *endoneurial* microvascular network consisting not only of capillaries (Fig. 2-2), but also of arterioles and venules.[6,7,70,71] The endoneurial vascular bed constitutes a continuous network throughout the length of the fascicles. Due to the numerous anastomoses in all directions, the endoneurial capillary circulation is little influenced by limited mobilization of a nerve trunk.[70] Due to the barrier action of the perineurium, the endoneurial blood flow is surprisingly well

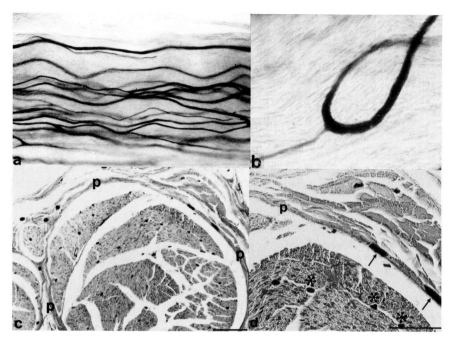

Figure 2-2. Microangiograms of a rabbit vagus nerve (India ink-perfused). (a) The longitudinal pattern of intraneural vessels in a fascicle (100 m thick nonstained section; length of bar 0.1 mm). (b) Loop formation of an endoneurial vessel (80 m thick nonstained section; length of bar 60 m). (c) Cross section of fascicles showing intraneural vessels (black spots) in all layers of the nerve (p indicates perineurium). The appearance of spaces between bundles of nerve fibers are artifacts. (d) Detail of c. Note the transversely cut capillaries (*) located in the endoneurial space as well as the vessels in the perineurium (arrows); c and d are transverse sections, 10 m thick, stained with hematoxylin and eosin. Length of bars 0.1 mm.

preserved even when extensive intraneural dissections, such as neurolysis, are performed.[112]

The Blood-Nerve Barrier

The fascicles and their contents can, in many respects, be regarded as extensions of the central nervous system (CNS) to the periphery. The perineurium has been regarded as an extension from the pia-arachnoid mater of the CNS.[119] Also certain structural and functional characteristics of vessels in the CNS are seen in the peripheral nervous system. The barrier to certain substances circulating in the blood, including macromolecules (the blood-brain barrier), is expressed also in peripheral nerves as a "blood-nerve barrier". The permeability of intraneural blood vessels to proteins in the microcirculation has been demonstrated in numerous studies involving the use of dyes and fluorescent and radioactive tracers.[70,101-104,132] While such substances easily pass through the endothelium of the *epineurial* blood vessels, there is no or minimal passage through the walls of *endoneurial* microvessels. The structural base for this blood-nerve barrier

is formed by so-called tight junctions between extremely closely opposed endothelial cells. The "blood-nerve barrier" is—together with the corresponding diffusion barrier in the perineurium—essential for the maintenance of the specialized endoneurial environment.

The Nerve Fiber

Nerve fibers can be myelinated or unmyelinated. In both types a chain of Schwann cells, arranged end to end, surrounds the axons, but the relationship between Schwann cells and axons are fundamentally different in myelinated and unmyelinated fibers. In unmyelinated fibers one Schwann cell can enclose a great number of axons, while in the myelinated fiber one axon is associated with only one Schwann cell at any one level. The membrane of the Schwann cell is wrapped spirally around the axon, thus producing a sheath of alternating layers of lipid and protein, the myelin sheath.[59] Along the myelinated fiber the Schwann cells meet each other at the nodes of Ranvier where fingerlike cellular processes allows an exchange between extra- and intracellular ions, an important process in the so-called saltatory propagation of impulses from node to node.

Effects of Compression

The severity of the nerve lesions induced by acute or chronic compression is a result of the *magnitude* as well as the *duration* of the compressive trauma. The onset of symptoms as well as the rate of recovery may be variable and reflects the pathophysiologic basis of the lesion. Nerve fibers show varying susceptibility to compression depending on their size and location in the fascicles, as well as the location of the fascicle within the nerve trunk. Large fibers are more susceptible to ischemia and compression[30,37] than small fibers are, and fibers situated circumferentially in fascicles suffer more than fibers located more centrally in the fascicle.[2,106,121] Similarly, nerve fibers located in superficial fascicles are affected more than fibers located in central fascicles. In addition, the construction of the nerve trunk at the compressed level affects response to compression: large fascicles in a small amount of epineurium are more vulnerable to compression than are several small fascicles embedded in a large amount of epineurium.

The basic pathophysiology of acute as well as chronic compression lesions is controversial; ischemia as well as mechanical factors have been proposed as primary underlying causes for impaired function. The issue is a difficult one, since all compression forces by definition include an ischemic factor secondary to the obliteration of microvessels in the nerve. Generally, slight or moderate compression, resulting in functional disorders immediately reversible following decompression, are based on a microvascular insufficiency, while mechanical factors, resulting in local myelin damage, might constitute primary etiologic factors in lesions requiring a longer time to recover.

Effects of Compression on Intraneural Microvascular Flow

The effects of local experimental compression have been studied in animals using various types of miniature compressive devices. Rydevik et al.[114] found, in an intravital microscopic study, that external compression at 20 to 30 mm Hg induced a retardation of the venular blood flow in the epineurium. When the cuff pressure was increased, the blood flow was also reduced in endoneurial capillaries. A cuff pressure of 80 mm Hg was followed by a complete stasis of all intraneural blood flow in the compressed nerve segment (ischemia). Rydevik's data was recently confirmed by Ogata and Naito[99] using the hydrogen washout technique. By the use of perfusion techniques, Bentley and Schlapp[8] found that compression of 60 to 65 mm Hg produced circulatory arrest at least in the superficial vessels of compressed nerve segments. Matsumoto[81] found a decreased intrafascicular blood flow (hydrogen washout technique) in dog sciatic nerves when the nerves were compressed at 45 to 50 mm Hg, while a pressure of around 120 mm Hg resulted in complete circulatory arrest.

Axonal Transport and Nerve Compression

It was reported already in 1948 by Weiss and Hiscoe[133] that constriction of a nerve resulted in swelling and accumulation of fluid proximal to the lesion. Weiss and Hiscoe felt that this was an effect of obstruction of the moving axoplasm inside fibers. Theoretically, one might expect compression to interfere with axonal transport by a direct mechanical blocking effect or secondary to obliteration of intraneural vessels resulting in anoxia. In experimental studies, where nerves were locally compressed by an inflated cuff, it has been shown that limited compression can inhibit axonal transport. *Fast* axonal transport, as studied by transport of proteins labelled with ^{3}H-leucine, in rabbit vagus nerves remained normal during compression at 20 mm Hg for two hours, while an accumulation proximal to the compressed segment was found after eight hours compression at the same pressure level.[20,21] A pressure of 30 mm Hg for two hours was followed by a complete or partial inhibition. Block of fast axonal transport induced by 50 mm Hg was reversible within 24 hours.[113] Reversal of transport blockage usually occurred within three days after compression at 200 mm Hg for two hours and within seven days after compression at 400 mm Hg for two hours.[113] In similar studies, carried out on the sciatic nerve of rats with streptozotocin-induced diabetes, fast axonal transport was more markedly inhibited than in control animals.[22] These data indicate that nerves of diabetic animals might be more susceptible to compression trauma than nerves of control animals.

Effects of graded compression on *slow* axonal transport was studied by Dahlin & McLean[20] using the rabbit vagus model. Compression at 20 mm Hg applied for eight hours did not cause any accumulation of slowly transported materials, while a pressure of 30 mm Hg applied for eight hours, was followed by an incomplete but marked accumulation of slowly transported proteins.

These results indicate that comparatively low pressures may interfere with fast as well as slow axonal transport, thereby inducing possible interference with the provision of cytoskeletal elements to the distal axon and axolemma constituents, as well as with transmittor substances required for synaptic function. The low pressure levels are of special interest, since similar pressures have been monitored in the carpal tunnel of patients with carpal tunnel syndrome.[38] The same low pressures may also affect *retrograde* axonal transport: in experiments with rabbit vagus nerve it was shown that even pressures of 20 to 30 mm Hg applied for eight hours induced inhibition of the retrograde transport.[23] Compression at 200 mm Hg for eight hours induced a more marked inhibition of retrograde axonal transport (Fig. 2-3). Dahlin et al.[24] observed also morphologic changes in the sensory nerve cell bodies in the nodose ganglion after compression of the vagus nerve at these low pressures. A pressure of 30 mm Hg induced a decrease in nuclear volume density, an eccentricity of the nucleus, and dispersal of the Nissl substance (chromatolysis) in the cell bodies when studied seven days after the injury (Fig. 2-4). This type of change has previously been known to occur only after more severe lesions to nerve trunks such as crush and transection (see, for example, Liebermann[62,63] and Barron[5]).

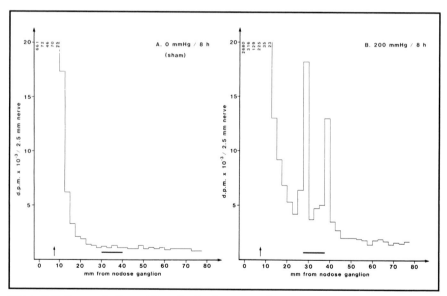

Figure 2-3. Demonstration of the effects of compression on anterograde and retrograde axonal transport. The figure shows the profile of radiolabeled proteins in rabbit vagus nerves 24 hours after radiolabeling of the cell bodies in nodose ganglion. The nerves were compressed at 0 mm Hg (sham;A) and 200 mm Hg (B) for the final eight hours. The black bars indicate site of compression and the vertical arrows indicate ligature to exclude slow axonal transport. Sham compression caused no inhibition of axonal transport, while compression at 200 mm Hg induced a marked inhibition of axonal transport around the distal (retrograde transport) as well as the proximal (anterograde transport) edge of the compressed segment.

Effects on Nerve Fiber Structure

Compression of a nerve trunk may cause damage by the direct pressure as well as by shearing forces associated with the redistribution of the tissue from compressed to noncompressed areas. It is known from several experimental studies that such redistribution of tissue, often occurring under the border zones (edges) of a compressive device, is dangerous with respect to fiber injury while a *uniform* pressure on nerve fibers causes little

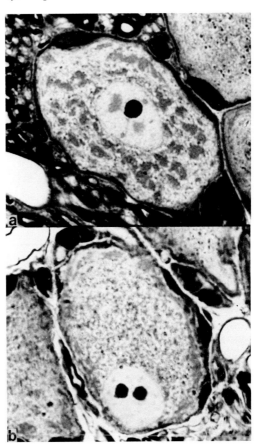

Figure 2-4. Nerve cell bodies from nodose ganglion of rabbits seven days after compression of the vagus nerve. (a) Shows a normal nerve cell with abundant Nissl substance and a central nucleus seven days after sham compression for two hours. (b) Shows a nerve cell with dispersed Nissl substance (chromatolysis) and an eccentric nucleus seven days after compression at 30 mm Hg for two hours (methylene blue and Azur II; × 1200).

or no damage. In experiments by Grundfest and Cattell[46] where segments of excised frog nerves were enclosed in a pressure chamber, the nerves could be subjected to pressures up to one thousand atmospheres before conduction failed.[45,46] Of more relevance for clinical situations, however, are experiments in which nerves are subjected to external pressure by local inflatable miniature cuffs or tourniquets around whole extremities. In such situations, nerve fiber injuries do not occur directly *under* the tourniquet or cuff, but they are frequent beneath the edges where the shearing forces are maximal. In studies, including the application of inflatable tourniquets around extremities of primates,[33,98] it was found that these lesions were based upon displacement of nodes of Ranvier toward uncompressed parts of the nerve.

The paranodal myelin was stretched on one side of the node and invaginated on the other. Such nodal displacement, occurring under proximal as well as distal border zones of the tourniquet, was followed by segmental demyelination and a subsequent conduction block, reversible within weeks or months. The local demyelination observed by those authors was directly referred to mechanical pressure from the tourniquet. In experimental studies by Powell and Myers where nerves were compressed by miniature inflatable cuffs, similar changes have been associated with local Schwann cell necrosis appearing prior to the demyelination.[106] It was pointed out by Powell and Myers[106] that local ischemia was the most probable pathogenic mechanism contributing to the observed paranodal demyelination.

Intraneural Edema Following Compression

Compression with consequent subtotal or total ischemia might induce damage to all intraneural tissue components including Schwann cells,[106] nerve fibers,[70,71] and intraneural microvessels.[70,71] Microvascular injury may be associated with increased permeability to proteins, and ischemic periods may, therefore, be followed by an intraneural edema when blood flow is restored. Local swelling with a "no reflow phenomenon" is well-known to occur in muscle tissue following ischemic periods (see reviews by Mubarak and Hargens[85] and Matsen[80]). Such "closed compartment syndromes" may be followed by severe ischemic damage to nerve and muscle tissue. In nerve, such phenomena may be critical because of the unyielding properties and barrier function of the perineurial sheath.

The intrafascicular vessels are very resistant to *ischemia* per se. As much as six hours complete ischemia may be followed by microvascular restoration with no or minimal thrombosis formation.[70,71] This remarkable phenomenon might be related to a local release of plasminogen activators from the endothelium of endoneurial blood vessels.[104b,110] Ischemic periods of longer duration (eight hours or more) are, however, followed by a marked endoneurial edema associated with a "no reflow phenomenon" in the fascicles—a "miniature closed compartment syndrome" (see subsequent discussion). In experimental animals such endoneurial edema is followed by irreversible loss of nerve function.[70,71]

When a nerve is subjected to local compression, both the magnitude and duration of the applied pressure are of importance for occurrence and distribution of the intrafascicular edema following release of the pressure. Changes in intraneural microvascular permeability have been studied in rabbit tibial nerves after local compression at 50, 200, and 400 mm Hg induced by a miniature cuff.[111] Compression at 50 mm Hg for two hours induced an edema that was restricted to the epineurium. The edema was prevented from reaching the endoneurial space because of the barrier properties of the perineurial sheath. Compression for two hours at higher pressure (200 to 400 mm Hg) was followed by marked microvascular injury at the edges of the compressed segment, as indicated by leakage of intravenously infused tracer substances (Fig. 2-5). There was a prominent endoneurial edema at the edges while no such edema was observed *centrally* in the compressed segments. Compression at 200 mm Hg for two hours and 400 mm Hg for 15 minutes was followed by edema in *some* fascicles *at the edges*, while after a longer duration of compression, edema was apparent in *all* fascicles. When compression at 200 mm Hg was applied for four and six hours, endoneurial edema was observed also in the *center* of the compressed segment. The data demonstrate that the *magnitude* as well as *duration* of pressure is of importance for occurrence of intraneural

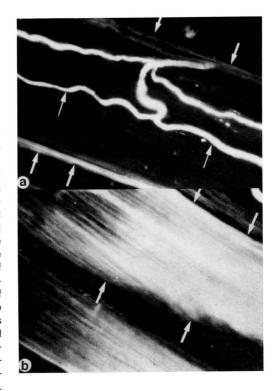

Figure 2-5. Fluorescence microscopic appearance of a segment of a compressed rabbit tibial nerve. Evans blue albumin (EBA) was injected intravenously immediately after compression at 400 mm Hg for two hours and longitudinal sections were prepared. (a) Central part of the compressed segment. The outlines of the fascicle are indicated by thick arrows. The blood-brain barrier was unaffected, as indicated by the fact that the red (here: white) EBA-complex has perfused the endoneurial capillaries (thin arrows) in a fascicle and the dye complex is strictly confined to the vessels' lumina. The nerve tissue has a green fluorescence (here: grayish-black). (b) Edge of the compressed segment. Compression increased permeability of the endoneurial vessels leading to endoneurial edema formation as indicated by the diffuse orange-red fluorescence (white) in the endoneurial space. Reproduced by permission of B. Rydevik and G. Lundborg. Scand. J. Plast. Reconstr. Surg. 11: 179-187, 1977.

edema, and that vascular lesions are most prominent at the *edges* of the compressed zone. As already stated, the nerve fiber injury also occurs at the edges of the compressed nerve segment. Such a phenomenon, in which the compression injury is most pronounced at the edges of the compressed segment, can be referred as "the edge effect".

In Rydevik's experiments,[114] compression at 80 mm Hg for two hours was followed by immediate microvascular recovery, while nerves compressed at 400 mm Hg for the same time showed no or very slow intraneural blood flow in the previously compressed segments when observed three or even seven days later. This "no reflow phenomenon" is based upon a massive intraneural edema in the compressed nerve segment as well as a direct mechanical injury to intraneural microvessels at the border zones of compression, preventing a reperfusion of the compressed segment.[115]

The endoneurial edema occurring in nerves of experimental animals following local compression by a pneumatic miniature cuff has been studied and quantified by Lundborg et al.[76] and Powell and Myers.[106] Normally the tissue fluid pressure (endoneurial fluid pressure [EFP]) inside a fascicle is slightly positive (2.0 ± 1.0 cm H20).[64,67,86,87] By the use of a micropipette technique, elevation in the EFP following compression was studied after one and 24 hours,[76] and the histologic and ultrastructural appearance of nerve fibers and endoneurial contents were followed for periods up to 28 days after release of pressure.[106] Severe endoneurial edema with a fourfold increase in EFP was observed one hour after compression at 80 mm Hg for four hours and a threefold increase of EFP was observed after compression at 30 mm or 80 mm Hg for eight hours. The same values could be recorded 24 hours after the operation, and endoneurial edema could be histologically verified up to 28 days after the compression period.[106] Microscopic analysis revealed pathologic changes of subperineurial fibers with demyelination even in nerves subjected to a pressure of only 10 mm Hg. Following compression at 80 mm Hg for two hours, abnormalities of Schwann cells including swelling and disintegration of cytoplasmic contents were observed throughout the 28-day period. The authors concluded that the Schwann cell damage might account for some of the paranodal changes observed, since death of the Schwann cell is inevitably followed by disintegration of the myelin sheath.

The increase in EFP, occurring parallel to the occurrence of an endoneurial edema,[86,88-90] is essential for understanding the pathophysiology of acute and chronic nerve compression lesions. A sustained increase in endoneurial fluid pressure may damage nerve fibers,[64,66,86] and changes in electrolyte composition of the endoneurial fluid may impair nerve function.[53,92] An increase in EFP may interfere with endoneurial capillary blood flow, although there will be no total collapse of the endoneurial capillaries:[65] a threefold increase in endoneurial fluid pressure has been found associated with a significant reduction in nerve blood flow.[91] An endoneurial edema may also increase the diffusion distance for oxygen from the endoneurial capillaries to the axons, which may induce endoneurial hypoxia.[91] The hypoxia may even affect different parts of the endoneurial space to a variable extent. In galactose neuropathy, with an endoneurial edema and an increase in EFP, the oxygen tension is significantly lower subperineurially than centrally in the fascicle.[68] An endoneurial edema cannot escape through the perineurium because of the perineurial diffusion barrier, and the increase in EFP may therefore last for a long time. An endoneurial edema may be subjected to fibroblast invasion and an intraneural scar may form, which is an irreversible condition.

Ischemia Versus Compression—Human Experiments

Lewis et al.[61] used a special device to apply a pressure of 60 to 70 mm Hg over the radial or median nerves of humans. They found that this pressure was sufficient to induce a local conduction block, and the authors concluded that occlusion of small intraneural microvessels was the cause of the block. The same authors also used inflatable cuffs around the upper arm to induce local conduction block. It was found that a cuff pressure of 150 mm Hg induced a conduction block at the same rate as a pressure of 300 mm Hg. These observations were taken as indications that ischemia of the compressed segment constituted the underlying cause of conduction block rather than mechanical changes of the nerve fibers. This theory was supported by other experiments in which the inflated cuff around the upper arm was maintained until complete sensory loss occurred in the hand, at which time a second cuff was inflated proximal to the first one. Sensation did not recover in the hand following release of the distal cuff until the second proximal cuff was deflated to reestablish microcirculation in the distal previously compressed segment.

The effects of controlled pressure on human median nerves have recently been studied by the use of a model developed by Lundborg et al.[75] In these experiments a wick catheter was introduced into the carpal tunnel to continuously monitor the tissue fluid pressure in the canal close to the median nerve. The hand of the volunteer was placed in an external compression device allowing a piece of molded rubber to be pressed toward the palmar aspect of the wrist. In that way, a local, controlled pressure could be applied to the median nerve. Motor and sensory nerve conduction were followed during the compression. It was found that a pressure of 30 mm Hg induced mild neurophysiologic changes and symptoms in the hand, including paresthesia, but complete blockage of motor and sensory conduction was found at first at a tissue fluid pressure of 40 to 50 mm Hg or more.[39,40,75] In these cases the sensory nerve conduction rapidly deteriorated and the amplitudes disappeared completely after 25 to 50 minutes, while motor action potentials usually could be followed for another 10 to 30 minutes.

In these experiments, 40 to 50 mm Hg represented a critical pressure level when intraneural microvessels were obliterated, the consequent ischemia being followed by a complete local conduction block. That ischemia and not the mechanical pressure per se was the critical factor was verified in combination experiments in which conduction block in the median nerve at wrist level was induced by local, external compression of 60 mm Hg. After disappearance of sensory fiber conduction, a tourniquet was inflated around the upper arm to a pressure exceeding the systolic blood pressure, after which the local pressure at the median nerve at the wrist was released. Although the pressure on the previously compressed median nerve segment had been released, function did not recover; ischemia was sustained by the inflated cuff around the upper arm. When the tourniquet was deflated, sensory and motor function at wrist level was immediately restored.

The significance of ischemia in this type of local conduction block was also verified in experiments in which the experimental model just described was applied to *hypertensive* patients (see earlier discussions). In these cases, sensory conduction was blocked at pressures of 60 to 70 mm Hg—a pressure threshold 20 mm Hg higher than the 40 to 50 mm Hg previously found in the normotensive subjects.[126]

Chronic Nerve Compression

The signs and symptoms seen in *chronic nerve compression lesions* represent a combined effect of a persistent inflammatory reaction in the nerve and a direct mechanical injury to the nerve fibers. Repeated compression, stretching, and friction are factors contributing to increased vascular permeability, chronic edema, and scarring. Impaired intraneural microvascular flow as well as repeated mechanical trauma to the fibers may result in myelin damage and axonal degeneration. The importance of mechanical nerve fiber damage per se in these lesions has been emphasized by Ochoa[96] and Gilliatt,[41] while the significance of microvascular insufficiency ultimately resulting in fiber damage has been stressed by others.[106,123]

Various experimental models have been developed in order to study the pathoanatomy and pathophysiology of chronic nerve entrapment. Guinea pigs, when they grow older, acquire a naturally developing entrapment lesion of the ulnar and median nerves under the transverse carpal ligament at the wrist.[4,34a,35,78,97] This naturally developed carpal tunnel syndrome offers an opportunity to study the pathology of chronic nerve entrapment, and the histologic and ultrastructural appearance of these nerves has been analyzed in detail. A consistent finding was an asymmetry of the myelin sheath on either side of the entrapment site. The sheath appeared to be thinned at the end of the internodal segment close to the center of the lesion, while it was thickened and swollen toward the edges of the lesion, giving an impression of tadpoles or sperm swimming from the center of the lesion. Electron microscopic studies have shown that the terminal loops of the inner myelin lamellae were detached from the axolemma at the node, with retraction of the myelin along the internode and the corresponding excess of myelin at the other end of the internode. In advanced stages the lesion included prominent paranodal demyelination with partial exposure of the axon, and in the most severe cases the damage was severe enough to induce wallerian degeneration. The "tadpole lesion" has also been found in the median nerve of man at wrist level and in the ulnar nerve at elbow level[49,93] as well as in the lateral cutaneous nerve of the thigh in meralgia paresthetica.[54,96]

Chronic nerve entrapment has also been experimentally created by using various types of locally applied devices. Narrow tubes have been placed around nerves of young animals, resulting in a gradual constriction of the nerve as the animal grows.[2,27] In these experiments, bulbous swellings of the nerve proximal as well as distal to the compressed segment were seen, which could be referred to obstruction of anterograde and retrograde axonal transport as well as local intraneural edema formation. MacKinnon et al.[77] "banded" the sciatic nerve of adult rats with longitudinally cut silicone tubes of various diameters. Well-fitting tubes induced a state of chronic irritation resulting in epineurial and perineurial fibrosis, deterioration of the blood-nerve barrier and damage to the large myelinated fibers located peripherally in the fascicles. Horiuchi[51] and Nemoto[94] induced controlled compression of longer duration to dog sciatic nerves by the use of specially designed spring clips. Compression at around 30 mm Hg resulted in a flattening of the compressed site, while adjacent portions both proximally and distally showed distinct swellings characterized by a prominent intraneural edema.

The effect of compression at *several levels* has also been studied experimentally.[94,118] Seiler et al.[118] induced chronic compression of rat sciatic nerves by a well-fitting silicone tube (see earlier discussion). A "double crush lesion" was created by placing a second tube around the tibial nerve of the same animal four months after the application of the proximal tube. Neurophysiologic evaluation performed four months later revealed a significant prolongation of motor latency between the four-month "double crush" sciatic nerve and the eight-month single-banded sciatic nerve, while no difference could be found between the latency of the eight-month single-banded nerve and its control nonbanded sciatic nerve on the contralateral side.

Nemoto[94] used a spring clip model to induce chronic compression of about 30 mm Hg at two different levels of dog sciatic nerves. Electrophysiologic assessment 10 weeks later showed that a proximal compression significantly increased the vulnerability of the distal part of the nerve to additional compression.

Stages of Nerve Compression Injury

Theoretical and Clinical Considerations

Since susceptibility to compression among nerve fibers varies depending on size[30,37,120] and intrafascicular topography,[2,77,106,121] each nerve compression injury represents in fact a mixed lesion with a varying extent of damage to various fiber populations. Still, it has been found valuable to define stages of nerve compression injuries based on the nature of overall functional disorder and the rate of functional recovery[116,117] as well as the pathoanatomy of the tissue components of the nerve trunk.[122,124]

Physiologic (Metabolic) Conduction Block

The term **physiologic conduction block** refers to a local deprivation of oxygen based on a circulatory arrest, inhibiting impulse transmission in structurally intact nerve fibers. Such a block may be induced by slight local compression, for instance, pressure on the peroneal nerve when one leg is crossed over the knee of the opposite side. In such a situation the foot "goes to sleep," but the block is immediately reversible when the pressure is released. Another example is the conduction block induced by a cuff inflated to suprasystolic pressure around the upper arm.[61] The local ischemia, induced by pressure from the cuff, results in deterioration of motor and sensory conduction across the compressed nerve segment, but conduction is immediately restored as soon as the cuff is released. The time required for functional recovery is extended with longer duration of ischemia, and intraneural edema secondary to anoxic endothelium damage may contribute to an increase of recovery time. The critical time limit for ischemia when the local metabolic block is transferred into irreversible nerve fiber damage is set to six to eight hours.[29a,70,71]

Neurapraxia

Neurapraxia refers to another type of local conduction block in which axonal continuity is preserved and no degeneration takes place, but conduction over the compressed segment recovers only after weeks or months. The term was introduced by Seddon[116,117] and was based upon observations in multiple cases in which nerves were subjected to compression or stretching. This type of lesion is supposed to correspond to an acute, local myelin damage at the nodes of Ranvier as described by, for instance, Denny-Brown and Brenner[25] and Ochoa et al.[98] The block will persist until local myelin repair restores local excitability, a process usually requiring weeks or months. Since larger fibers are more vulnerable to compression than are thinner fibers, the true neurapraxia usually represents a mixed lesion. According to Seddon's original observations, neurapraxia usually includes complete motor paralysis while there is often much sparing of sensory and sympathetic functions—a fact based upon the representation of some afferent and sympathetic pathways among small unmyelinated fibers.

"Saturday night palsy," as well as radial nerve paralysis following fractures of the humerus, represent typical examples of neurapractic lesions. There is usually a complete paralysis of all muscles innervated by the radial nerve distal to the lesion, while there may be some sparing of sensation. Since axonal continuity is preserved, muscles innervated by the radial nerve can be activated by stimulation of the nerve distal to the lesion. Usually there is a spontaneous recovery within several weeks to months parallel to local repair and remodeling of the damaged myelin sheath. If there is no recovery within three to four months, local processes (e.g., entrapment in bone callus) may have prevented local nerve fiber repair, or the lesion was severe enough to induce nerve fiber degeneration.

Another classic example of a neurapractic lesion is the nerve function disorder sometimes seen after tourniquet application around the upper arm. Reported complications vary in severity from light sensibility disturbances to total three-nerve paralysis of the upper extremity, and the application time has varied from 15 minutes to 2.5 hours.[3,14,16,17,28,32,34,47,48,83,84,107,134] The frequency of nerve injuries seen after bloodfree field has been reported to be 1/5000 procedures.[83] From the literature it is clear that the nerve lesion is not based upon prolonged ischemia in the arm. On the contrary, pressure from the cuff has induced a compression lesion to the nerve structure at the level of the tourniquet, usually beneath the edges of the cuff. In the majority of reported cases there has been a calibration error with respect to the manometer (faulty gauges); the real pressures being applied varying from 350 to 1200 mm Hg.

Sunderland[122] has introduced a more detailed classification of nerve injuries, based upon the anatomic kind (type I-V). In this classification neurapraxia has been related to a Sunderland type I lesion, implying local myelin damage in preserved nerve fibers not presenting wallerian degeneration.

Axonotmesis

Axonotmesis implies a *loss of continuity* of axons, but with endoneurial tubes remaining intact. The lesion corresponds to an advanced compression or traction injury severe enough to interrupt continuity of axons, thereby inducing wallerian degeneration. The endoneurial tubes are preserved, and therefore functional recovery reflects the time required for the axons to regenerate in their original endoneurial tubes to the peripheral target. Since the growing axons are guided by their original tubes, the prognosis is good with respect to regeneration to correct targets. Surgery is not required as long as severe intraneural scarring is not complicating the situation. Axonotmesis corresponds to a type II lesion according to the Sunderland classification.

Neurotmesis

Neurotmesis indicates loss of continuity of axons as well as other elements of the nerve trunk including endoneurial tubes, perineurium, and epineurium. According to Seddon's original classification, neurotmesis is a term "used to describe a state of a nerve that has either been completely severed or is so disorganized by scar tissue that spontaneous recovery is out of the question".[117] Sunderland has divided corresponding lesions into three subgroups (types III-V). Type III implies loss of continuity of axons of endoneurial tubes, while the perineurium still is intact. In this situation continuity and orientation of endoneurial pathways are lost, and the lesion is often associated with intrafascicular fibrosis. The type IV lesion implies, in addition, loss of continuity of the perineurium with preserved epineurium, while the type V lesion indicates loss of continuity of the entire nerve trunk. Neurotmesis (Sunderland type III-V lesions) requires surgery if functional recovery is to be expected.

Conclusion

From the preceding discussions, it is apparent that acute as well as chronic nerve compression lesions are complex with respect to their pathophysiologic basis. Interference with intraneural microcirculation, axonal transport, and impulse transmission may together form a base for clinical signs and symptoms presented in early as well as advanced stages of nerve compression. The term "nerve compression injury" is, from the pathophysiologic standpoint, misleading, since it does not emphasize that intraneural inflammatory reactions as well as friction and stretching are essential etiologic factors.

Hypothetically, the various stages of the carpal tunnel syndrome (CTS) (see Chapter 6) nicely illustrate the involvement of etiologic and pathophysiologic factors. The early stage of CTS, characterized by nocturnal paresthesia, is based upon nocturnal intraneural microvascular insufficiency secondary to nocturnal increase in carpal tunnel tissue fluid pressure. The increase in tissue fluid pressure reflects exclusion of the muscle pump, redistribution of body fluid in horizontal body position and palmar flexion of the wrist. In addition, the decreased intraneural perfusion pressure occurring at night secondary to general decrease in blood pressure makes the median nerve more susceptible to external pressure (see Szabo et al.).[126] The symptoms are based on a local metabolic disorder in the nerve, resulting from oxygen deprivation secondary to impaired intraneural microcirculation. The symptoms are immediately reversible when wrist position, muscle pump, and body posture are normalized or when the transverse carpal ligament is cut.[31,50] In more advanced stages a persistent edema is induced in the nerve first in the epineurium, later in the endoneurium. A constant impairment of the microcirculation and an increase in endoneurial fluid pressure result in *constant* symptoms, but a decompression may still reverse this situation parallel to restoration of normal intraneural blood flow and drainage of the edema. At this stage there is probably a component of local fiber damage with myelin sheath lesions induced either by the pressure or secondary to ischemia in the nerve. Such a neurapractic lesion may require longer to recover, and function in the corresponding fiber populations may first appear several months after decompression. A long-standing intraneural edema may be invaded by fibroblasts and transferred into a scar. In this situation, some fibers may still suffer only from a metabolic disorder and some from severe myelin damage (neurapractic lesion), while other fibers may degenerate (axonotmesis). Decompression may be followed by extended and various patterns of recovery. Some improvement of sensibility may be noted already at the same day due to microvascular improvement, while other functional qualities may require months to years to recover. Intraneural scarring combined with fiber degeneration should be expected to result in some permanent functional loss.

The Double Crush Lesion

It is known from clinical investigations that there is an overrepresentation of carpal tunnel syndromes in patients suffering from cervical radiculopathy.[52,128] Upton and McComas[128] proposed a "double crush theory," implying that subsequent compressions of a nerve trunk might have a cumulative effect, making distal parts of a proximal compressed nerve more susceptible to compression. Current knowledge of the influence of graded compression on axonal transport (see earlier discussion) makes such a theory highly plausible, and probably the puzzling pictures of multientrapment cases could be explained in pathophysiologic terms. Anterograde axonal transport delivers necessary materials to the axon as well as to its terminals, and it is natural that interference with axonal transport therefore, may interfere with, for example, membrane composition in distal parts of the axon. A defective axonal membrane might exhibit an impaired resistance to external compression as compared to a healthy membrane. The studies by Dahlin et al.[23] on effects of compression at low pressures on *retrograde* axonal transport make theories suggesting membrane changes even more interesting. Pressures of the same magnitude as those recorded in the carpal tunnel of patients with carpal tunnel syndrome[38] have been shown to block retrograde axonal transport and to induce morphologic changes in corresponding nerve cell bodies in nodose ganglia.[24] The cell body response is probably an expression for a lack of neuronotrophic factors synthesized by Schwann cells or target tissues. Sick nerve cell bodies will not be able to manage an adequate *anterograde* axonal transport, and the proximal part of the axon may thereby suffer from a deficient supply of materials. In this way a *distal* nerve compression may hypothetically predispose for *proximal* compression lesions of the same nerve constituting a "reversed double crush syndrome." The theory can explain why a simple carpal tunnel release sometimes can reverse symptoms typical of an additional or proximal lesion as described by Carroll and Hurst.[18]

References

1. Adams WE: The blood supply of nerves. I. Historical review. J Anat (Lond) 76:323, 1942.
2. Aguayo A, Nair CPV, Midgley R: Experimental progressive compression neuropathy in the rabbit. Arch Neurol 24:358, 1971.
3. Aho K, Sainio K, Kianta M, Varpanen E: Pneumatic tourniquet paralysis. J Bone Joint Surg 65B:441, 1983.
4. Anderson MH, Fullerton PM, Gilliatt RW, Hern JE: Changes in the forearm associated with median nerve compression at the wrist in the guinea-pig. J Neurol Neurosurg Psychiatry 33:70, 1970.
5. Barron KD: Comparative observations on the cytologic reactions of central and peripheral nerve cells to axotomy. *In* CC Kao, RP Bunge, PJ Reier (Eds): Spinal Cord Reconstruction. New York, Raven Press, 1983, pp 7-40.
6. Bell MA, Weddell AGM: A morphometric study of intrafascicular vessels of mammalian sciatic nerve. Muscle Nerve 7:524, 1984.
7. Bell MA, Weddell AGM: A descriptive study of the blood vessels of the sciatic nerve in the rat, man and other mammals. Brain 107:871, 1984.
8. Bentley FH, Schlapp W: The effects of pressure on conduction in peripheral nerve. J Physiol (Lond) 102:72, 1943.
9. Bisby MA: Orthograde and retrograde axonal transport of labeled protein in motoneurons. Exp Neurol 50:628, 1976.
10. Bisby MA: Retrograde axonal transport. *In* L Hertz, S Federoff (Eds): [Adv Cell Neurobiol], vol 1. New York, Academic Press, 1980, pp 69.
11. Bisby MA: Functions of retrograde axonal transport. Fed Proc 41:2307, 1982.
12. Black MM, Lasek RJ: Slow components of axonal transport: two cytoskeletal networks. J Cell Biol 86:616, 1980.
13. Blunt JM: Functional and clinical implications of the vascular anatomy of peripheral nerves. Postgrad Med J 33:68, 1957.

14. Bolton C, McFarlane RM: Human pneumatic tourniquet paralysis. Neurol 28:787, 1978.

15. Brady ST, Lasek RJ: The slow components of axonal transport: movements, compositions and organization. *In* DG Weiss (ed): Axoplasmic Transport. Berlin/Heidelberg, Springer-Verlag, 1982, pp 206.

16. Bruner JM: Safety factors in the use of the pneumatic tourniquet for hemostasis in surgery of the hand. J Bone Joint Surg 33A:221, 1951.

17. Calderwood JW, Dickie WR: Tourniquet paresis complicating tendon grafting. Hand 4:53, 1972.

18. Carroll RE, Hurst LC: The relationship of thoracic outlet syndrome and carpal tunnel syndrome. Clin Orthop 164:149, 1982.

19. Cragg BG: What is the signal for chromatolysis? Brain Res 23:1, 1970.

20. Dahlin LB, McLean WG: Effects of graded experimental compression on slow and fast axonal transport in rabbit vagus nerve. J Neurol Sci 72:19, 1986.

21. Dahlin LB, Rydevik B, McLean WG, Sjostrand J: Changes in fast axonal transport during experimental nerve compression at low pressures. Exp Neurol 84:29, 1984.

22. Dahlin LB, Meiri KF, McLean WG, Rydevik B, Sjostrand J: Effects of nerve compression on fast axonal transport in streptozotocin-induced diabetes mellitus. An experimental study in the sciatic nerve of rats. Diabetol 29:181, 1986.

23. Dahlin LB, Sjostran J, McLean WG: Graded inhibition of retrograde axonal transport by compression of rabbit vagus nerve. J Neurol Sci 76:221, 1986.

24. Dahlin LB, Nordborg C, Lundborg G: Morphological changes in nerve cell bodies induced by experimental graded nerve compression. Exp Neurol. 95:611, 1987.

25. Denny-Brown D, Brenner C: Paralysis of nerve induced by direct pressure and by tourniquet. Arch Neurol Psychiatry 51:1, 1944.

26. Droz B: Synthetic machinery and axoplasmic transport: Maintenance of neuronal connectivity. *In* DB Tower (Ed): The Nervous System, vol 1. New York, Raven Press, 1975, pp 111.

27. Duncan D: Alterations in the structure of nerves caused by restricting their growth with ligatures. J Neuropathol Exp Neurol 7:261, 1948.

28. Durkin MA, Crabtree SD: Hazard of pneumatic tourniquet application. J R Soc Med 75:658, 1982.

29. Edshage S: Peripheral nerve suture. A technique for improved intraneural topography evaluation of some suture materials. Acta Chir Scand, (Suppl) 331:1-104, 1964.

29a. Eiken O, Nabseth DC, Mayer RF, Deterling RA Jr: Limb replantation. II. The pathophysiological effects. Arch Surg 88:54, 1964.

30. Erlanger J, Gasser HS: Electrical signs of nervous activity. Philadelphia, University of Pennsylvania Press, 1937.

31. Eversmann WW Jr, Ritsick JA: Intraoperative changes in motor nerve conduction latency in carpal tunnel syndrome. J Hand Surg 3:77, 1978.

32. Flatt AE: Tourniquet time in hand surgery. Arch Surg 104:190, 1972.

33. Fowler TJ, Danta G, Gilliatt RW: Recovery of nerve conduction after a pneumatic tourniquet: observations on the hind-limb of the baboon. J Neurol Neurosurg Psychiatry 35:638, 1972.

34. Fry D: Inaccurate tourniquet gauges. Br Med J 1:511, 1972.

34a. Fullerton PM, Gilliatt RW: Pressure neuropathy in the hind foot of the guinea-pig. J Neurol Neurosurg Psychiatry 30:18, 1967.

35. Fullerton PM, Gilliatt RW: Median and ulnar neuropathy in the guinea-pig. J Neurol Neurosurg Psychiatry 30:393, 1976.

36. Gainer H, Fink DJ: Covalent labelling techniques and axonal transport. *In* DG Weiss (Ed): Axoplasmic Transport. Berlin/Heidelberg, Springer-Verlag, 1982, pp 464.

37. Gasser HS, Erlanger J: The role of fiber size in the establishment of a nerve block by pressure or cocaine. Am J Physiol 88:581, 1929.

38. Gelberman RH, Hergenroeder PT, Hargens AR, Lundborg G, Akeson WH: The carpal tunnel syndrome. A study of carpal tunnel pressures. J Bone Joint Surg 63A:380, 1981.

39. Gelberman RH, Szabo RM, Williamson RV, Hargens AR, Yaru NC, Minteer-Convery MA: Tissue pressure threshold for peripheral nerve viability. Clin Orthop 178:285, 1983.

40. Gelberman RH, Szabo RM, Williamson RV, Dimick MP: Sensibility testing in peripheral nerve compression syndromes. An experimental study in humans. J Bone Joint Surg 65A:632, 1983.

41. Gilliatt RW: Physical injury to peripheral nerves. Physiologic and electrodiagnostic aspects. 1980, Mayo Clin Proc 56:361, 1981.

42. Grafstein B: The nerve cell body response to axotomy. Exp Neurol 48:32, 1975.

43. Grafstein B, Forman DS: Intracellular transport in neurons. Physiol Rev 60:1167, 1980.

44. Grafstein B, McQuarrie IG: Role of the nerve cell body in axonal regeneration. *In* CW Cotman (Ed): Neuronal Plasticity. New York, Raven Press, 1978, pp 155.

45. Grundfest H: Effects of hydrostatic pressures upon the excitability, the recovery and the potential sequence of frog nerve. Cold Spring Harbour Symp Quant Biol 4:179, 1936.

46. Grundfest H, Cattell M: Some effects of hydrostatic pressure on nerve action potentials. Am J Physiol 113:56, 1935.

47. Garde A, Stensman R: Total tre-nerv-pares efter operation i blodtomt falt—tourniquet paralysis. Lakartidningen (Sthlm) 70:4159, 1973.

48. Hamilton WK, Sokoll MD: Tourniquet paralysis. JAMA 199:37, 1967.

49. Harriman DG: Ischemia of peripheral nerve and muscle. J Clin Pathol, Suppl 30, 11:94, 1977.

50. Hongell A, Mattsson HS: Neurographic studies before, after, and during operation for median nerve compression in the carpal tunnel. Scand J Plast Reconstr Surg 5:103, 1971.

51. Horiuchi Y: Experimental study on peripheral nerve lesions—Compression neuropathy. J Jpn Orthop Assoc 57:789, 1983.

52. Hurst LC, Weissberg D, Carroll RE: The relationship of the double crush to carpal tunnel syndrome (an analysis of 1,000 cases of carpal tunnel syndrome). J Hand Surg 10B:202, 1985.

53. Jakobsen J: Peripheral nerves in early experimental diabetes. Expansion of the endoneurial space as a cause of increased water content. Diabetol 14:113, 1978.

54. Jefferson D, Eames RA: Subclinical entrapment of the lateral femoral cutaneous nerve: an autopsy study. Muscle Nerve 2:145, 1979.

55. Klemm H: Das Perineurium als Diffusionsbarriere gegnüber Peroxydase bei epi- und endoneuraler Applikation. Z Zellforsch Mikrosk Anat 108:431, 1970.

56. Korsching S, Auburger G, Heumann R, Scott J, Thoenen H: Levels of nerve growth factor and its mRNA in the central nervous system of the rat correlate with cholinergic innervation. EMBO J 4:1389, 1985.

57. Kristensson K, Olsson Y: Retrograde transport of horseradish peroxidase in transected axons. 3. Entry into injured axons and subsequent localization in perikaryon. Brain Res 115:201, 1976.

58. Kristensson K, Sjostrand J: Retrograde transport of protein tracer in the rabbit hypoglossal nerve during regeneration. Brain Res 45:175, 1972.

59. Kuczynski K: Functional micro-anatomy of the peripheral nerve trunks. Hand 6:1, 1974.

60. Levine J, Willard M: The composition and organization of axonally transported proteins in the retinal ganglion cells of the guinea-pig. Brain Res 194:137, 1980.

61. Lewis T, Pickering GW, Rothschild P: Centripetal paralysis arising out of arrested blood flow to the limb, including notes on a form of tingling. Heart 16:1, 1931.

62. Lieberman AR: The axon reaction: A review of principal features of perikaryal responses to axon injury. Int Rev Neurobiol 14:49, 1971.

63. Lieberman AR: Some factors affecting retrograde neuronal responses to axonal lesions. *In* R Bellairs, EG Gray (Eds): Essays on the Nervous System. Oxford, Clarendon Press, 1974, pp 71.

64. Low PA, Dyck PJ: Increased endoneurial fluid pressure in experimental lead neuropathy. Nature (Lond) 269:427, 1977.

65. Low PA, Dyck PJ, Schmelzer JD: Mammalian peripheral nerve sheath has unique responses to chronic elevations of endoneurial fluid pressure. Exp Neurol 70:300, 1980.

66. Low PA, Dyck PJ, Schmelzer JD: Chronic elevation of endoneurial fluid pressure is associated with low-grade fiber pathology. Muscle Nerve 5:162, 1982.

67. Low PA, Marchand G, Knox F, Dyck PJ: Measurement of endoneurial fluid pressure with polyethylene matrix capsules. Brain Res 122:373, 1977.

68. Low PA, Nukada H, Schmelzer JD, Tuck RR, Dyck PJ: Endoneurial oxygen tension and radial topography in nerve edema. Brain Res 341:147, 1985.

69. Lubinska L: Axoplasmic streaming in regenerating and in normal nerve fibers. *In* M Singer, JP Schade (eds): Mechanisms of Neural Regeneration. Progress in Brain Research 13: 1, Amsterdam, Elsevier Publishing Co., 1964, pp 1-71.

70. Lundborg G: Ischemic nerve injury. Experimental studies on intraneural microvascular pathophysiology and nerve function in a limb subjected to temporary circulatory arrest. Scand J Plast Reconstr Surg, Suppl 6, 1970.

71. Lundborg G: Structure and function of the intraneural microvessels as related to trauma, edema formation, and nerve function. J Bone Joint Surg 57A:938, 1975.

72. Lundborg G: The intrinsic vascularization of human peripheral nerves: Structural and functional aspects. J Hand Surg 4:34, 1979.

73. Lundborg G, Branemark P-I: Microvascular structure and function of peripheral nerves. Vital microscopic studies of the tibial nerve in the rabbit. Adv Microcirculation 1:66, 1968.

74. Lundborg G, Nordborg C, Rydevik B, Olsson Y: The effect of ischemia on the permeability of the perineurium to protein tracers in rabbit tibial nerve. Acta Neurol Scand 49:287, 1973.

75. Lundborg G, Gelberman RH, Minteer-Convery M, Lee YF, Hargens AR: Median nerve compression in the carpal tunnel—Functional response to experimentally induced controlled pressure. J Hand Surg 7:252, 1982.

76. Lundborg G, Myers R, Powell H: Nerve compression injury and increased endoneurial fluid pressure: A "miniature compartment syndrome." J Neurol Neurosurg Psychiatry 46:1119, 1983.

77. MacKinnon SE, Dellon AL, Hudson AR, Hunter DA: Chronic nerve compression—an experimental model in the rat. Ann Plast Surg 13:112, 1984.

78. Marotte LR: An electron microscope study of chronic median nerve compression in the guinea pig. Acta Neuropathol (Berl) 27:69, 1974.

79. Martin KH: Untersuchungen über die perineurale Diffusions-barriere an gefriergetrochneten Nerven. Z Zellforsch 64:404, 1964.

80. Matsen FA: Compartmental Syndromes. New York, Grune and Stratton, 1980.

81. Matsumoto N: An experimental study on compression neuropathy— determination of blood flow by a hydrogen washout technique. J Jpn Orthop Ass 57:805, 1983.

82. McLean WG, McKay AL, Sjostrand J: Electrophoretic analysis of axonally transported proteins in rabbit vagus nerve. J Neurobiol 14:227, 1983.

83. Middleton RW, Varian JP: Tourniquet paralysis. Aust NZ J Surg 44:124, 1974.

84. Moldaver J: Tourniquet paralysis syndrome. Arch Surg 68:136, 1954.

85. Mubarak SJ, Hargens AR: Compartment syndromes and Volkmann's contracture. Philadelphia, W.B. Saunders Co., 1981.

86. Myers RR, Powell HC: Endoneurial fluid pressure in peripheral neuropathies. *In* AR Hargens (Ed): Tissue Fluid Pressure and Composition. Baltimore, Williams and Wilkins, 1981, pp 193.

87. Myers RR, Powell HC, Costello ML, Lampert PW, Zweifach BW: Endoneurial fluid pressure: direct measurement with micropipettes. Brain Res 148:510, 1978.

88. Myers RR, Costello ML, Powell HC: Increased endoneurial fluid pressure in galactose neuropathy. Muscle Nerve 2:299, 1979.

89. Myers RR, Powell HC, Costello ML, Heckman HM, Shapiro HM: Endoneurial fluid pressure in peripheral neuropathies. Abstract, Second World Congress for Microcirculation. Microvasc Res 17:231, 1979.

90. Myers RR, Powell HC, Shapiro HM, Costello ML, Lampert PW: Changes in endoneurial fluid pressure, permeability and peripheral nerve ultrastructure in experimental lead neuropathy. Ann Neurol 8:392, 1980.

91. Myers RR, Mizisin AP, Powell HC, Lampert PW: Reduced nerve blood flow in hexachlorophene neuropathy: relationship to elevated endoneurial fluid pressure. J Neuropathol Exp Neurol 41:391, 1982.

92. Myers RR, Heckman HM, Powell HC: Endoneurial fluid is hypertonic. Results of microanalysis and its significance in neuropathy. J Neuropathol Exp Neurol 42:217, 1983.

93. Neary D, Eames RA: The pathology of ulnar nerve compression in man. Neuropathol Appl Neurobiol 1:69, 1975.

94. Nemoto K: An experimental study on the vulnerability of the peripheral nerve. J Jpn Orthop Ass 57:1773, 1983.

95. Nissl F: Uber die Veranderungen der Ganglienzellen am Facialiskern des Kaninchens nach Ausreissung der Nerven. Allg Z Psychiat 48:197, 1892.

96. Ochoa J: Nerve fiber pathology in acute and chronic compression. *In* GE Omer, M Spinner (Eds): Management of peripheral nerve problems. Philadelphia, W.B. Saunders Co., 1980, pp 487.

97. Ochoa J, Marotte L: The nature of the nerve lesion caused by chronic entrapment in the guinea-pig. J Neurol Sci 19:491, 1973.
98. Ochoa J, Fowler TJ, Gilliatt RW: Anatomical changes in peripheral nerves compressed by a pneumatic tourniquet. J Anat 113:433, 1972.
99. Ogata K, Naito M: Blood flow of peripheral nerve; effects of dissection, stretching and compression. J Hand Surg 11B:10, 1986.
100. Oldfors A: Permeability of the perineurium of small nerve fascicles: an ultrastructural study using ferritin in rats. Neuropathol Appl Neurobiol 7:183, 1981.
101. Olsson Y: Studies on vascular permeability in peripheral nerves. 1. Distribution of circulating fluorescent serum albumin in normal, crushed and sectioned rat sciatic nerve. Acta Neuropathol (Berl) 7:1, 1966.
102. Olsson Y: Studies on vascular permeability in peripheral nerves. 2. Distribution of circulating fluorescent serum albumin in rat sciatic nerve after local injection of 5-hydroxytryptamine, histamine and compound 48/80. Acta Physiol Scand 69, Suppl 284, 1966, pp 1.
103. Olsson Y, Reese TS: Inaccessibility of the endoneurium of mouse sciatic nerve to exogenous proteins. Anat Rec 163:318, 1969.
104. Olsson Y, Reese TS: Permeability of vasa nervorum and perineurium in mouse sciatic nerve studied by fluorescence and electron microscopy. J Neuropathol Exp Neurol 30:105, 1971.
104b. Peterson, HI, Risberg, B, Stenberg, B, Selander, D: Peripheral nerve vessel fibrinolysis. Bibl. Anat. 20:322, 1981.
105. Pilar G, Landmesser L: Axotomy mimicked by localized colchicine application. Science 177:1116, 1972.
106. Powell HC, Myers RR: Pathology of experimental nerve compression. Lab Invest 55:91, 1986.
107. Prevoznik SJ: Injury from use of pneumatic tourniquets. Anesthesiol 32:177, 1970.
108. Purves D: Functional and structural changes in mammalian sympathetic neurones following colchicine application to post-ganglionic nerves. J Physiol 259:159, 1976.
109. Purves D, Nja A: Effect of nerve growth factor in synaptic depression following axotomy. Nature (Lond) 260:535, 1976.
110. Risberg B: Fibrinolysis and tourniquet. Lancet 2:360, 1977.
111. Rydevik B, Lundborg G: Permeability of intraneural microvessels and perineurium following acute, graded experimental nerve compression. Scand J Plast Reconstr Surg 11:179, 1977.
112. Rydevik B, Lundborg G, Nordborg C: Intraneural tissue reactions induced by internal neurolysis. An experimental study on the blood-nerve barrier, connective tissue and nerve fibers of rabbit tibial nerve. Scand J Plast Reconstr Surg 10:3, 1976.
113. Rydevik B, McLean WG, Sjöstrand J, Lundborg G: Blockage of axonal transport induced by acute, graded compression of the rabbit vagus nerve. J Neurol Neurosurg Psychiatry 43:690, 1980.
114. Rydevik B, Lundborg G, Bagge U: Effects of graded compression on intraneural blood flow. An in vivo study on rabbit tibial nerve. J Hand Surg 6:3, 1981.
115. Rydevik B, Hansson HA, Dahlin LB, Lundborg G: Intraneural microvascular injury following acute, graded nerve compression. An ultrastructural study in rabbit tibial nerve and rat sciatic nerve. To be published.
116. Seddon HJ: Three types of nerve injury. Brain 66:237, 1943.

117. Seddon H: Surgical disorders of the peripheral nerves. London, Churchill Livingstone, 1972, pp 34.
118. Seiler WA, Schlegel R, MacKinnon SE, Dellon AL: Double crush syndrome: Experimental model in the rat. Surg Forum 34:596, 1983.
119. Shanthaveerappa TR, Bourne GH: The perineural epithelium: Nature and significance. Nature (Lond) 199:577, 1963.
120. Shyu BC, Dahlin LB, Danielsen N, Andersson S: Effects of nerve compression or ischemia on conduction properties of myelinated and unmyelinated nerve fibers. Acta Physiol. Scand. Submitted.
121. Spinner M, Spencer PS: Nerve compression lesions of the upper extremity. A clinical and experimental review. Clin Orthop 104:46, 1974.
122. Sunderland S: Nerves and Nerve Injuries. 1st ed. London, Churchill Livingstone, 1968.
123. Sunderland S: The nerve lesion in the carpal tunnel syndrome. J Neurol Neurosurg Psychiatry 39:615, 1976.
124. Sunderland S: Nerves and Nerve Injuries, 2nd ed. London, Churchill Livingstone, 1978.
125. Sunderland S, Bradley KC: The cross-sectional area of peripheral nerve trunks devoted to nerve fibers. Brain 72:428, 1949.
126. Szabo RM, Gelberman RH, Williamson RV, Hargens AR: Effects of increased systemic blood pressure on the tissue fluid pressure threshold of peripheral nerve. J Orthop Res 1:172, 1983.
127. Thomas PK, Olsson Y: Microscopic anatomy and function of the connective tissue components of peripheral nerve. *In* PJ Dyck, PK Thomas, EH Lambert, R Bunge (Eds): Peripheral Neuropathy, vol 1. Philadelphia, W.B. Saunders Co., 1984, pp 97.
128. Upton AR, McComas AJ: The double crush in nerve entrapment syndromes. Lancet 2:359, 1973.
129. Varon S, Adler R: Nerve growth factors and control of nerve growth. Curr Top Dev Biol 16:207, 1980.
130. Varon S, Adler R: Trophic and specifying factors directed to neuronal cells. Adv Cell Neurobiol 2:115, 1981.
131. Waggener JD, Bunn SM, Beggs J: The diffusion of ferritin within the peripheral nerve sheath: An electron microscopy study. J Neuropathol Exp Neurol 24:430, 1965.
132. Waksman BH: Experimental study of diphtheritic polyneuritis in the rabbit and guinea pig. III. The blood-nerve barrier in the rabbit. J Neuropathol Exp Neurol 20:35, 1961.
133. Weiss P, Hiscoe HB: Experiments on the mechanism of nerve growth. J Exp Zool 107:315, 1948.
134. Wheeler DK, Lipscomb PR: A safety device for a pneumatic tourniquet. J Bone Joint Surg 46A:870, 1964.

CHAPTER 3

Measurement of Tissue Fluid Pressure As Related to Nerve Compression Syndromes

Alan R. Hargens, Ph.D.

The wick catheter technique for measuring tissue pressure was developed when I was a graduate student of P.F. Scholander at Scripps Institution of Oceanography, UCSD during 1966 to 1971. Previous needles and catheters used for measuring interstitial fluid pressure required saline infusion in order to maintain patency of the probe. This requirement precluded measurements of negative fluid pressure in tissue, a concept that Arthur Guyton pioneered in the early 1960's. Although Guyton's capsule[12] provided very dynamic measurements of tissue fluid pressure, it was very large and required implantation for six weeks prior to any determinations. The wick catheter was developed to provide immediate, equilibrium measurements of tissue fluid pressure without saline infusion (Fig. 3-1). Microscopic channels of free fluid between the wick fibers maintained catheter patency and offered a relatively large pick-up area for sensing changes in tissue pressure.

Pete Scholander's dream of a floating laboratory to study physiologic adaptations throughout the world became a reality in 1965 with the christening of the R/V Alpha Helix. The maiden voyage of this NSF-supported research vessel was to the Great Barrier Reef of Australia where plants living in sea water and "air-breathing" fishes were studied. The Alpha Helix's second major expedition was to the Amazon River Basin and it was here we developed the wick technique.[43] A simple catheter system made from plastic tubing, a cotton wick, glass tube, and custom manometer were designed especially for field-type research "where electronic gadgetry was useless," according to Scholander. The system was thoroughly tested to ensure that it accurately measured hydrostatic fluid pressures only,

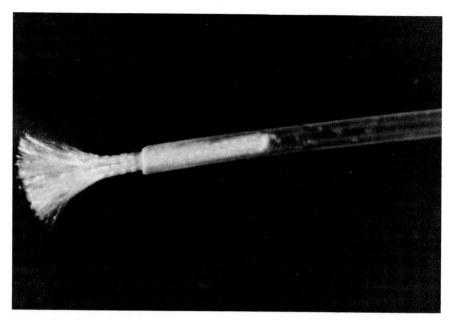

Figure 3-1. Close-up view of wick catheter tip showing microscopic wick fibers that provide contact with tissue fluids and maintain catheter patency without saline. (From Adair et al., 1983.)

especially under conditions of negative fluid pressures where other techniques were found inoperative. The wick technique was also tested in model systems of dehydration, for example, in monitoring development of negative pressure in starch suspensions during water evaporation. These initial studies were extended to measurement of fluid pressure in subcutaneous, peritoneal, and muscle tissues (Fig. 3-2) during the Amazon expedition.

The basic principles for measuring tissue fluid pressure in animals were applied and refined for intracompartmental studies in humans. For example, intramuscular fluid pressures in the forearm could be measured instantaneously using the glass capillary technique or continuously using a pressure transducer (Fig. 3-3). Revisions of the original technique included use of braided suture for wick material, smaller catheter tubing and improved techniques to minimize trauma during insertion, heparinized saline to prevent coagulation, and sterilization of all system components to minimize risks of infection. Over time, we developed a "wick kit" that included a pressure transducer, minirecorder, wick catheters, and all other items necessary for sterile measurements of intracompartmental pressure. Later, we helped Drs. Rorabeck and Castle develop and test a "slit catheter" that is based upon the wick principle and offers higher frequency of response for exercise studies.[30] We and our research residents were on call to make emergency measurements in patients with suspected acute compartment syndromes within the San Diego and Orange County areas (over 150 cases

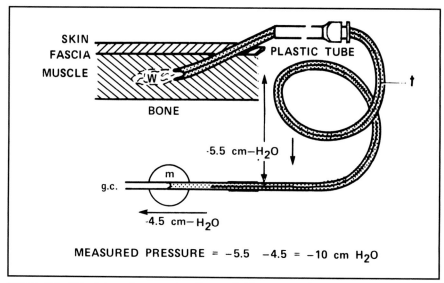

Figure 3-2. Principles of measuring tissue fluid pressure in muscle using the wick technique. Wick *w* is held within tubing by thread *t*. Glass capillary *G.C.* is adjusted vertically until read-out meniscus *m* is stationary, indicating equilibrium is reached. In this case, intramuscular fluid pressure equals hydrostatic height (—5.5 cm H_2O) plus capillarity (—4.5 cm H_2O) to give —10 cm H_2O.

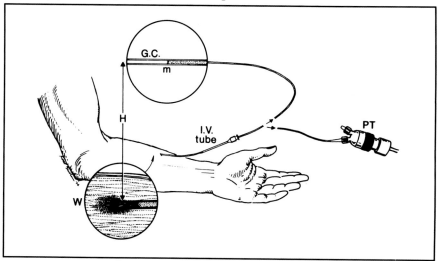

Figure 3-3. Wick catheter for measuring intracompartmental (volar forearm) fluid pressure. The sterile, heparinized catheter is connected to a read-out glass capillary tube *G.C.* where the meniscus *m* is held stationary by adjusting its hydrostatic height *h* above the wick *w*. Meniscus movement is followed microscopically. Subtracting the capillary of the glass tube *G.C.* from the equilibrium height *h* yields muscle fluid pressure in cm H_2O. Alternatively, the wick catheter can be connected to a pressure transducer *PT* zeroed to the wick's hydrostatic level *w*. The IV tube shields the wick catheter during the latter's entry into muscle. (From Hargens et al., 1977.)

of these patients were positive). Over 2000 studies of intramuscular pressure were undertaken in patients and volunteers at UCSD over the past 10 years and only one infection occurred using our technique.

Tissue Fluid Pressures in Myoneural Compression Syndromes

Compartment Syndromes

A compartment syndrome is a condition characterized by high muscle pressure, myoneural pain, paresthesia, paresis, pink skin color, and presence of distal pulse (the six ps of a compartment syndrome). The syndrome is induced by high tissue pressure within a confined region of skeletal muscle, causing sufficient ischemia to compromise myoneural structures. Elevated pressure is produced by internal swelling or external compression on muscle and may occur in almost any region of the body (Fig. 3-4). Muscle compartments of the leg are involved most frequently, but compartment syndromes are reported in thigh, buttock, shoulder, arm, and hand muscles as well.[30] Typically, muscles involved in this ischemic process are enclosed within relatively impermeable, noncompliant osseofascial boundaries that preclude spontaneous dissipation of tamponade within the involved compartment. Therefore, surgical decompression by fasciotomy is required to renew adequate blood flow through ischemic tissues. If intracompartmental pressure remains elevated for a sufficiently long period of time without fasciotomy, necrosis of intracompartmental tissues will result. The well-known clinical entity of Volkmann's contracture may thus occur if prompt diagnosis and treatment of the jeopardized limb are not undertaken.

Acute Compartment Syndrome: Compartment syndromes are commonly divided into two forms, acute and chronic, based on etiology and reversibility. An acute compartment syndrome develops when intramuscular pressure exceeds capillary blood pressure for a prolonged period of time. In this setting, immediate decompression is necessary to prevent myoneural necrosis and Volkmann's contracture. Acute compartment syndromes are produced by trauma, arterial injury, arterial reconstruction, extreme exertion, or prolonged limb compression.

Chronic Compartment Syndrome: A second form of the syndrome is defined as a chronic (exertional) compartment syndrome, also termed recurrent compartment syndrome by some authors. This condition occurs when exercise increases intramuscular pressure sufficiently to cause ischemia, pain, and, on some occasions, decreased sensibility or neurologic dysfunction. Commonly, these symptoms disappear when the activity is stopped and reappear during the next exercise activity. However, if muscular activity is maintained despite pain, neurologic deficit, and persistent tamponade, a chronic compartment syndrome can precipitate an acute compartment syndrome, which then requires immediate fasciotomy.

Volkmann's Contracture: The natural history of an untreated compartment syndrome involving a limb produces a deformity known as Volkmann's

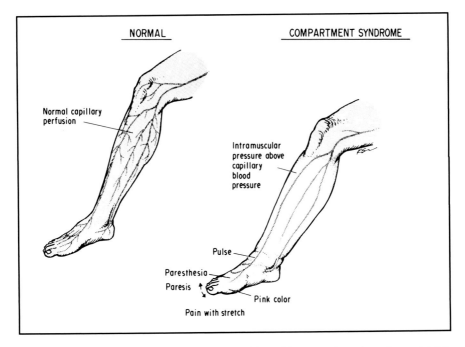

NORMAL   COMPARTMENT SYNDROME

Normal capillary
perfusion

Intramuscular
pressure above
capillary
blood
pressure

Pulse

Paresthesia

Paresis

Pink color

Pain with stretch

Figure 3-4. Comparison of normal leg (*left*) and leg with compartment syndrome (*right*). When tissue fluid pressure within one or more muscle compartments rises above capillary blood pressure (30-40 mm Hg), ischemia occurs and blood flow is confined solely to large vessels and collateral circulations. (From Hargens et al., 1984.)

contracture. First described by Volkmann in the 1880s, this contracture was thought to result from tight dressings or casts applied to a traumatized extremity. Now, however, internal and external causes of elevated pressure are known to occur. An untreated acute compartment syndrome will cause muscle necrosis, atrophy, and fibrous tissue replacement several weeks after the initial traumatic insult. Volkmann's contracture represents the final stage of myoneural necrosis and atrophy.

Other Terms and Associated Conditions: Whereas compartment syndrome usually relates to localized or limited myoneural ischemia, a crush syndrome represents the systemic manifestations of more severe muscle necrosis.[31,39] Muscle infarctions associated with crush syndromes produce myoglobinuria, extracellular fluid loss, and acidosis/hyperkalemia. In severe cases these manifestations produce renal failure, shock, and cardiac arrhythmia, respectively.

Several debilitating conditions mimic the symptoms of compartment syndromes (pain, neurologic deficit, or subcutaneous edema). However, elevated intracompartmental pressure is absent in these conditions, and thus, there is none of the intrinsic muscle ischemia that characterizes all compartment syndromes. These conditions include stress fracture, arterial injury (compensated occlusion), direct nerve contusion, cellulitis, snake bite, and shin splints.[35]

The sequelae of an unrelieved acute compartment syndrome are devastating, ranging from functional deficits to death (e.g., crush syndrome). Despite an increased awareness of the problem by physicians, compartment syndromes remain poorly managed for the following reasons: despite many reports of compartment syndromes in the literature, compartment syndrome pathophysiology has not been fully clarified; physicians are not always well informed; and the accepted indications for decompressive fasciotomy based on clinical findings alone are rather subjective. We believe accurate measurements of intracompartmental pressure by the wick or slit catheter enable the physician to evaluate compartment syndromes more objectively. Hopefully, prompt diagnosis of compartment syndromes will help clarify the etiology, prevent major functional deficits and enhance our understanding of the conditions.

Pathophysiology: A compartment syndrome develops when intramuscular pressure is sufficiently elevated to compromise nutritional blood flow to tissues within the involved compartment. Capillary blood flow may be obstructed by external compression (prolonged limb compression caused by comatose posture and associated with alcohol or drug abuse, tight bandage or cast, burn eschar) or internal swelling (hemorrhage, increased capillary permeability related to toxic substances, or postischemic swelling). Internal swelling may be related to interstitial or intracellular edema. Historically, many mechanisms (venous obstruction, arterial occlusion or spasm, exertion) were proposed to explain compartment syndrome pathogenesis. Today, however, these diverse mechanisms are replaced by one pathogenic factor: increased compartment pressure, sufficiently elevated to compromise blood perfusion of tissues.[27]

The pathogenesis of compartment syndromes is related to fluid accumulation in extracellular or intracellular spaces. Such accumulation increases intracompartmental volume, which as a consequence of low fascial compliance, raises intracompartmental pressure to levels up to 100 mm Hg. After reaching a threshold pressure (sufficiently high to cause myoneural ischemia) and threshold time (sufficiently long to produce irreversible injury), myoneural necrosis results (Fig. 3-5). Acute ischemia alone can raise capillary permeability and produce interstitial edema, thus raising intracompartmental pressure above the threshold level and causing the self-perpetuating cycle of ischemia followed by more postischemic swelling. Furthermore, a posttraumatic vascular leak may increase intracompartmental volume and pressure, thus initiating the vicious edema-ischemia cycle. Therefore, a multifactorial etiology for compartment syndrome pathogenesis is apparent.

Etiology: As based upon our experience with over 150 patients with a positive diagnosis, acute compartment syndromes are caused by the following conditions (in order of frequency): fractures, contusions, postischemic swelling, comatose limb compression, burns, bleeding diathesis (hemophilia, anticoagulants), and other causes (exertion, venomous snake bites). Tibial fractures are the most common cause of compartment syndrome. Moreover, surgical procedures involving the tibia

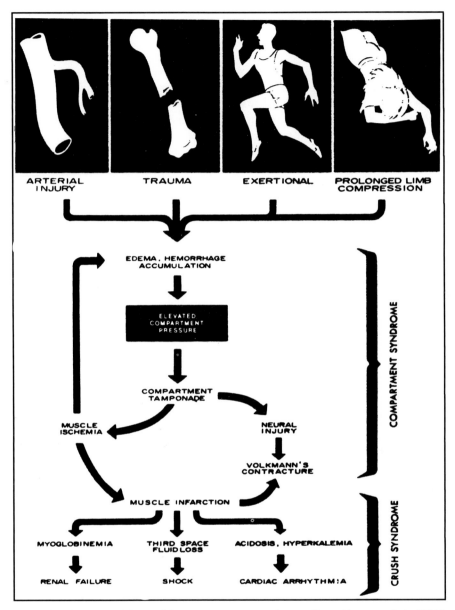

Figure 3-5. Pathophysiology of the compartment syndrome. (From Hargens et al., 1984.)

(e.g., donor site for grafts, tibial tubercle advancements, tibial osteotomies, tibial lengthening) are known to cause compartment syndromes.

A frequently overlooked cause of compartment syndrome is postischemic swelling produced by vascular occlusion. In this case, acute arterial occlusion caused by artery laceration, thrombosis, or embolization causes ischemia. After arterial repair or clot removal, circulation is restored, but postischemic swelling, intracompartmental tamponade, and further ischemia occur, especially if the initial ischemia lasted over six hours. Frequently, this cause of compartment syndrome yields poor results because of the extended ischemic period of arterial obstruction coupled with postischemic swelling.

Acute compartment syndromes can be classified according to increased or decreased intracompartmental volume, edema or hemorrhage accumulation, and miscellaneous causes (Table 3-1). Although venomous snake bites are a possible cause of compartment syndrome, our experience with patients in Southern California indicates that edema associated with snake venom is most often confined to subcutaneous spaces, and therefore, antivenin therapy without fasciotomy is usually the treatment of choice.[16] This research, primarily led by Steve Garfin, has helped prevent unnecessary surgery on patients with venomous snake bites.

Diagnosis

Acute Compartment Syndrome: The clinical indications of a compartment syndrome are related to the specific muscles involved. Swelling and tenseness over the involved compartment are the earliest signs of an acute compartment syndrome. However, edema sometimes present in the subcutaneous tissues will mask any underlying compartmental tamponade. Furthermore, because palpation over the involved compartment is only a very gross indication of elevated pressure, a tissue fluid pressure technique should be employed whenever a question arises regarding the presence of compartment syndrome. Our technique will be described later.

Compartment syndromes of the leg are often differentiated in conscious, cooperative patients by sensory deficit, pain with stretch, and muscular weakness (Table 3-2). Sensory deficit is the most reliable early finding in our experience.[33] Initially, the sensory deficit may consist of paresthesia only. Without decompression, however, this subjective finding will progress to objective hypoesthesia or even anesthesia. Pain with passive stretch of involved muscles is a common finding, but is also subjective in nature. Following fracture or contusion, it may be difficult to separate out any increase in pain due to ischemia. Pain with stretch may be absent in later stages of an acute compartment syndrome. Muscle weakness or paresis may occur but is difficult to interpret, because it may result from nerve compression, muscle ischemia, or guarding due to severe pain. Distal pulses and normal skin color are usually deceptively present in compartment syndromes of the leg. Deep vein thrombosis, tenosynovitis, stress fracture, osteomyelitis, and cellulitis may cause some swelling in limbs, but these conditions rarely cause compartment syndromes.

Differential diagnosis of compartment syndrome, nerve injury, and arterial injury is very important, because their treatments are quite different (Table 3-3). Sometimes two or more of these conditions exist at the same time, making differential diagnosis very difficult. Nerve injury with fracture or contusion is usually neurapraxia, which is followed clinically without

---

Table 3-1. Classification of Acute Compartment Syndrome

I. Decreased compartment size
  A. Constrictive dressings and casts
  B. Closure of fascial defects
  C. Thermal injuries and frostbite
II. Increased compartment contents
  A. Primarily edema accumulation
    1. Postischemic swelling
      a. Arterial injuries
      b. Arterial thrombosis or embolism
      c. Reconstructive vascular and bypass surgery
      d. Replantation
      e. Prolonged tourniquet time
      f. Arterial spasm
      g. Cardiac catheterization and angiography
      h. Ergotamine ingestion
    2. Prolonged immobilization with limb compression
      a. Drug overdose with limb compression
      b. General anesthesia with knee-chest position
    3. Thermal injuries and frostbite
    4. Exertion
    5. Venous disease
    6. Venomous snakebite
  B. Primarily hemorrhage accumulation
    1. Hereditary bleeding disorders (e.g., hemophilia)
    2. Anticoagulant therapy
    3. Vessel laceration
  C. Combination of edema and hemorrhage accumulation
    1. Fractures
      a. Tibia
      b. Forearm
      c. Elbow (*e.g.*, supracondylar)
      d. Femur
    2. Soft tissue injury
    3. Osteotomies (*e.g.,* tibia)
  D. Miscellaneous
    1. Intravenous infiltration (*e.g.,* blood, saline)
    2. Popliteal cyst
    3. Long leg brace

(Mubarak SJ, Hargens AR: Compartment Syndromes and Volkmann's Contracture, p. 75. Philadelphia, WB Saunders, 1981)

surgical intervention. Arterial injury produces absent pulses, lower skin temperature, and poor color. Pain with stretch, muscular weakness, and hypoesthesia may also occur with arterial injury. On the other hand, compartment syndromes usually manifest intact distal pulses unless an

Table 3-2. Typical Findings of Acute Compartment Syndromes of the Leg

Compartment	Sensory Deficit	Muscle Weakness	Pain with Stretch	Pedal Pulses
Anterior	Deep peroneal nerve	Tibialis anterior, toe extensors	Foot and toe flexion	Intact
Lateral	Superficial and deep peroneal nerves	Pereneus longus and brevis	Foot inversion	Intact
Superficial posterior	Sural nerve	Gastrocnemius, soleus	Foot dorsi-flexion	Intact
Deep posterior	Tibial nerve	Tibialis posterior, toe flexors	Toe extension	Intact

(Mubarak SJ, Hargens AR: Diagnosis and management of compartment syndromes. In Symposium on Trauma to the Leg and Its Sequelae, American Academy of Orthopaedic Surgeons, p 330. St Louis, CV Mosby, 1981)

Table 3-3. Differential Diagnosis for a Closed Limb Injury with Neurovascular Deficits: Typical Findings and Treatment

Diagnosis	Pain with Stretch	Paresis or Paralysis	Paresthesia or Anesthesia	Increased Compartmental Pressure	Pulses Intact	Treatment
Compartment syndrome	Yes	Yes	Yes	Yes	Yes	Fasciotomy
Arterial injury	Yes	Yes	Yes	No	No	Repair or remove thrombosis
Nerve contusion (neura-praxia)	No	Yes	Yes	No	Yes	Observe

(Mubarak SJ, Hargens AR: Diagnosis and management of compartment syndromes. In Symposium on Trauma to the Leg and Its Sequelae, American Academy of Orthopaedic Surgeons, p. 332. St. Louis, CV Mosby, 1981)

arterial injury or degenerative process occurs concomitantly. In some cases, Doppler flow studies, arteriography, and intracompartmental pressure tests are required to differentiate neurapraxia, arterial injury, and compartment syndrome.

Measurement of Intracompartmental Pressure: Because high intracompartmental pressure is the underlying pathogenic factor common to all acute compartment syndromes, its measurement is often required, especially in patients who are uncooperative (children), unresponsive, or comatose.

Several clinical techniques for monitoring intracompartmental pressure are available today. However, some techniques are preferred over others in terms of accuracy, safety, and cost.

The needle injection technique of Whitesides and coworkers[47] is simple in design and least expensive, but measurements by one physician or technician often differ from those of another by 20 mm Hg to 30 mm Hg, a degree of reproducibility far below other techniques available. Similarly, a noninvasive technique[48] using a blood pressure cuff and hydrostatic pressure differences is not sufficiently accurate for diagnosis of compartment syndromes. Neither of these techniques allows continuous monitoring of intracompartmental pressure, a feature desirable for following the clinical course of an acute compartment syndrome, adequacy of fasciotomy, and pressure during muscle contraction. Moreover, any injection of saline will cause overestimation of true intracompartmental pressure, and we believe these techniques should be used only when other more accurate techniques are not available.

The continuous infusion technique of Matsen and associates[28] has the advantage of long-term (up to three days) monitoring of tissue pressure. Plugging or coagulation around the infusion needle tip is rarely a problem. The principal disadvantages of this technique are the necessity of extra infusion equipment and the risk of improperly adjusting the rate of saline infusion to a high setting, thus creating or exacerbating a compartment syndrome. This technique typically responds more slowly to pressure changes during exercise studies of chronic compartment syndromes.

The wick catheter technique was originally developed as a basic science tool for studies of fluid balance in a variety of Amazon River animals.[43] Its subsequent development for clinical use[13,32] allowed continuous equilibrium measurements of tissue fluid pressure in compartment syndromes. Advantages of this technique include a relatively large area for sensing tissue fluid pressure, avoidance of saline infusion (equilibrium measurements are thus obtained), and continuous monitoring of pressure (Fig. 3-6). Disadvantages include possible coagulation around the catheter tip, especially if the wick fibers are packed too tightly in the catheter tip, and relatively slow response to pressure changes during exercise studies. Overall, the wick technique is simple, accurate to ± 1 mm Hg, and reliable for diagnosis of compartmental tamponade (Fig. 3-7).

The slit catheter technique[34,42] represents an attempt to improve the wick catheter by a more open catheter tip (Fig. 3-8). This design allows a higher frequency response to intracompartmental pressure changes. The slit catheter is less prone to coagulation, but air bubbles form more easily around the tip, which may reduce response time and invalidate a measurement. Obviously, the slit catheter tip is easier to manufacture. Overall, however, the wick and slit catheters are equally accurate and reliable for diagnosis of acute compartment syndrome.

Thresholds of Pressure and Time for Fasciotomy: Based on several clinical studies,[30,32,33] and animal experiments,[14,15,17] decompressive fasciotomy is recommended for normotensive patients with positive clinical findings and

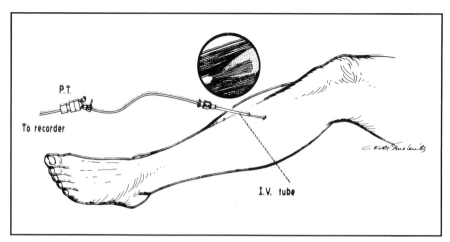

Figure 3-6. Wick catheter for measuring intracompartmental pressure. The sterile, heparinized-saline-filled catheter is connected to a pressure transducer (PT) for continuous monitoring of anterior compartment pressure in this leg. Catheter insertion is facilitated by prior sterile insertion of an intravenous placement unit using local anesthesia. The IV tube is pulled back after entry of the wick catheter into muscle. A close-up of the wick tip is depicted above the insertion site. (From Hargens et al., 1984.)

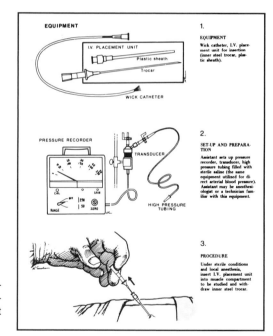

Figure 3-7. Equipment and stepwise procedure for the wick catheter technique. (From Hargens et al., 1984.)

intracompartmental pressures over 30 mm Hg when duration of increased pressure is unknown or thought to be eight hours or more since the initial traumatic event. Undoubtedly there exists a broad spectrum of tolerance to compartmental tamponade and ischemia among patients. However, considering the disastrous results of an unrelieved acute compartment

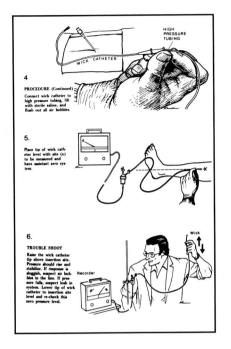

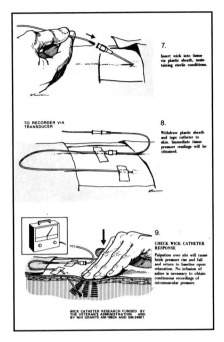

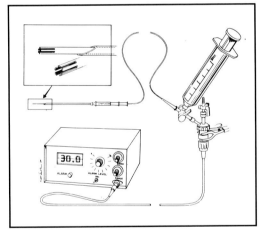

Figure 3-8. Slit catheter system for measurement of intracompartmental pressure. (From Mubarak and Hargens, 1981.)

syndrome, we recommend that any compartment with stable or rising pressures over 30 mm Hg be decompressed if clinical indications are positive. When clinical signs of a compartment syndrome are difficult to obtain (e.g., uncooperative or unconscious patient), fasciotomy should be performed on any compartment with pressure over 30 mm Hg. Recent animal and clinical experiments indicate that in some instances, the previously indicated threshold for fasciotomy should be revised. Under conditions of low blood pressure, the fasciotomy pressure and time thresholds fall to 20 mm Hg and six hours, respectively.[50]

Tissue Pressure Thresholds for Nerve Dysfunction

The mechanism by which acute compression affects the function of peripheral nerve is not completely understood. The pathophysiology of nerve compression syndromes is related to both the magnitude and the duration of pressure. However, other factors such as nerve anatomy, systemic blood pressure, and cardiovascular disease may modify the pressure-duration thresholds for nerve dysfunction. Recognition of these factors has important implications for treatment of nerve compression lesions.

The pathophysiology of acute and chronic nerve compression syndromes is an issue of considerable theoretical and clinical relevance. The clinical findings associated with chronic nerve entrapment, including the carpal tunnel syndrome, are well known.[2,23,40,44] A very interesting clinical model for acute nerve compression is the compartment syndrome. As indicated in the previous section, its diagnosis, prognosis, and treatment often depend on the determination of a critical pressure threshold at which neurologic conduction is interrupted and nerve fiber viability is jeopardized.

Experimental studies in our laboratory have focused upon: (1) carpal canal pressures in normal volunteers and patients with carpal tunnel syndrome,[8] (2) the relative importance of ischemia versus mechanical deformation in early peripheral nerve compression,[25] (3) the critical threshold pressure for peripheral nerve conduction,[10] and (4) the clinical sensibility testing system most appropriate for evaluating and following

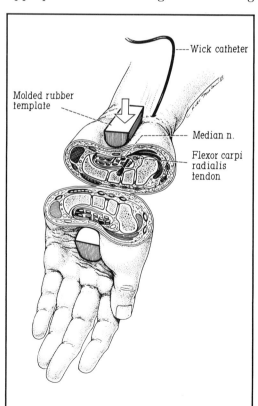

Figure 3-9. Local compression is applied over the median nerve by a molded rubber template. The wick catheter is inserted adjacent to the flexor carpi radialis tendon at the level of the proximal wrist. (From Gelberman et al., 1986.)

Wick catheter

Molded rubber template

Median n.

Flexor carpi radialis tendon

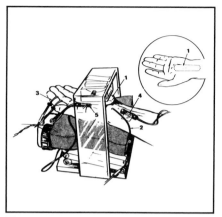

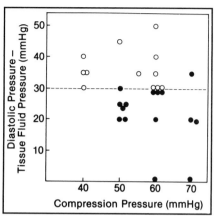

Figure 3-10. Apparatus for controlled external compression of the carpal canal. Localized pressure was applied to the carpal canal by adjusting level of lower platform toward fixed roof of compression device. (1) Molded rubber placed on the palmar aspect of the wrist. (2) Wick catheter in carpal canal just ulnar to flexor carpi radialis tendon. (3) Self-retaining spring ring digital electrode for recording the stimulating (sensory conduction tests). (4) Bar surface electrode for stimulating median nerve 3 cm proximal to wrist. (5) Bar surface electrode on thenar eminence for recording motor response. (From Gelberman et al., 1983.)

Figure 3-11. Relationship between diastolic blood pressure minus tissue fluid pressure, and the tissue fluid pressure (compression pressure) that blocks median nerve conduction. Summary of all tests performed at compression pressures of 40-70 mm Hg. Open circles signify no nerve conduction block. Solid points signify complete conduction block. (From Szabo et al., 1983.)

patients with acute and chronic compressive neuropathies.[9,45] Each of our initial studies utilized a human model for median nerve compression of the carpal canal (Fig. 3-9).

The acute carpal tunnel syndrome model is very useful for studying the effects of compression on human nerve because the median nerve is superficial in the wrist and very accessible to controlled localized pressure. Electrical and sensory tests of the median nerve are sensitive and reliable. Our volunteers consisted of 25 healthy subjects without any history of diabetes, alcoholism, hand trauma, symptoms of carpal tunnel syndrome or peripheral neuropathy. In addition, nine hypertensive subjects were tested.[45] A sterile wick catheter was introduced into the carpal canal as previously described.[8] After measurement of the resting pressure, the hand was placed within a specially designed external compression device and localized pressure was applied over the carpal canal using a piece of molded rubber placed on the palmar aspect of the wrist (Fig. 3-10). The wrist rested on a layer of foam, leaving several large dorsal veins free from compression. Thus, adequate venous drainage from the hand was ensured. Compression was gradually applied to the wrist, while tissue fluid pressure was continuously measured by the wick catheter. Different levels of pressure between 30 and 90 mm Hg were used in each subject. The catheter was withdrawn when the desired pressure level was reached. Motor and sensory

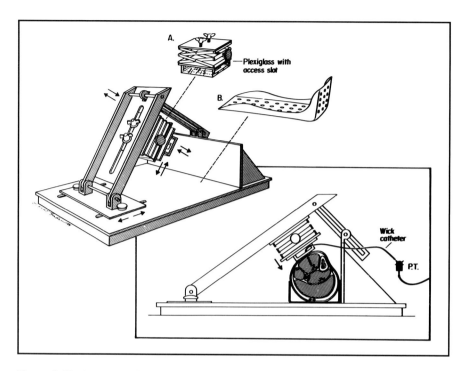

Figure 3-12. Apparatus for short-term studies of anterior compartment compression in human subjects. Compression device employs an adjustable Plexiglas plate (20 cm long, 9 cm wide) attached to a lab jack *A* so that various levels of external compression are applied to the anterior compartment. Intramuscular pressure level around the deep peroneal nerve is monitored continuously by a wick catheter connected to a pressure transducer *P.T.* and recorder. (From Hargens et al., 1987.)

latencies of the median nerve at the wrist were studied by a TECA electromyograph at 10-minute intervals during compression and during the recovery phase after release of compression. A nerve stimulator delivered a rectangular pulse of 0 to 1 millisecond duration at the rate of 1 per second to the median nerve (supramaximal intensity). Each subject was questioned as to subjective changes such as numbness, tingling, or pain throughout the experiment. In the first 16 subjects, the Weber two-point discrimination test was performed on each digit using a dull-pointed eye caliper[46] applied in a longitudinal axis with care taken to avoid blanching the skin.[7,37] In addition, the strength of the abductor pollicis brevis was tested manually and graded on a scale from 0 to 5.[26] The remaining subjects were also tested by a 256 cps tuning fork, by the moving two-point discrimination test as described by Dellon[5,6] and by Semmes-Weinstein monofilaments (von Frey pressure test).[24,38,46] Six subjects were also tested with a fixed-frequency (120 Hz) variable amplitude vibrometer (Bio-Thesiometer, Biomedical Instrument Co., Newbury, OH) to assess vibratory threshold.[6] Each experiment was terminated when, after the release of compression, both subjective sensation and neurophysiologic tests returned to their baseline values. Compression was maintained for no less than 30 min and no longer than 240 min.

The major conclusions of our studies of carpal canal compression were:

1. In 16 normotensive volunteers, compression at 50 to 90 mm Hg induced a rapid, complete sensory conduction block that consistently preceded a motor block by 10-30 minutes. Two-point discrimination remained normal until the last stages of preserved sensory fiber conduction. Using a tourniquet model, ischemic rather than mechanical deformation was the primary cause of nerve dysfunction.[5]

2. Again, in a second series of nine normotensive human subjects, some functional loss occurred at a tissue fluid pressure of 40 mm Hg but motor and sensory responses were blocked completely at 50 mm Hg. Semmes-Weinstein monofilaments and the 256-cycle vibratory test were more sensitive and demonstrated more gradual changes than two-point discrimination tests.[9]

3. Nine hypertensive subjects (130 to 190 mm Hg systolic and 90 to 110 mm Hg diastolic) had compression thresholds of 60 to 70 mm Hg for nerve dysfunction, as compared to 40 to 50 mm Hg for nine normotensive subjects (100 to 120 mm Hg systolic and 60 to 75 mm Hg diastolic). The tissue pressure threshold for all normotensive and hypertensive subjects (Fig. 3-11) was consistently 30 mm Hg below diastolic blood pressure (approximately 45 mm Hg below mean arterial blood pressure), again supporting the concept that ischemia is the primary factor for blocking conduction in nerve compression syndromes.[45]

Recently, we extended these studies of carpal canal compression to external compression of the anterior compartment.[19] A new apparatus was developed to compress selectively the anterior compartment (Fig. 3-12). Thirty-five normal volunteers were studied in order to determine short-term thresholds of local tissue pressure that produce significant neuromuscular dysfunction. Local tissue fluid pressure adjacent to the deep peroneal nerve was elevated by our compression apparatus and continuously monitored for 2 to 3 hours by the wick or slit catheter technique (Fig. 3-13). Elevation of tissue fluid pressure to within 30 to 40 mm Hg of diastolic blood pressure (approximately 40 mm Hg absolute pressure in our subjects) elicited a consistent progression of neuromuscular deterioration, assessed quantitatively (Fig. 3-14), including in order: (1) gradual loss of sensation as determined by Semmes-Weinstein monofilaments (Fig. 3-15), (2) subjective complaints, (3) reduced nerve conduction velocity (Fig. 3-16), (4) decreased action potential amplitude of the extensor digitorum brevis muscle, and (5) motor weakness of muscles within the anterior compartment. Generally, higher intracompartmental pressures caused more rapid deterioration of neuromuscular function. Two subjects placed in the apparatus with compression levels of 0 and 30 mm Hg maintained normal neuromuscular function for three hours.

Short-term external compression of human muscle compartment is a highly relevant model for studying pressure-time thresholds for compartment syndromes in clinical terms. Intramuscular blood flow[36] and nerve

Figure 3-13. The wick or slit catheter is placed adjacent to the deep peroneal nerve at midanterior compartment level under sterile conditions. (1) Insertion needle is directed at 45° angle to skin surface. (2) As shown here, slit catheter is passed through insertion needle and the latter is retracted. Sensibility is tested in the first web space of the foot. (From Hargens et al., 1987.)

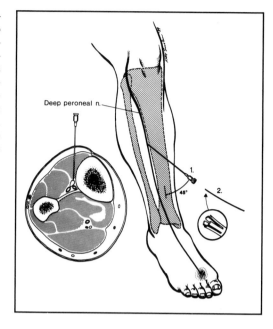

Figure 3-14. Placement of stimulating and recording electrodes for electrophysiologic studies during compression of the anterior compartment: (1) external sensory branch of superficial peroneal nerve: (*a*) record sensory NCV with stimulus at ankle; (*b*) point of stimulation for sensory branch of peroneal nerve; (*c*) extensor digitorum brevis: recording point for motor response to peroneal nerve with stimulation at ankle, fibular neck or popliteal fossa; (*d*) point of ankle stimulation of peroneal motor NCV; (*e,f*) points of stimulation at the fibular neck and popliteal fossa for peroneal motor NCV; (*g*) tibialis anterior: recording point for motor response to tibial nerve with stimulation at ankle or popliteal fossa; (*i,j*) points of stimulation for tibial nerve at ankle, and popliteal fossa. *W* is wick catheter. (From Hargens et al., 1987.)

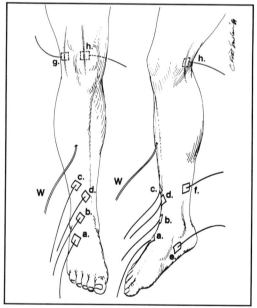

function[10,25,28] are both reduced in proportion to the magnitude of tissue pressure. Furthermore, pressure thresholds for peripheral nerve dysfunction can be correlated with arterial blood pressure,[28,45] and external compression models allow objective analyses of various techniques for neurologic examination of compartment syndrome and other nerve compression syndromes.[9] The validity of these models in terms of compartment syndrome

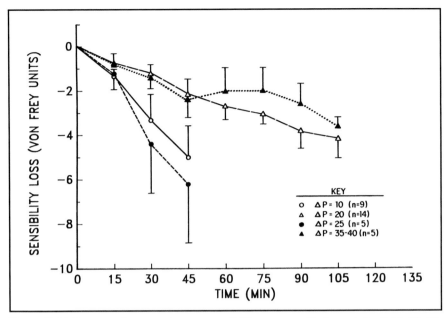

Figure 3-15. Decreased peroneal nerve sensibility occurs with time at Ps of 10, 20, 25, and 35-40 mm Hg. ΔP = diastolic blood pressure minus tissue fluid pressure near peroneal nerve. n = number of human subjects. In ΔP groups of 10 and 20 mm Hg, sensation was lost completely after 45 minutes of compression. (From Hargens et al., 1987.)

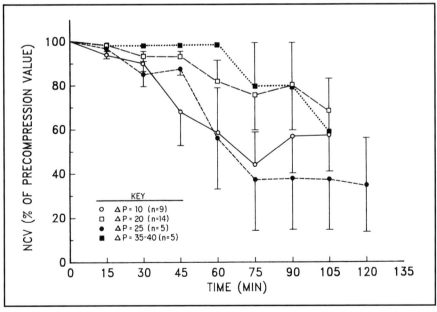

Figure 3-16. Decreased nerve conduction velocity (NCV) with time at ΔPs of 10, 20, 25 and 35-40 mm Hg. ΔP = diastolic blood pressure minus tissue fluid pressure near peroneal nerve. n = number of human subjects. (From Hargens et al., 1987.)

pathophysiology is supported by recent studies which indicate that limb compression associated with drug or alcohol abuse[39] and use of anti-shock trousers[3,49] causes acute compartment syndromes. Of course, external compression studies of normal human subjects are necessarily limited to periods of two to three hours. It is noteworthy that neuromuscular function in all of our volunteers returned to normal one hour after compression release, and our subjects experienced no untoward effects from this study.

Matsen and coworkers[28] studied effects of compressing the leg by a segmental air splint but only three normal subjects were examined. Moreover, their study was somewhat limited because local tissue pressure around the peroneal nerve was not measured. Using our compression device on two cadaver legs, we found that deep muscle pressures near the peroneal nerve are about 20 mm Hg less than those measured by Matsen and coworkers[28] at a depth of 1 cm. As previously indicated, we investigated local extenal compression of the carpal canal in nine healthy volunteers (normal blood pressure) and nine hypertensive patients and found that the threshold tissue fluid pressure for median nerve dysfunction was consistently 30 mm Hg below diastolic pressure in all subjects.[45] The findings of this leg compression study agree with those obtained using the carpal canal model. Although local tissue pressure was continuously monitored and controlled around the median nerve, our carpal canal model did not involve compression of skeletal muscle. Subsequently, we developed a model whereby the anterior compartment of human subjects is compressed externally by a plate while local tissue pressure adjacent to the peroneal nerve is continuously monitored. This is necessary because the distribution of tissue pressures beneath any compression device is nonuniform[4] with bone and other tissue anisotropy providing shelter from high external pressure.[20]

In terms of defining a threshold tissue pressure at which neuromuscular function is acutely jeopardized, our leg compression results for 35 normal subjects indicate that sensibility and nerve conduction velocity are decreased when compression levels are within 30 to 40 mm Hg of diastolic blood pressure. Nerve conduction and anterior compartment motor function are diminished when tissue fluid pressure approaches within 25 mm Hg of diastolic pressure. Of the four neuromuscular functions examined in this study, however, sensibility and nerve conduction velocity are considered the most sensitive in terms of criteria for evaluating the effects of external compression.[9] It is noteworthy that higher compression levels caused more rapid (15 to 45 minutes) loss of neuromuscular function in almost all subjects. The duration of compression is important as well, because individuals with relatively low levels of anterior compartment compression demonstrated dysfunction only after one to two hours. Although our results suggest that intracompartmental pressures approaching 30 to 40 mm Hg of diastolic pressure produce significant neuromuscular dysfunction, it is still possible that lower pressure thresholds exist for longer durations of nerve compression (e.g., 3 to 10 or more hours).

Despite increasing clinical experience and scientific data concerning the pathophysiology of acute compartment syndromes, controversy persists with reference to pressure thresholds that require fasciotomy in patients. Based upon several clinical studies[30,32,33] and animal experiments,[14,15,17] decompressive fasciotomy is recommended for patients with positive clinical findings and intracompartmental pressures over 30 mm Hg when the duration of increased pressure is unknown or thought to be eight hours or more since the initial traumatic event. Undoubtedly, there exists a broad spectrum of tolerance to compartmental tamponade and ischemia among patients. Therefore, when clinical signs of an acute compartment syndrome are not present, it is possible to defer fasciotomy until pressures reach 40 to 50 mm Hg in normotensive patients, as based upon our present results with the leg compression model.

As monitored by ^{31}P-NMR spectra techniques, Heppenstall and collaborators[22] also note that blood pressure plays an important role in determining the threshold intramuscular pressure at which ischemia occurs. These investigators emphasize the additive effect of ischemia and local muscle trauma on the lowering of fasciotomy thresholds for acute compartment syndromes.[21] Their important experiments indicate that a lower mean arterial pressure and local muscle trauma both make muscle more susceptible to necrosis associated with increased intracompartmental pressure. However, the pressure thresholds for fasciotomy recommended by Heppenstall and colleagues (20 to 30 mm Hg below *mean arterial pressure* in the nontraumatized anterior compartment) are too high as based upon results in this study as well as our clinical experience over the past 12 years in more than 150 acute compartment syndromes. They usually employ mean arterial pressure, calculated as diastolic pressure plus one-third (systolic pressure minus diastolic pressure), as the arterial pressure component of their ΔP term. On the other hand, because mean arterial pressure is a calculated parameter, we have preferred use of diastolic blood pressure in our studies of ΔP thresholds for acute neuromuscular dysfunction. Reduced capillary perfusion caused by elevated intramuscular pressure is considered the primary problem in the pathophysiology of compartment syndromes.[14,41] Therefore, although mean arterial pressure or diastolic pressure may give some indication of perfusion pressure at the precapillary level, capillary pressures often do not correlate directly with arterial pressures.[51] Consequently, the concept of a ΔP (mean arterial pressure minus intramuscular pressure or diastolic pressure minus intramuscular pressure) may not always be valid.

Our previous canine studies indicated that muscle damage began to appear at an absolute intracompartmental pressure of 30 mm Hg[17] or at a ΔP of approximately 50 mm Hg (diastolic blood pressure minus tissue pressure). We subsequently showed that compartment syndromes with pressures of 30 to 40 mm Hg were reversible if sustained for only eight hours and that muscle function subsequently normalized after a 30-day period.[29] Nevertheless, we still employ 30 mm Hg as one indication for fasciotomy *when other clinical signs are present*. Briefly, our reasoning takes into account that (1) direct muscle trauma is usually sustained, and (2) periods of hypotension and lower tolerance to elevated intramuscular are commonly encountered in multitrauma patients. Both factors predispose compartmental tissues to ischemic necrosis. Moreover, because the greater risk involves ischemic contracture with its attendant major long-term disability, we believe it is prudent to recommend a conservative pressure threshold of 30 mm Hg absolute tissue pressure so that the error term favors too many fasciotomies rather than ischemic necrosis and Volkmann's contracture.

It is possible, of course, for the experienced physician to modify the fasciotomy criteria in individual clinical cases. In alert and cooperative patients, for example, the clinical criteria of elevated intramuscular pressure (myoneural pain, paresthesia, paresis, pink skin color, and presence of distal pulse) are usually detectable and confirm the diagnosis of an acute compartment syndrome. Therefore, it is reasonable to observe a patient carefully over time in spite of elevated compartment pressures, if perfusion is adequate for muscle and nerve viability. This requires hourly observations in a hospital setting with continuous tissue pressure monitoring. Increasing pressure with time accompanied by the development of increased tenseness, pain, and neurologic deficits will mandate fasciotomy. Stable or declining pressure without those signs in a normotensive patient with minor tissue damage, localized to a single extremity, is obviously more likely to resolve without the need for fasciotomy than those in a comatose, hypotensive, multiple trauma victim with extensive tissue damage.

Therefore, the question of a pressure threshold for fasciotomy has no single answer. There is no critical pressure value for all patients with impending compartment syndrome. We emphasize clinical criteria in the alert, cooperative, localized-injury patient population. We supplement these observations with measurements of intracompartmental pressure, but when clear clinical signs are absent, we delay fasciotomy until pressures reach 40 mm Hg. Finally, cases between these extremes will continue to challenge clinical judgment. It will be necessary for each clinician to act upon his or her experience and judgment appropriately. In this context, it is always wise to bear the risk factors in mind: a fasciotomy produces a scar, but ischemic necrosis may cause loss of limb.

Acknowledgements

The research and clinical progress that is outlined in this chapter was only made possible by a team effort of many colleagues, fellows, residents, students and staff at the University of California, San Diego, and the Veterans Administration Medical Center, San Diego. Their contributions, combined with continued research support from the Veterans Administration; National Institute of Arthritis and Musculoskeletal and Skin Diseases; National Heart, Lung and Blood Institute; National Institute of General Medical Sciences; NASA; NSF; and the National Geographic Society, are gratefully appreciated.

References

1. Adair TH, Hogan RD, Hargens AR, Guyton AC: Techniques in the measurement of tissue fluid pressure and lymph flow. *In* Techniques in the Life Sciences, edited by R.J. Linden. County Clare, Ireland, Elsevier Scientific Publishers Ireland Ltd, Volume P3/1:1, 1983.

2. Adamson JE, Srouji SJ, Horton CE, Malkick RA: The acute carpal tunnel syndrome. Plast Reconstr Surg 47:332, 1971.

3. Brotman S, Browner BD, Cox EF: MAS trousers improperly applied causing a compartment syndrome in lower-extremity trauma. J Trauma 22:598, 1982.

4. Dahlin LB, Rydevik B, Lundborg G, Hargens AR, Skalak R: Distribution of tissue fluid pressure beneath a pneumatic tourniquet. Trans, 30th Ann Orthop Res Soc 9:362, 1984.

5. Dellon AL: The moving two-point discrimination test: Clinical evaluation of the quickly adapting fiber/receptor system. J Hand Surg 3:474, 1978.

6. Dellon AL: Evaluation of sensibility and re-education of sensation in the hand. Baltimore, Williams and Wilkins, pp 95, 1981.

7. Gelberman RH, Urbaniak JR, Bright DS, Levin LS: Digital sensibility following replantation. J Hand Surg 3:313, 1978.

8. Gelberman RH, Hergenroeder PR, Hargens AR, Lundborg GN, Akeson WH: The carpal tunnel syndrome: A study of carpal canal pressures. J Bone Joint Surg 63A:632, 1983.

9. Gelberman RH, Szabo RM, Williamson RV, Dimick MP: Sensibility testing in peripheral—nerve compression syndromes—A human experimental study in humans. J Bone Joint Surg 65A:632, 1983.

10. Gelberman RH, Szabo RM, Williamson RV, Hargens AR, Yaru NC, Minteer-Convery MA: Tissue pressure threshold for peripheral nerve viability. Clin Orthop 178:285, 1983.

11. Gelberman RH, Szabo RM, Hargens AR: Pressure effect on human peripheral nerve. *In* Tissue Nutrition and Viability, edited by A.R. Hargens, New York, Springer-Verlag, pp 161, 1986.

12. Guyton AC: A concept of negative interstitial pressure based on pressures in implanted perforated capsules. Circ Res 12:399, 1963.

13. Hargens AR, Mubarak SJ, Owen CA, Garetto LP, Akeson WH: Interstitial fluid pressure in muscle and compartment syndromes in man. Microvas Res 14:1, 1977.

14. Hargens AR, Akeson WH, Mubarak SJ, Owen CA, Evans KL, Garetto LP, Gonsalves MR, Schmidt DA: Fluid balance with canine anterolateral compartments and its relationship to compartment syndromes. J Bone Joint Surg 60A:499, 1978.

15. Hargens AR, Romine JS, Sipe JC, Evans KL, Mubarak SJ, Akeson WH: Peripheral nerve-conduction block by high muscle-compartment pressure. J Bone Joint Surg 61A:192, 1979.

16. Hargens AR, Garfin SR, Mubarak SJ, Castilonia RR, Russell FE: Edema associated with venomous snake bites. Recent Advances in Microcirculatory Research, Bibli Anat 20:267, 1981.

17. Hargens AR, Schmidt DA, Evans KL, Gonsalves MR, Cologne JB, Garfin SR, Hagan PL, Akeson WH: Quantitation of skeletal-muscle necrosis in a model compartment syndrome. J Bone Joint Surg 63A:631, 1981.

18. Hargens AR, Mortensen WW, Gershuni DH, Crenshaw AG, Lieber RL, Akeson WH: Long-term measurement of muscle function in the dog hindlimb using a new apparatus. J Ortho Res 1:284, 1984.

19. Hargens AR, Botte MJ, Gelberman RH, Rhoades CE, Akeson WH, Swenson MR: Intracompartmental pressure thresholds for peroneal nerve dysfunction in humans. J Bone Joint Surg, Submitted 1988.

20. Hargens AR, McClure AG, Skyhar MJ, Lieber RL, Gershuni DH, Akeson WH: Local compression patterns beneath pneumatic tourniquets applied to arms and thighs of human cadavera. J Orthop Res, 5:247, 1987.

21. Heppenstall RB, Shenton DW, Sapega AA, Chance B, Hazelgrove JC: Compartment syndrome: A bioenergetic study using 31 P-NMR Spectroscopy. Trans, 30th Ann Orthop Res Soc 9:330, 1984.

22. Heppenstall RB, Scott RJ, Shenton DW, Chance B: Compartment syndrome: The critical role of blood pressure in the establishment of muscle ischemia and the increased susceptability of the traumatized compartment. Trans, 31st Ann Orthop Res Soc 10:370, 1985.

23. Hunter JM, Schneider LH, Mackin EJ, Bell JA: Rehabilitation of the hand. St. Louis, C.V. Mosby, pp 273, 1978.

24. Levin S, Pearsell G, Ruderman RJ: Von Frey's method of measuring pressure sensibility in the hand: An engineering analysis of the Weinstein-Semmes pressure anesthesiometer. J Hand Surg 3:211, 1978.

25. Lundborg G, Gelberman RH, Minteer-Convery M, Lee YF, Hargens AR: Median nerve compression in the carpal tunnel: Functional response to experimentally induced controlled pressure. J Hand Surg 7:252, 1982.

26. Manual of Orthopaedic Surgery, Chicago, American Orthopaedic Association, 1972.

27. Matsen FA III: Compartmental syndrome: A unified concept, Clin Orthop 113:8, 1975.

28. Matsen FA III, Mayo KA, Krugmire RB, Sheridan GW, Kraft GH: A model compartment syndrome in man with particular references to the quantification of nerve function. J Bone Joint Surg, 59A:648, 1977.

29. Mortensen WW, Hargens AR, Gershuni DH, Crenshaw AG, Garfin SR, Akeson WH: Long-term muscle function after an induced compartment syndrome in the canine hindlimb. Clin Orthop 195:289, 1985.

30. Mubarak SJ, Hargens AR: Compartment Syndromes and Volkmann's Contracture. Philadelphia, W.B. Saunders, 1981.

31. Mubarak SJ, Owen CA: Compartmental syndrome and its relations to the crush syndrome: A spectrum of disease. Clin Orthop 113:81, 1975.

32. Mubarak SJ, Hargens AR, Owen CA, Garetto LP, Akeson WH: The wick catheter technique for measurement of intramuscular pressure: A new research and clinical tool. J Bone Joint Surg 58A:1016, 1976.

33. Mubarak SJ, Owen CA, Hargens AR, Garetto LP, Akeson WH: Acute compartment syndromes: Diagnosis and treatment with the aid of the wick catheter. J Bone Joint Surg 60A:1091, 1978.

34. Mubarak SJ, Hargens AR, Lee YF, Lundblad A-K, Castle GSP, Rorabeck CH: Slit catheter—A new technique for measuring tissue fluid pressure and quantifying muscle contraction. Trans 27th Ann Meeting Orthop Res Soc 6:34, 1981.

35. Mubarak SJ, Gould RN, Lee YF, Schmidt DA, Hargens AR: The medial tibial stress syndrome: A cause of shin splints. Am J Sports Med 10:201, 1982.

36. Ogata K, Whiteside LA: Effects of external compression on blood flow to muscle and skin. Clin Orthop 168:105, 1982.

37. Omer GE Jr: Injuries to nerves of the upper extremity. J Bone Joint Surg 56A:1615, 1974.

38. Omer GE Jr: Sensibility testing. *In* Management of peripheral nerve problems G.E. Omer Jr. and M Spinner (eds.). Philadelphia, W.B. Saunders, pp 3, 1980.

39. Owen CA, Mubarak SJ, Hargens AR, Rutherford L, Garetto LP, Akeson WH: Intramuscular pressure with limb compression. Clarification of the pathogenesis of the drug-induced compartment syndrome/crush syndrome. N Eng J Med 300:1169, 1979.

40. Phalen GS: The carpal-tunnel syndrome. Clinical evaluation of 598 hands. Clin Orthop 83:29, 1972.

41. Reneman RS, Slaaf DW, Lindbom L, Tangelder GJ, Arfors KE: Muscle blood flow disturbances produced by simultaneously elevated venous and total muscle tissue pressure. Microvasc Res 20:307, 1980.

42. Rorabeck CH, Castle GSP, Hardie R, Logan J: Compartmental pressure measurements: An experimental investigation using the slit catheter. J Trauma 21:446, 1981.

43. Scholander PF, Hargens AR, Miller SL: Negative pressure in the interstitial fluid of animals. Science 161:321-328, 1968.

44. Sunderland S: The nerve lesion in the carpal tunnel syndrome. J Neurol Neurosurg Psychiatry 39:615, 1976.

45. Szabo RM, Gelberman RH, Williamson RV, Hargens AR: Effects of increased systemic blood pressure on the tissue fluid pressure threshold of peripheral nerve. J Orthop Res 1:172, 1983.

46. Werner JL, Omer GE Jr: Evaluating cutaneous pressure sensation of the hand. Am J Occup Ther 24:347, 1970.

47. Whitesides TE Jr, Haney TC, Morimoto K, Hirada H: Tissue pressure measurements as a determinant for the need of fasciotomy. Clin Orthop 113:43, 1975.

48. Willey RF, Corall RJM, French EB: Noninvasive method for the measurement of anterior tibial compartment pressure. Lancet 1:595, 1982.

49. Williams TM, Knopp R, Ellyson JH: Compartment syndrome after antishock trouser use without lower extremity trauma. J Trauma 22:595, 1982.

50. Zweifach SS, Hargens AR, Evans KL, Smith RK, Mubarak SJ, Akeson WH: Skeletal muscle necrosis in pressurized compartments associated with hemorrhagic hypotension. J Trauma 20:941, 1980.

51. Zweifach BW, Kovalcheck S, DeLano F, Chen P: Micropressure-flow relationships in a skeletal muscle of spontaneously hypertensive rats. Hypertension 3:601, 1981.

CHAPTER 4

Electrodiagnosis in Upper Extremity Nerve Compression

James S. Lieberman, M.D.
Robert G. Taylor, M.D.

Electrodiagnostic techniques have a very significant role in the evaluation and diagnosis of patients suspected of having nerve compression syndromes, and in monitoring progress following treatment.

The techniques available for electrodiagnostic (EDX) study are electromyography (EMG) and nerve conduction study (NCS). The EMG is a slightly invasive procedure requiring placement of needle electrodes into the muscles to be studied. The information that can be obtained is: (1) presence or absence of the spontaneous activity that confirms loss of axons; and (2) the size, duration, and number of the voluntary motor unit action potentials (MUAPs) that can suggest whether an abnormality is due to a neuropathic or myopathic etiology. Large, long duration MUAPs represent loss of axons with reinnervation of some additional muscle fibers by surviving axons, while small MUAPs suggest a myopathic or ischemic etiology in which muscle fibers, not axons, are lost. In general, for a nerve lesion to show abnormalities on EMG, the problem must have been severe enough and present long enough for axons to have been lost in order for the abnormal spontaneous activities that characterize denervation (fibrillation potentials, positive sharp wave potentials) to appear. In addition, significant time must pass for axon collateral sprouting to occur before the characteristic MUAP of a chronic neuropathic process can be seen.

Nerve conduction studies are usually of considerably more value in assessing compressive neuropathies than EMG. The major exception is nerve compression at a site so proximal that stimulation of the nerve proximal to the suspected lesion is not possible. In those conditions the EMG is the only EDX procedure available. In order for sensory nerve conduction studies to be able to identify abnormality of function, it is necessary to be able to stimulatge, or record from, the nerve proximal to the suspected lesion. For motor nerve conduction studies, it must be possible to stimulate the nerve proximal to the site of compression and record from a muscle innervated by that nerve distal to the site of suspected compression.

In nerve conduction studies, the variables observed are: (1) nerve conduction velocity (NCV); (2) latencies, including the distal motor (DML) and distal sensory (DSL) latencies; (3) the amplitude of the sensory nerve action potential (SNAP or N wave), or the compound muscle action potential (CMAP or M wave). Deviation from normal of these variables is the basis for evaluation of suspected compression neuropathies.

To determine conduction velocity for a motor nerve it is necessary to stimulate the nerve at two different sites and record the evoked CMAP from a muscle that is innervated by that nerve, but distal to both sites of stimulation. The latencies and amplitudes are measured directly on the oscilloscope screen. The nerve conduction velocity is calculated by dividing the distance between the two stimulating electrodes by the difference between the two latencies. It is necessary to subtract the latency for the distal segment because the axons become much smaller in diameter in the distal regions, and as the nerve enters the muscle the axon diameters can become very small, with resultant reduction in conduction velocity. In addition, synaptic delay and muscle conduction time decrease velocity distally. Nerve conduction velocities are directly proportional to the diameter of the axons, but, for the major limb segments, the diameter variation is of minimal significance.

Conduction velocity of sensory or mixed nerve can be determined by stimulating a nerve trunk at one point and recording the SNAP as it passes along the nerve under a recording electrode at a remote point, either proximal or distal to the point of stimulation used to activate the nerve. For sensory nerve conduction studies the technique can be either orthodromic (distal to proximal) or antidromic (proximal to distal).

The velocity at which the depolarization impulse travels along a nerve may be slowed across the segment of a nerve that is compressed, when compared to velocities for the segments proximal or distal to the impaired segment. The velocity may also be slowed distal or proximal to the site of compression, but to a lesser degree than for the involved segment. Slowing of nerve conduction velocity distal or proximal to the site of compression is not an acute change, and weeks or months may be required before this change will be observed. In other cases, axonal loss seems to be the most significant feature, and a decreased CMAP or SNAP is present without evidence of slowed conduction.

The cause of slowed conduction across an involved segment of nerve may be focal demyelination or transient ischemia.[135] It is not known whether ischemia can produce long-term slowing of conduction without loss of axons, which would result in reduced amplitude of the evoked responses.

There are many books and handbooks available to describe the specific procedures for performing EMG and motor and sensory nerve conduction studies. The reader should consult those references for details of specific techniques.[11,18,48,80,95] Problems with techniques and interpretation can permit significant errors, particularly in NCS studies.[81] Normal values for any NCS vary from laboratory to laboratory. Therefore, this chapter will usually not give actual test values.

The electrodiagnostic findings in the various nerve compression syndromes are described below, in detail, for each upper extremity nerve.

Median Nerve
Carpal Tunnel Syndrome

Carpal tunnel syndrome (CTS) is the most common entrapment neuropathy and the most thoroughly studied electrodiagnostically. While electromyography has a role in the evaluation of the patient with CTS, nerve conduction studies are more useful for the diagnosis of CTS. The initial step in the electrodiagnostic evaluation of CTS consists of routine motor and sensory conduction studies. If these routine studies are normal, several more specialized studies are available when a high index of clinical suspicion is present.

Motor Conduction Studies. In 1956, Simpson[128] reported slowing of median nerve motor conduction across the carpal tunnel. This has also been clearly shown by several other investigators.[9,136,137] A prolonged distal motor latency (DML) of the median nerve is considered one of the important diagnostic findings in CTS. Reports of the sensitivity of the DML in CTS vary from extremes of 39.4[130] to 90.7 percent,[22] when only DML slowing or an absent CMAP response are considered. However, most studies report a sensitivity in the range of 60 to 70 percent for motor conduction studies.[70,79,123,136,137] The amplitude of the compound muscle action potential (CMAP) may also be impaired,[76] but this finding is not specific for CTS, and represents axon loss somewhere in the median nerve or its root supply. While not of great value for diagnosis of CTS, the CMAP amplitude may be important for therapeutic decisions (see later discussion).

In addition to a prolonged DML, a slowed median forearm motor conduction velocity may be observed in CTS. This is reported in 11 to 35 percent of cases in various studies.[8,123,130,136] The slowing of median forearm motor conduction is thought to be secondary to either retrograde fiber degeneration or selective involvement of large fibers by the compressive lesion.[131]

Finally, in a few cases the DML may be abnormal when sensory conduction studies are normal. This is the reverse of the usual situation, and may be due to selective involvement of motor fibers or an anatomic variant in the course of motor fibers through the carpal tunnel.[66]

Special Motor Conduction Calculations. Two calculated values, the residual latency[84] and the terminal latency index[126] are reported to improve the sensitivity of motor conduction studies in CTS. The principals of these calculations are beyond the scope of this chapter. Comparison of these calculated values to sensory palmar stimulation in CTS clearly shows the sensory studies to be more sensitive.[29,130]

Sensory Conduction Studies

Finger-to-Wrist. Sensory conduction studies are generally more sensitive than motor conduction studies in the diagnosis of CTS. The routinely performed study is measurement of the distal sensory latency (DSL) from index finger-to-wrist. This may be done by either orthodromic or antidromic techniques. A prolonged DSL or slowed sensory conduction velocity from finger-to-wrist is reported in 35 to 93 percent of cases, while absence of the sensory nerve action potential (SNAP) is reported in 0 to 55 percent of cases in various series.[8,22,70,79,130,136] The overall sensitivity of finger-to-wrist sensory conduction studies varies from 63 to 98 percent, although most series report an overall sensitivity of about 85 percent or greater for finger-to-wrist sensory studies.[8,22,70,123,136] Studies of SNAP amplitude show a diminished SNAP in 3 to 88 percent of cases.[8,70,92,130] A diminished SNAP amplitude by itself has no value for localizing the lesion at the wrist.

A slow median nerve sensory conduction velocity in the forearm has been reported in 3 to 9 percent of patients.[8,130] However, data in this area are sparse. The presumed explanation would be similar to that given already for motor conduction slowing in the forearm.

Palm-to-Wrist. A further refinement in CTS electrodiagnosis is the measurement of the sensory latency from palm-to-wrist. This measurement was first made using orthodromic techniques,[8,9,147] but antidromic techniques were soon described.[38] Recently there have been a number of reports using these techniques.[28,75,104,105,152]

The principle underlying the palm-to-wrist technique is that the shorter the segment studied, the greater the effect of the lesion on NCS. In CTS, nerve conduction is presumed to be normal distal to the carpal tunnel. This normal segment (palm-to-finger) in the finger-to-wrist studies, dilutes the effect of the focal lesion in the palm-to-wrist segment. Thus, the palm-to-wrist techniques are more sensitive than finger-to-wrist techniques in CTS evaluation. In addition, the palm-to-wrist techniques add more specificity to CTS diagnosis. In distal neuropathy the palm-to-wrist segment may be normal while the finger-to-palm segment is slowed. Thus, an abnormal finger-to-wrist latency could be due to peripheral neuropathy, not CTS. Although very valuable, the palm-to-wrist and finger-to-palm techniques are technically more difficult and are not necessary if routine techniques show abnormality and peripheral neuropathy can be ruled out by other means (see later discussion). As an example of the value of palmar techniques, Kimura[77] reported an abnormal palm-to-wrist DSL in 20 percent of hands in which routine studies were normal.

Other Nerve Conduction Techniques

Serial Stimulation. Kimura[79] has reported a technique for studying both the DML and DSL for the median nerve using serial stimulation sites at 1 cm increments from 4 cm proximal to 6 cm distal to the distal wrist crease. This technique may well provide the highest sensitivity in CTS; however, it is technically difficult and time consuming,[130] and, therefore, is probably not suitable for routine use. This technique presumes that serial increments in distance will produce relatively uniform changes in latency. In CTS there are focal areas of excessive latency change.

Median/Median, Median/Ulnar, Median/Radial Comparisons. A number of studies have shown a relatively fixed relationship between bilateral median DML and DSL, and median/ulnar DML and DSL when done at the same distances. Thomas et al.[36] suggests that the median nerve DMLs would have a difference of less than 1.0 msec between the two sides, while the ipsilateral median DML and ulnar DML should have less than 1.8 msec difference. They consider values in excess of these to be abnormal and consistent with CTS or impaired function on the side with the longer DSL.

In further extensive studies, Felsenthal[34,37] has shown that the difference in DSL for median nerves bilaterally, or median and ulnar nerves in the same or different hands should not exceed 0.5 msec. Similarly, he[34] shows that the median/median DML difference should not exceed 0.6 msec, while the median/ulnar DML difference for the same or opposite hands should not exceed 1.0 msec. Felsenthal and Spindler[37] further contend that median/ulnar DSL difference values are equally sensitive to palmar stimulation in the diagnosis of CTS.

Johnson et al.[64] report that median and ulnar DSL values to the ring finger were 0.3 msec or less in 93 percent of hands and 0.6 msec or less in all control hands. By contrast, in CTS cases the range of DSL difference was 1.0 to 2.1 msec (mean 1.46 msec). This is an extension of the other median/ulnar comparison studies.

Stevens[130] reports that with *palmar* stimulation median and ulnar sensory latency differences should not exceed 0.2 msec. He considers this to be of value when palmar stimulation gives normal results for the median nerves.

In an interesting recent study, Johnson et al.[65] report that median and radial DSL values to digit 1 were within 0.2 msec in 93 percent of hands. CTS patients had a 100 percent incidence of a median/radial DSL difference of 1.0 msec or greater. They consider this test to be of value in CTS diagnosis.

Finally, Loong and Seah[91] have compared median and ulnar SNAP amplitudes. In their study, the ratio of the median (index finger) SNAP amplitude to ulnar (small finger) SNAP amplitude was greater than one in all controls, and less than one in 91 percent of CTS cases. They suggest that this determination is a sensitive test for CTS. This ratio is not generally used, however.

In considering the value of the various commparison values just described, one must rememmber that CTS is bilateral in 55 to 61 percent of cases.[4,130] Thus, median/median comparison will have a high rate of false negative results. In addition, distal ulnar nerve involvement in association with CTS is reported in 6.4 to 46 percent of cases[9,11,123] in various series. In bilateral CTS, one recent study[11] reports an 88 percent incidence of distal ulnar nerve involvement. While the results of this most recent study[11] have not been confirmed by others, the median/ulnar difference tests must be viewed with these data in mind. Concomitant ulnar and median nerve involvement would lead to false negative; however, excessive median/ulnar differences are abnormal.

Multifinger DSL Measurements. In the occasional patient with CTS, the DSL is abnormal in only one or two branches.[9] Therefore, it is useful to measure the DSL to other than the index finger especially when symptoms are prominent in other than the index finger.

Provocative or Stress Tests. A change in median nerve DML or DSL with wrist flexion for two minutes was reported in 1980.[122] In this study median DML or DSL were never increased more than 0.1 msec in controls. In patients with CTS, a change of DML or DSL of 0.2 msec or more was considered abnormal. This occurred in 16 of 40 CTS hands, two of which had normal routine studies.

In a more recent study,[98] both wrist flexion and extension for 5 and 10 minutes resulted in an increase in DML and DSL in controls and in patients with CTS. The greatest increase was with flexion for 5 minutes. The increase in DML and DSL never exceeded normal values for controls, while the increase was much greater for CTS patients. Three of four patients with a normal DSL showed an increase in DSL to above the normal range. The results of these two studies suggest that stress tests may be of some value in evaluating CTS patients with normal values on other studies. More confirmation is needed, however, to determine the exact value of stress testing with normal routine test values.

Changing DSL Criteria

A very recent study suggests that the normal values for median nerve DSL can be changed to reflect improved techniques and equipment.[20] In this study the values reported suggested that the upper limit of DSL latency for that laboratory could be reduced to 3.3 msec from 3.7 msec. This would result in increased numbers of abnormal results in CTS cases. The data from this study have not been confirmed by other investigators.

Needle Electromyography. Needle electromyography in CTS is useful to determine the severity of the lesion. Abnormalities such as the presence of fibrillations or positive sharp wave potentials are indicators of axonal injury, which suggests a more severe lesion. Abnormal spontaneous activity is reported in 18 to 50 percent of cases.[9,130,136]

In addition to indicating axonal injury, EMG is useful in differentiating CTS from radiculopathy, more proximal median neuropathy, and polyneuropathy. The coexistence of CTS and radiculopathy (the double crush)[142] is reported with an incidence of 14 to 18 percent in two recent series.[11,40] Without needle EMG as a routine part of the evaluation of CTS patients, the double crush would not be recognized.

Differentiation of CTS from Peripheral Neuropathy. In all cases of suspected CTS it is necessary to rule out polyneuropathy as a cause of the slowing of distal median nerve conduction. Therefore, most laboratories study ulnar nerves as well as median nerves in CTS cases. However, because of frequent concomitant ulnar involvement, it would be preferable to do sural, peroneal, or radial nerve studies to rule out peripheral neuropathy in CTS cases. In addition, the use of palmar stimulation may be helpful in this regard, as already noted.

Electrodiagnostic Results as an Indication for Surgery. There is no electrodiagnostic finding that is an absolute indicator of the need for surgical intervention. A decreased SNAP or CMAP amplitude or the presence of fibrillation potentials or positive sharp waves in median intrinsic musculature suggests more severe median nerve involvement with axonal injury. In such cases, surgery may be needed. Although a significantly prolonged DML or DSL may suggest the need for surgery, it is important to remember that the median nerve DML and DSL may not correlate well with symptomatology.[130]

Electrodiagnostic Studies and Treatment. Following surgical decompression, there may be rapid improvement in median nerve conduction (i.e., within 15 to 30 minutes).[30,56] However, this could not be confirmed in another study.[155] After the initial rapid improvement in conduction, there is a slower phase of improving conduction over many weeks to months.[9,51] However, some degree of slowing may persist for years or permanently, even in an asymptomatic patient. In general, patients with more severe conduction changes show greater initial improvement in conduction,[50] and younger patients show more improvement in conduction than older ones.[100] A total failure of improvement in conduction three months or more postsurgery suggests an erroneous diagnosis or possibly a failure to decompress the nerve adequately.

The results of electrodiagnostic tests after conservative treatment of CTS are poorly studied. Goodman and Gilliatt[50] found variable results after splinting. Goodman and Foster[49] reported that following steroid injection to the carpal tunnel, nerve conduction abnormalities improved, but the improvement often was followed by relapse.

Proximal Median Nerve Lesions

Anterior Interosseous Nerve. Needle electromyography provides the most useful information in anterior interosseous nerve lesions. The EMG diagnosis depends upon seeing evidence of denervation in the three muscles supplied by the nerve: pronator quadratus, flexor pollicis longus and the median innervated portion of flexor digitorum profundus.[108]

Routine motor and sensory conduction studies are usually normal in anterior interosseous nerve lesions.[9,41,108,110] There is one report of a nerve conduction velocity technique for the anterior interosseous nerve,[16] but this is not a standard technique in most laboratories. In addition, Nakano et al.[108] described a prolonged latency from elbow to pronator quadratus in five of seven cases. All seven of these patients had an increased duration of the CMAP.

Pronator Syndrome

In pronator syndrome, EMG is, again, usually more valuable than nerve conduction testing. The EMG diagnosis depends upon finding denervation in median innervated muscles in the arm and hand. Conventional wisdom states that the pronator teres itself is spared in this syndrome.[146] However, this is not always the case.[1]

Routine median nerve conduction studies may be normal or show slowing across the elbow or in the forearm.[9,107] Nerve conduction studies are often normal early in the clinical course.

Ligament of Struthers Syndrome

Very little is reported about the electrodiagnostic findings in this condition. There is a single case study[88] with EMG findings suggestive of a radiculopathy of C7 and C8 with slowed median nerve conduction across the elbow. There is also an additional case report with slowed median nerve conduction across the elbow and EMG abnormalities in all median nerve muscles, including pronator teres.[132] Since the median nerve branch to pronator teres leaves the nerve proximal to the elbow, the pronator teres EMG should be abnormal in ligament of Struthers compression but normal in pronator entrapment.[146] Obviously from data already given,[1] this is not always going to be the case.

Ulnar Nerve

Guyon's Canal

Distal ulnar nerve compressive lesions are considerably less common than ulnar nerve lesions at the elbow, and very uncommon compared to the incidence of CTS, despite the data already cited for concomitant distal ulnar nerve involvement in CTS.[9,11,123]

A number of classifications of distal ulnar nerve lesions have been proposed, dividing the lesions into three to five categories.[102,111,127,154] There are three basic lesion types: (1) mixed motor and sensory; (2) pure motor; and (3) pure sensory.

Little has been published on electrodiagnostic tests for distal ulnar nerve lesions.[23] The expected electrodiagnostic findings in the various lesion types are as follows:[102,111,154]

Mixed Motor and Sensory Lesions. In this situation one would expect prolonged distal motor latencies to both the hypothenar muscles and the first dorsal interosseous. In addition, sensory conduction would be abnormal in the distal ulnar nerve. Needle EMG would show evidence of denervation in all ulnar innervated hand muscles if axonal degeneration had occurred. CMAP and SNAP amplitudes would also be affected following axonal loss.

Pure Motor Lesions. In these lesions, the ulnar nerve distal motor latency would be prolonged to either the first dorsal interosseous or both the hypothenar muscles and first dorsal interosseous, depending upon whether the lesion was distal or proximal to the branch to the hypothenar muscles.

Sensory conduction studies would be normal. EMG would show evidence of denervation in the involved ulnar musculature. If the lesion were distal enough, a normal EMG would be seen in intrinsic muscles distal to the hypothenar branch but proximal to the actual lesion site. Again, if axonal loss is present, the CMAP amplitude would be affected.

Pure Sensory Lesions. This is the least common type. Motor conduction studies and EMG would be normal. The only positive electrodiagnostic finding would be an abnormality of sensory conduction. SNAP amplitude would be diminished more often than conduction would be slowed.

When distal ulnar sensory conduction is abnormal, it is helpful to investigate sensory conduction in the dorsal sensory branch of the ulnar nerve. While this branch is not routinely studied, there are two reports of its value.[59,74] The dorsal sensory branch leaves the ulnar nerve proximal to the ulnar styloid. This branch is not involved in distal (wrist) lesions of the ulnar nerve. With elbow lesions, it may show an abnormality of sensory conduction that is equal to that in the sensory branch to the little finger.[102]

It is also important to realize that the ipsilateral DML difference to first dorsal interosseous versus abductor digiti minimi should not exceed 2 msec.[112] In addition, the latency difference between hands to first dorsal interosseous should not exceed 1.3 msec,[112] while latencies for abductor digiti minimi of contralateral hands should be within 1 msec of each other.[102] The CMAP amplitude for the first dorsal interosseous should be at least 6 mV while that for abductor digiti minimi should be at least 4 mV.[102,112]

Ulnar Nerve

Compression at the Elbow (Cubital Tunnel)

Ulnar compressive neuropathy occurs most often at the elbow. This is the second most common focal neuropathy for which electrodiagnostic evaluation is sought. The electrodiagnostic evaluation relies heavily on motor conduction studies and to a lesser degree on sensory conduction studies.

Motor Nerve Conduction Studies. As with CTS, the first demonstration that ulnar nerve lesions at the elbow could be localized by nerve conduction velocity techniques was provided by Simpson in 1956.[128] Since that report, assessment of ulnar motor conduction across the elbow has become the standard diagnostic technique. As a general rule, the motor conduction study is carried out using the abductor digiti minimi for recording. Some laboratories record to first dorsal interosseous,[60] flexor carpi ulnaris, and flexor digitorum profundus as well.[35,113] The principle behind recording from alternative sites is the possibility that only fibers to a particular muscle group may be affected by the compressive lesion. Recording from alternative muscles is not a common practice in EMG laboratories, however.

What constitutes an abnormal value for ulnar nerve motor conduction velocity across the elbow is controversial. The NCV of the ulnar nerve across the elbow is significantly influenced by elbow position.[12,54,82] With the elbow extended, NCV values are slower than those assessed with the elbow flexed. The use of either the flexed or extended elbow position is acceptable as long as the method is standardized, and normal values reflect the elbow position used. As an example, Checkles et al.[12] report their normal across elbow NCV as 52 to 74 msec (mean 62.7 msec) with elbow flexed compared to 34 to 66 msec (mean 49.9 msec) with the elbow extended. Similar results are reported by Kincaid et al.[82]

The purpose of the motor conduction velocity study is to detect focal slowing across the elbow. Another approach is to demonstrate disproportionate slowing across the elbow even though all values may be normal. As an example, Eisen[24] suggests that a drop in NCV of 10 msec or more across the elbow in relation to above-elbow and below-elbow velocities is significant. Payan[113] also used disproportionate slowing in his study. Overall, the diagnostic success rate for motor conduction velocity testing revealing focal slowing or disproportionate slowing varies from 68 to 86 percent for focal slowing to 32 to 87 percent for disproportionate slowing.[24,69,101,109,113] In addition to routine studies, Miller[101] advocates serial stimulation techniques (inching) to differentiate between cubital tunnel compression and compression at a more proximal site.

In addition to changes in conductive velocity, ulnar nerve lesions at the elbow produce changes in the CMAP. Significant axonal loss from a proximal lesion can produce a significantly reduced CMAP from wrist stimulation. However, this is a nonlocalizing finding. Amplitude changes that are localizing include the demonstration of a focal conduction block in the elbow region with a resultant focal amplitude drop. Some drop in amplitude with above elbow stimulation is acceptable (up to 2 mV).[151] Amplitude drops of 25 percent[116] and 30 to 40 percent[101] are reported as being diagnostically helpful.

Sensory Conduction Studies. Sensory nerve conduction studies are more sensitive than motor conduction studies in ulnar nerve lesions at the elbow. However, they are technically more difficult and often require mixed nerve techniques[57] or near-nerve needle techniques[113] to study other than the finger to wrist segment. In general, using routine techniques, it is not unusual to see no sensory response or a very low amplitude SNAP on wrist stimulation in ulnar neuropathy at the elbow. In this situation, more proximal studies are not possible.

The most common sensory conduction abnormality seen is a decrease in amplitude of the SNAP recorded finger to wrist. In more severe cases, no SNAP is obtained. These amplitude changes are nonlocalizing because they are obtained from distal stimulation. Assistance in localization can be obtained by doing sensory conduction studies to the dorsal sensory branch (see earlier discussion). If both the finger-wrist and dorsal sensory branch are involved, the lesion is proximal to the latter. If only the distal study is abnormal, the lesion is *probably* distal to the dorsal sensory branch, although selective sparing of the dorsal sensory fibers could occur in an elbow lesion.[151]

Sensory conduction abnormalities are reported in 50 to 94 percent of cases using distal conduction techniques[24,101,109,113] and in 58 to 93 percent of cases using proximal techniques.[109,113] Using a combination of motor and sensory conduction testing, an overall diagnostic success rate of 91 to 96 percent is reported.[24,101,109,113]

Needle Electromyography. EMG studies may be of value in ulnar nerve lesions at the elbow. Abnormal findings in ulnar muscles of the forearm as well as the hand help to localize the lesion to a proximal site. The presence of denervation in the flexor carpi ulnaris suggests that the lesion may be proximal to the cubital tunnel, since the branch to this muscle frequently comes off proximal to the tunnel. With denervation demonstrable only in hand muscles, no localization is possible. Generally, abnormal spontaneous activity such as fibrillations occur in forearm muscles in 50 percent or less of cases.[5,24,26,101,113] The EMG is of no help in localization in a large number of cases.

Overview of Electrodiagnostic Findings. Wilbourn[151] characterizes focal ulnar nerve lesions at the elbow as being of the non-axon loss or axon loss type, and further characterizes each group by mild, moderate, or severe involvement.

According to Wilbourn,[151] all three subgroups of non-axon loss lesions produce focal slowing and thus they can be localized to the elbow region. In addition, lesions with mild axon loss can often be localized.

By contrast, lesions with moderate axon loss are difficult to localize as are those with severe axon loss, in many cases. Since moderate to severe axon loss lesions are common, it is not unusual for the electromyographer to be unable to localize the lesion to the elbow despite obvious abnormality in the ulnar nerve.

Electrodiagnostic Results After Surgery. Improvement in electrodiagnostic abnormalities after surgery are reported in a number of studies.[93,103,114] All parameters including conduction velocity, evoked potential emplitude, and an improvement in the EMG contraction pattern are reported.

Radial Nerve Lesions

Compressive lesions of the radial nerve occur primarily at the spiral groove (Saturday night palsy), or at the arcade of Frohse (posterior interosseous nerve). In addition, there may be compression of the sensory nerve at the wrist. Although electrodiagnostic findings are reported for lesions at all three sites, radial nerve syndromes are not as thoroughly studied as those involving the median and ulnar nerve.

Sensory Nerve Lesions at the Wrist

Methodology for recording sensory conduction in the distal portions of the superficial radial nerve has been reported by several authors.[21,33,94,96,124,141] While these techniques vary, radial sensory conduction studies are easily done.

In distal compressive lesions of the superficial radial nerve, abnormalities expected include a diminished or absent SNAP or slowing of sensory conduction.

Arcade of Frohse

There are few studies that detail methodology for motor conduction studies of the posterior interosseous nerve. While some attention has been paid to this segment of the radial nerve,[32,43,47,61,62,119,141] only two studies deal with this segment in detail.[32,119] In one case study,[47] a conduction block was the only abnormality demonstrated. A more recent study of two cases demonstrated slowing of posterior interosseous nerve conduction, which recovered after surgery.[32] No amplitude data are presented in this latter report. With significant axon loss, the EMG would be expected to show denervation in muscles supplied by the posterior interosseous nerve.

Spiral Groove

Despite the relatively common occurrence of spiral groove compression, there is only one report that studies this condition with meticulous attention to technical factors.[138] This study revealed focal slowing at the site of compression, with normal conduction velocities and CMAP amplitudes from stimulation below the level of the lesion. In addition, there was marked reduction of the CMAP, and there was SNAP with stimulation proximal to the lesion. EMG abnormalities demonstrating denervation are seen in the brachioradialis and more distal radial innervated muscles if axon loss is present. Typically the triceps is normal. In Trojaborg's[138] study, electrophysiologic improvement was seen in six to eight weeks in association with the clinical improvement.

Lateral Antebrachialcutaneous Nerve

Compression of the lateral antebrachialcutaneous nerve may occur where this terminal branch of the musculocutaneous nerve passes between biceps brachii and brachialis.[3,7,36,53] Sensory conduction techniques for this nerve are reported by several authors.[58,129,139] Felsenthal et al.[36] report a decrease in amplitude of the SNAP in three cases, with a prolongation of the latency in one case. In their report on technique, Spindler and Felsenthal[129] reported that amplitudes should not differ by more than 30 percent on side to side comparisons.

Sensory conduction techniques are available for the medial cutaneous (Antebrachial) nerve of the forearm as well.[58,117,118] This may be of value in the evaluation of injuries or compression in this nerve, and in differentiating medial cord lesions from ulnar nerve lesions in the proximal arm.[118]

Nerve Compression in the Shoulder Area

Nerve conduction velocity techniques exist for the study of motor conduction in the axillary, musculocutaneous, suprascapular, accessory, and long thoracic nerves.[2,13,14,25,31,42,52,72,83,87,115,139] The majority of these studies utilize latency rather than nerve conduction velocity methods because only a single stimulus site is available. Abnormalities may occur in latency or in CMAP amplitude. In unilateral lesions, side-to-side comparisons are valuable but great care must be taken to ensure that distances are equivalent. EMG evaluation of the muscles supplied by the preceeding nerves is easily obtained and may be of equal or greater value in assessing lesions of these nerves.

Thoracic Outlet Syndrome

The subject of the electrodiagnostic evaluation of thoracic outlet syndrome (TOS) is extremely controversial, as is the entire subject of TOS. For simplicity, TOS can be classified as vascular or neurogenic in etiology.[149] In general, vascular TOS would not be expected to show electrodiagnostic changes and is not especially controversial. It is with the neurogenic category that most of the controversy arises.

Wilbourn[149] classifies neurogenic TOS into four groups: (1) classical, true, or motor; (2) atypical; (3) droopy shoulder; and (4) disputed type. Atypical TOS is probably not really TOS, but rather plexus involvement by compression from a known source such as a backpack. Droopy shoulder TOS is a recently described syndrome[133] in which there are no electrodiagnostic findings.

Classical (motor) neurogenic TOS is a primarily motor syndrome with muscle wasting as a prominent feature.[44] In this condition there is a characteristic electrodiagnostic picture[45,148,149] consisting of a diminished amplitude of the median motor CMAP and the ulnar sensory SNAP. The median sensory SNAP is normal, while the ulnar motor CMAP may be normal or low in amplitude. Needle EMG in this condition reveals evidence of chronic denervation (MUAP's of large amplitude and prolonged duration, reduced number of MUAP's, normal recruitment) with very little evidence of abnormal spontaneous activity (fibrillations, positive sharp waves). Occasional proximal nerve conduction slowing or prolongation of the F wave are reported, but results are variable and of little help in diagnosis or localization. It must be remembered that this is a very uncommon condition.

The majority of suspected TOS cases are of the disputed neurogenic type. Patients in this category would be expected to have intermittent neurologic symptomatology without evidence of fixed neurologic deficits, and certainly not the marked atrophy seen in classical neurogenic TOS. With respect to this category, there are proponents who believe it to be a common disorder, and skeptics who question the existence of TOS of this type.[149] In this context it is not surprising that electrodiagnostic results are also controversial.

The major controversy in electrodiagnosis in this group of TOS patients concerns whether or not there is slowing of ulnar nerve conduction from Erb's point to the axilla. Urschel et al.[143] and Caldwell et al.[10] reported that ulnar nerve conduction across the thoracic outlet was slow in a great proportion of patients with this type of TOS. These reports also suggested that patients with NCV values of less than 60 msec required surgery, and that conduction improved postoperatively. These findings have received some confirmation in other reports.[86,120] However, most investigators have been unable to corroborate these findings.[15,17,46,85,90,121,125]

Needle EMG in this disputed type of TOS produces little useful information. Lower motor neuron (denervation) EMG abnormalities are reported in only 14 percent of 459 patients in one report.[153] In another study,[19] the characteristic EMG abnormality is said to be an increase in long duration polyphasic potentials. Such a nonspecific abnormality should not be used to diagnose any specific condition.

The use of F wave latencies for the evaluation of TOS has been suggested.[27,144] However, other reports[78,125,150] suggest that F waves are normal. Root stimulation of C8 with recording over the abduction digiti minimi has also been suggested for TOS diagnosis.[6] However, there have been no actual studies of this technique's value in TOS.

Finally, the use of somatosensory evoked potentials has been suggested for evaluation of TOS.[63,157] As with many procedures already noted, another study found no somatosensory evoked potential abnormalities in a series of TOS patients.[106]

In conclusion, there is no electrodiagnostic test that is undeniably of value in the evaluation of patients with the so-called disputed type of neurogenic TOS.

Other Brachial Plexus Compressive Lesions

Lesions of the brachial plexus are more difficult to evaluate electrodiagnostically than more peripheral nerve lesions. This is because of complex anatomy in the region, the limited accessibility of the plexus, and the multiple tests which must be employed.

Generally speaking, acute compressive lesions of the brachial plexus produce findings which are similar to those seen in traumatic plexus injuries. Such plexus injuries produce axonal loss. Therefore, the expected electrodiagnostic findings are reduced amplitude CMAP's and SNAP's on nerve conduction testing, in association with evidence of denervation on needle EMG. The SNAP is usually more involved than the CMAP, and actual nerve conduction velocities are usually normal or only minimally involved.[39] With motor conduction studies, the musculocutaneous nerve shows the highest incidence of abnormality.[39]

In idiopathic brachial neuritis, one study reported diffusely slow nerve conduction velocities in 71% of the cases.[145] However, subsequent studies have failed to corroborate this finding.[39,99] In the study by Flaggman and Kelly,[39] the findings in idiopathic brachial neuritis were similar to those seen in acute compressive lesions.

In more chronic compressive lesions such as those secondary to tumor infiltration or low-grade chronic extrinsic compression, focal slowing of conduction or evidence of a conduction block may occur.[140]

More esoteric nerve conduction studies, such as F wave determinations and root stimulation, have been reported as being of value in brachial plexus lesions.[71,73,97] However, their exact role in the evaluation of plexopathy remains to be determined.

Finally, there have been a number of reports concerning the value of somatosensory evoked potentials in assessing brachial plexus lesions.[67,68,89,156] Proponents of their use feel that they can differentiate amounts of pre- and postganglion involvement in a given plexus injury by comparing the amplitudes of the N9, N13, and N20 potentials. A more recent report, however, casts some doubt on the usefulness of median nerve somatosensory evoked potentials in the evaluation of plexus lesions.[134]

Compartment Syndromes

The electrodiagnostic evaluation of suspected compartment syndromes is quite different from the evaluation of typical chronic nerve compression syndromes, since the compartment syndromes are very acute problems and functional loss can be rapidly progressive unless treatment is prompt and corrective. In our opinion the best electrodiagnostic monitor of impaired function in compartment syndromes is frequent (every few hours) EMG of the muscles within the compartment and monitoring of the CMAP from muscles within the compartment if the nerve to those muscles can be stimulated proximal to the compartment.

On EMG, when compartment pressures reach levels that jeopardize survival of the muscle fibers, the muscle fibers will have reduced ability to maintain their resting membrane potential and the insertional activity evoked by movement of the examining electrode can be significantly reduced. Serial monitoring of the CMAP evoked from muscles within the compartment may also show progressive decline in amplitude with serial studies, unless the damaging pressures are corrected.

Electrodiagnostic procedures are not a substitute for monitoring compartment pressures. However, these procedures: (1) can be of assistance when techniques and equipment for monitoring of compartment pressure are not available; (2) they can assist by providing evidence of functional status of the muscles and nerve within the compartment when pressure studies are equivocal; and (3) they can be of considerable assistance to help monitor recovery of function following treatment.

References

1. Aiken BM, Moritz MJ: Atypical electromyographic findings in pronator teres syndrome. Arch Phys Med Rehabil 68:173, 1987.
2. Alfonsi E, Moglia A, Sandrini G, Pisoni MR, Arrigo A: Electrophysiological study of long thoracic nerve conduction in normal subjects. Electromyogr Clin Neurophysiol 26:63, 1986.
3. Bassett FH, Nunley JA: Compression of musculocutaneous nerve at elbow. J Bone Joint Surg 64:1050, 1982.
4. Bendler EM, Greenspun B, Yu J, Erdman WJ: The bilaterality of carpal tunnel syndrome. Arch Phys Med Rehabil 77:362, 1977.

5. Benecke R, Conrad B: Value of electrophysiological examination of flexor carpi ulnaris muscle in diagnosis of ulnar nerve lesions at elbow. J Neurol 223:207, 1980.

6. Braddom RL: Motor conduction in Practical Electromyography. Johnson EW (ed): Baltimore, Williams and Wilkins, 1980, pp 16.

7. Braddom RL, Wolfe C: Musculocutaneous nerve injury after heavy exercise. Arch Phys Med Rehabil 59:290, 1978.

8. Buchthal F, Rosenfalck A: Sensory conduction from digit to palm and from palm to wrist in the carpal tunnel syndrome. J Neurol Neurosurg Psychiatry 34:243, 1971.

9. Buchthal F, Rosenfalck A, Trojaborg W: Electrophysiological findings in entrapmment of the median nerve at wrist and elbow. J Neurol Neurosurg Psychiatry 37:340, 1974.

10. Caldwell JW, Crane CR, Krusen EM: Nerve conduction studies: An aid in the diagnosis of thoracic outlet syndrome. South Med J 64:211, 1971.

11. Cassvan A, Rosenberg A, Rivera LF: Ulnar nerve involvement in carpal tunnel syndrome. Arch Phys Med Rehabil 67:290, 1986.

12. Checkles NS, Russakov AD, Piero DL: Ulnar nerve conduction velocity—Effect of elbow position on measurement. Arch Phys Med Rehabil 52:362, 1971.

13. Cherington M: Accessory nerve: Conduction studies. Arch Neurol 18:708, 1968.

14. Cherington M: Long thoracic nerve: Conduction study. Dis Nerv Syst 33:49, 1972.

15. Cherington M: Ulnar conduction velocity in thoracic-outlet syndrome. N Engl J Med 194:1185, 1976.

16. Craft S: Motor conduction of the anterior interosseous nerve. Phys Ther 57:1143, 1977.

17. Daube JR: Nerve conduction studies in the thoracic outlet syndrome. Neurology 25:347, 1975.

18. DeLisa JA, Mackenzie K: Manual of Nerve Conduction Velocity techniques. New York, Raven Press, 1982.

19. DiBenedetto M: Thoracic outlet slowing. Electromyogr Clin Neurophysiol 17:191, 1977.

20. DiBenedetto M, Mitz M, Klingbeil GE, Davidoff D: New criteria for sensory nerve conduction especially useful in diagnosing carpal tunnel syndrome. Arch Phys Med Rehabil 67:586, 1986.

21. Downie AW, Scott RT: Improved technique for radial nerve conduction studies. J Neurol Neurosurg Psychiatry 30:332, 1967.

22. Duensing F, Lowitzsch K, Thorwirth V, Vogel P: Neurophysiologische Befunde beim Karpaltunnelsyndrom. Z Neurol 206:267, 1974.

23. Ebeling P, Gilliatt RW, Thomas PK: A clinical and electrical study of ulnar nerve lesions in the hand. J Neurol Neurosurg Psychiatry 23:1, 1960.

24. Eisen A: Early diagnosis of ulnar nerve palsy. Neurology 24:256, 1974.

25. Eisen A, Bertrand G: Isolated accessory nerve palsy of spontaneous origin. Arch Neurol 27:496, 1972.

26. Eisen A, Danon J: The mild cubital tunnel syndrome. Neurology 24:608, 1974.

27. Eisen A, Schomer D, Melmed C: The application of F-wave measurements in the differentiation of proximal and distal upper limbs entrapments. Neurology 27:662, 1977.

28. Escobar PL, Goka RS: Carpal tunnel syndrome. Palmar sensory latencies to 3rd digit and wrist. Orthop Rev 14:633, 1985.

29. Evans BA, Daube JR: A comparison of three electrodiagnostic methods of diagnosing carpal tunnel syndrome. Muscle Nerve 7:565, 1984.
30. Eversmann WW Jr, Ritsick JA: Intraoperative changes in motor nerve conduction latency in carpal tunnel syndrome. J Hand Surg 3:77, 1978.
31. Fahrer H, Ludin HP, Mumenthaler M, Neiger M: The innervation of the trapezius muscle. An electrophysiological study. J Neurol 207:183, 1974.
32. Falck B. Hurme M: Conduction velocity of the posterior interosseous nerve across the arcade of Frohse. Electromyogr Clin Neurophysiol 23:567, 1983.
33. Feibel A, Foca FJ: Sensory conduction of radial nerve. Arch Phys Med Rehabil 55:314, 1974.
34. Felsenthal G: Median and ulnar distal motor and sensory latencies in the same normal subject. Arch Phys Med Rehabil 58:297, 1977.
35. Felsenthal G, Brockman PS, Mondell DL, Hilton EB: Proximal forearm ulnar nerve conduction techniques. Arch Phys Med Rehabil 67:440, 1986.
36. Felsenthal G, Mondell DL, Reischer MA, Mack RH: Forearm pain secondary to compression syndrome of lateral cutaneous nerve of forearm. Arch Phys Med Rehabil 65:139, 1984.
37. Felsenthal G, Spindler H: Carpal tunnel syndrome diagnosis. (letter to editor) Arch Phys Med Rehabil 60:90, 1979.
38. Felsenthal G, Spindler H: Palmar conduction time of median and ulnar nerves of normal subjects and patients with carpal tunnel syndrome. Am J Phys Med 58:131, 1979.
39. Flaggman PD, Kelly JJ Jr: Brachial plexus neuropathy. An electrophysiologic evaluation. Arch Neurol 37:160, 1980.
40. Frith RW, Litchy WJ: Electrophysiologic abnormalities of peripheral nerves in patients with cervical radiculopathy. Muscle Nerve 8:613, 1985.
41. Gardner-Thorpe C: Anterior interosseous nerve palsy: Spontaneous recovery in two patients. J Neurol Neurosurg Psychiatry 37:1146, 1974.
42. Gassel MM: Test of nerve conduction to muscles of shoulder girdle as aid in diagnosis of proximal neurogenic and muscular disease. J Neurol Neurosurg Psychiatry 27:200, 1964.
43. Gassel MM, Diamantopulos E: Pattern of conduction times in the distribution of the radial nerve. Neurology 14:222, 1964.
44. Gilliatt RW, LeQuesne PM, Logue V, Sumner AJ: Wasting of the hand associated with cervical rib or band. J Neurol Neurosurg Psychiatry 33:615, 1970.
45. Gilliatt RW, Willison RG, Dietz V, Williams IR: Peripheral nerve conduction in patients with a cervical rib and band. Ann Neurol 4:124, 1978.
46. Ginzburg M, Lee M, Ginzburg J, Alba A: Median and ulnar nerve conduction determinations in the Erb's point-axilla segment in normal subjects. J Neurol Neurosurg Psychiatry 41:444, 1978.
47. Goldman S, Honet JC, Sobel R, Goldstein AS: Posterior interosseous nerve palsy in the absence of trauma. Arch Neurol 21:435, 1969.
48. Goodgold J, Eberstein A: Electrodiagnosis of Neuromuscular Diseases. 3rd ed. Baltimore, Williams and Wilkins, 1983.
49. Goodman HV, Foster JB: Effect of local corticosteroid injection on median nerve conduction in carpal tunnel syndrome. Ann Phys Med 6:287, 1962.
50. Goodman HV, Gilliatt RW: The effect of treatment on median nerve conduction in patients with the carpal tunnel syndrome. Ann Phys Med 6:137, 1961.

51. Goodwill CJ: The carpal tunnel syndrome: Long-term followup showing relation of latency measurements to response to treatment. Ann Phys Med 8:12, 1965.

52. Green RF, Brien M: Accessory nerve latency to middle and lower trapezius. Arch Phys Med Rehabil 66:23, 1985.

53. Hale BR: Handbag paresthesia. Lancet 2:470, 1976.

54. Harding C, Halar E: Motor and sensory ulnar nerve conduction velocities: Effect of elbow position. Arch Phys Med Rehabil 64:227, 1983.

55. Hartz CR, Linscheid RL, Gramse RR, Daube JR: Pronator teres syndrome: Compressive neuropathy of median nerve. J Bone Joint Surg 63A:885, 1981.

56. Hongell A, Mattsson HS: Neurographic studies before, after, and during operation for median nerve compression in the carpal tunnel. Scand J Plast Reconstr Surg 5:103, 1971.

57. Ioppolo A, Granger CV: A technique for demonstrating nerve entrapment in the ulnar groove. Electromyogr 12:273, 1972.

58. Izzo KL, Aravabhumi S, Jafri A, Sobel E, Demopoulos JT: Median and lateral antebrachial cutaneous nerves: Standardization of technique, reliability and age effects on healthy subjects. Arch Phys Med Rehabil 66:592, 1985.

59. Jabre JF: Ulnar nerve lesions at the wrist: New technique for recording from the sensory dorsal branch of the ulnar nerve. Neurology 30:873, 1980.

60. Jabre J, Wilbourn AJ: The EMG findings in 100 consecutive ulnar neuropathies. Acta Neurol Scand (Suppl 73) 60:91, 1979.

61. Jebsen RH: Motor conduction velocity of distal radial nerve. Arch Phys Med Rehabil 47:12, 1966.

62. Jebsen RH: Motor conduction velocity in proximal and distal segments of the radial nerve. Arch Phys Med Rehabil 47:597, 1966.

63. Jerrett SA, Cuzzone LJ, Pasternak BM: Thoracic outlet syndrome. Arch Neurol 41:960, 1984.

64. Johnson EW, Kukla RD, Wongsam PE, Piedmont A: Sensory latencies to the ring finger: Normal values and relation to the carpal tunnel syndrome. Arch Phys Med Rehabil 62:206, 1981.

65. Johnson EW, Sipski M, Lammertse T: Median and radial sensory latencies to digit I: Normal values and usefulness in carpal tunnel syndrome. Arch Phys Med Rehabil 68:140, 1987.

66. Johnson RK, Shrewsbury MM: Anatomical course of the thenar branch of the median nerve—Usually in a separate tunnel through the transverse carpal ligament. J Bone Joint Surg 52A:269, 1970.

67. Jones SJ: Investigation of brachial plexus traction lesions by peripheral and spinal somatosensory evoked potentials. J Neurol Neurosurg Psychiatry 42:107, 1979.

68. Jones SJ, Wynn Parry CB, Landi A: Diagnosis of brachial plexus traction by sensory nerve action potentials and somatosensory evoked potentials. Injury 12:376, 1981.

69. Kaesar HE: Erregungleitungsstoerngen bei ulnarisparesen, Dtsch. Z. Nervenheilk. 185:231, 1963.

70. Kaesar HE: Diagnostiche Probleme beim karpaltunnelsyndrom, Dtsch. Z. Nervenheilk 185:453, 1963.

71. Kaplan PE: F waves as an electrodiagnostic confirmation of brachial plexus neuropathies of the upper trunk. Electromyogr Clin Neurophysiol 18:527, 1978.

72. Kaplan PE: Electrodiagnostic confirmation of long thoracic nerve palsy. J Neurol Neurosurg Psychiatry 43:50, 1980.

73. Kaplan PE: A motor conduction velocity across the upper trunk and the lateral cord of the brachial plexus. Electromyogr Clin Neurophysiol 22:315, 1982.
74. Kim D, Kalantri A, Guha S, Wainapel SF: Dorsal cutaneous ulnar nerve conduction. Arch Neurol 38:321, 1981.
75. Kim LYS: Palmar digital nerve stimulation to diagnose carpal tunnel syndrome. Orthop Rev 12:59, 1983.
76. Kimura I, Ayyar DR: The carpal tunnel syndrome: Electrophysiological aspects of 639 symptomatic extremities. Electromyogr Clin Neurophysiol 25:151, 1985.
77. Kimura J: A method for determining median nerve conduction velocity across the carpal tunnel. J Neurol Sci 38:1, 1978.
78. Kimura J: Clinical value and limitations of F wave determination: A comment. Muscle Nerve 1:248, 1978.
79. Kimura J: The carpal tunnel syndrome: Localizations of conduction abnormalities within the distal segment of the median nerve. Brain 102:619, 1979.
80. Kimura J: Electrodiagnosis in Diseases of Nerve and Muscle: Principles and practice. Philadelphia, F.A. Davis, 1983.
81. Kimura J: Principles and pitfalls of nerve conduction studies. Ann Neurol 16:415, 1984.
82. Kincaid JC, Phillips LH, Daube JR: The evaluation of suspected ulnar neuropathy at the elbow: Normal conduction study values. Arch Neurol 43:44, 1986.
83. Kraft GH: Axillary musculocutaneous and suprascapular nerve latency studies. Arch Phys Med Rehabil 53:383, 1972.
84. Kraft GH, Halvorson GA: Median nerve residual latency: Normal value and use in diagnosis of carpal tunnel syndrome. Arch Phys Med Rehabil 64:221, 1983.
85. Kremer RM, Ahlquist RE: Thoracic outlet compression syndrome. Am J Surg 130:612, 1975.
86. Krogness K: Ulnar trunk conduction studies in the diagnosis of thoracic outlet syndrome. Acta Chir Scand 139:597, 1973.
87. Krogness K: Serial conduction studies of the spinal accessory nerve used as a prognostic tool in a lesion caused by lymph node biopsy. Acta Chir Scand 140:7, 1974.
88. Laha RK: Entrapment of median nerve by supracondylar process of the humerus. J Neurol Neurosurg Psychiatry 46:252, 1977.
89. Landi A, Copeland SA, Wynn Parry CB, Jones SJ: The role of somatosensory evoked potentials and nerve conduction studies in the surgical management of brachial plexus injuries. J Bone Joint Surg 62B:492, 1980.
90. Lascelles RG, Mohr PD, Neary D, Bloor K: The thoracic outlet syndrome. Brain 100:601, 1977.
91. Loong SC, Seah CS: Comparison of median and ulnar sensory nerve action potentials in the diagnosis of the carpal tunnel syndrome. J Neurol Neurosurg Psychiatry 34:750, 1971.
92. Ludin H, Tackmann W: Sensory Neurography. New York, Thieme-Stratton, 1980.
93. Lugnegard H, Walheim G, Wennberg A: Operative treatment of ulnar neuropathy in the elbow region. Acta Orthop Scand 48:168, 1977.
94. Ma DM, Kim SH, Speilholz N, Goodgold J: Sensory conduction study of distal radial nerve. Arch Phys Med Rehabil 62:562, 1981.

95. Ma DM, Liveson JA: Nerve Conduction Handbook. Philadelphia, F.A. Davis, 1983.
96. Mackenzie K, DeLisa JA: Distal sensory latency of the superficial radial nerve in normal adult subjects. Arch Phys Med Rehabil 62:31, 1981.
97. MacLean IC, Taylor RS: Nerve root stimulation to evaluate brachial plexus conduction. Arch Phys Med Rehabil 56:551, 1975.
98. Marin EL, Vernick S, Friedmann LW: Carpal tunnel syndrome: Median nerve stress test. Arch Phys Med Rehabil 64:206, 1983.
99. Martin WA, Kraft GH: Shoulder girdle neuritis: A clinical and electrophysiological evaluation. Milit Med 139:21, 1974.
100. Melvin JL, Johnson EW, Duran R: Electrodiagnosis after surgery for the carpal tunnel syndrome. Arch Phys Med Rehabil 49:502, 1968.
101. Miller RG: The cubital tunnel syndrome: Diagnosis and precise localization. Ann Neurol 6:56, 1979.
102. Miller RG: Ulnar neuropathy in the hand. American Association of Electromyography and Electrodiagnosis, Rochester, Minnesota, Course E, 1986, pp 7.
103. Miller RG, Hummel EE: The cubital tunnel syndrome: Treatment with simple decompression. Ann Neurol 7:567, 1980.
104. Mills KR: Orthodromic sensory action potentials from palmar stimulation in the diagnosis of carpal tunnel syndrome. J Neurol Neurosurg Psychiat 48:250, 1985.
105. Monga TN, Shanks GL, Poole BJ: Sensory palmar stimulation in the diagnosis of carpal tunnel syndrome. Arch Phys Med Rehabil 66:598, 1985.
106. Morales-Blanquez G, Delwaide PJ: The thoracic outlet syndrome: An electrophysiological syndrome. Electromyogr Clin Neurophysiol 22:255, 1982.
107. Morris HH, Peters BH: Pronator syndrome: Clinical and electrophysiological features in seven cases. J Neurol Neurosurg Psychiat 39:461, 1976.
108. Nakano KK, Lundergran C, Okihiro MM: Anterior interosseous nerve syndromes. Arch Neurol 34:477, 1977.
109. Nishihira T, Oh SJ: Ulnar neuropathy: An improved method of diagnosis. Arch Phys Med Rehabil 57:602, 1976.
110. O'Brien MD, Upton ARM: Anterior interosseous nerve syndrome. J Neurol Neurosurg Psychiatry 35:531, 1972.
111. Oh SJ: Clinical Electromyography: Nerve Conduction Studies. Baltimore, University Park Press, 1984.
112. Olney RK, Wilbourn AJ: Ulnar nerve conduction study of the first dorsal interosseous muscle. Arch Phys Med Rehabil 66:16, 1985.
113. Payan J: Electrophysiological localization of ulnar nerve lesions. J Neurol Neurosurg Psyuchiatry 32:208, 1969.
114. Payan J: Anterior transposition of the ulnar nerve: An electrophysiological study. J Neurol Neurosurg Psychiatry 33:157, 1970.
115. Petrera JE, Trojaborg W: Conduction studies along the accessory nerve and follow-up of patients with trapezius palsy. J Neurol Neurosurg Psychiatry 47:630, 1984.
116. Pickett JB, Coleman LL: Localizing ulnar nerve lesions to the elbow by motor conduction studies. Electromyogr Clin Neurophysiol 24:343, 1984.
117. Pribyl R, You SB, Jantra P: Sensory nerve conduction velocity of the median antebrachial cutaneous nerve. Electromyogr Clin Neurophysiol 19:41, 1979.
118. Reddy MP: Conduction studies of the medial cutaneous nerve of the forearm. Arch Phys Med Rehabil 64:209, 1983.

119. Rosen I, Werner CO: Neurophysiological investigation of posterior interosseous nerve entrapment causing lateral elbow pain. EEG Clin Neurophysiol 50:125, 1980.

120. Sadler TR, Rainer GW, Twombley G: Thoracic outlet compression: Application of positional arteriographic and nerve conduction studies. Am J Surg 130:704, 1975.

121. Sanders RJ, Monsour JW, Gerber WF, Adams WR, Thompson N: Scalenectomy versus first rib resection for treatment of the thoracic outlet syndrome. Surgery 85:109, 1979.

122. Schwartz MS, Gordon JA, Swash M: Slowed nerve conduction with wrist flexion in carpal tunnel syndrome. Ann Neurol 8:69, 1980.

123. Sedal L, McLeod JG, Walsh JL: Ulnar nerve lesions associated with the carpal tunnel syndrome. J Neurol Neurosurg Psychiatry 36:118, 1973.

124. Shahani B, Goodgold J, Spielholz NI: Sensory nerve action potentials in radial nerve. Arch Phys Med Rehabil 48:602, 1967.

125. Shahani BT, Potts F, Juguilon A, Young RR: Electrophysiological studies in "thoracic outlet syndrome." EEG Clin Neurophysiol 50:172, 1980.

126. Shahani BT, Young RR, Potts F, Maccabee P: Terminal latency index (TLI) and late response studies in motor neuron disease (MND) peripheral neuropathies and entrapment syndromes. Acta Neurol Scan (suppl) 73:118, 1979.

127. Shea JD, McClain EJ: Ulnar nerve compression syndromes at and below wrist. J Bone Joint Surg 51A:1095, 1969.

128. Simpson JA: Electrical signs in the diagnosis of carpal tunnel and related syndromes. J Neurol Neurosurg Psychiatry 19:275, 1956.

129. Spindler HA, Felsenthal G: Sensory conduction in the musculocutaneous nerve. Arch Phys Med Rehabil 59:20, 1978.

130. Stevens JL: AAEE minimonograph #26: The electrodiagnosis of carpal tunnel syndrome. Muscle Nerve 10:99, 1987.

131. Stoehr M, Petruch F, Scheglmann K, Schilling K: Retrograde changes of nerve fibers with carpal tunnel syndrome: An electroneurographic investigation. J Neurol 218:287, 1978.

132. Suryani L: Median nerve compression by Struthers ligament. J Neurol Neurosurg Psychiatry 46:1047, 1983.

133. Swift TR, Nichols FT: The droopy shoulder syndrome. Neurology 34:212, 1984.

134. Synek VM: Validity of median nerve somatosensory evoked potentials in the diagnosis of supraclavicular brachial plexus lesions. EEG Clin Neurophysiol 65:27, 1986.

135. Szabo RM, Gelberman RH: Peripheral nerve compression: Etiology, critical pressure threshold and clinical assessment. Orthopedics 7:1461, 1984.

136. Thomas JE, Lambert EH, Cseuz KA: Electrodiagnostic aspects of the carpal tunnel syndrome. Arch Neurol 16:635, 1967.

137. Thomas PK: Motor nerve conduction in the carpal tunnel syndrome. Neurology 10:1045, 1960.

138. Trojaborg W: Rate of recovery in motor and sensory fibers of the radial nerve: Clinical and electrophysiological aspects. J Neurol Neurosurg Psychiatry 33:625, 1970.

139. Trojaborg W: Motor and sensory conduction in the musculocutaneous nerve. J Neurol Neurosurg Psychiatry 39:890, 1976.

140. Trojaborg W: Electrophysiological findings in pressure palsy of the brachial plexus. J Neurol Neurosurg Psychiatry 40:1160, 1977.

141. Trojaborg W, Sindrup EN: Motor and sensory conduction in different segments of radial nerve in normal subjects. J Neurol Neurosurg Psychiat 32:354, 1969.

142. Upton ARM, McComas AJ: The double crush in nerve entrapment syndromes. Lancet 2:359, 1973.

143. Urschel HC, Razzuk MA, Wood RE, Parekh M, Paulson DL: Objective diagnosis (ulnar nerve conduction velocity) and current therapy of the thoracic outlet syndrome. Ann Thorac Surg 12:608, 1971.

144. Weber RJ, Piero DL: F wave evaluation of thoracic outlet syndrome: A multiple regression derived F wave latency predicting technique. Arch Phys Med Rehabil 59:464, 1978.

145. Weikers NJ, Mattson RM: Acute paralytic brachial neuritis: A clinical electrodiagnostic study. Neurology 19:1153, 1969.

146. Wertsch JJ, Melvin J: Median nerve anatomy and entrapment syndromes: Review. Arch Phys Med Rehabil 63:623, 1982.

147. Wiederholt WC: Median nerve conduction velocity in sensory fibers through carpal tunnel. Arch Phys Med Rehabil 51:328, 1970.

148. Wilbourn AJ: Case Report #7: True neurogenic thoracic outlet syndrome. American Association of Electromyography and Electrodiagnosis, Rochester, Minnesota, 1982.

149. Wilbourn AJ: Thoracic outlet syndrome. American Association of Electromyography and Electrodiagnosis, Rochester, Minnesota, Course D, 1984, pp 28.

150. Wilbourn AJ: Slowing across the thoracic outlet with thoracic outlet syndrome: Fact or fiction. Neurology 34:143, 1984.

151. Wilbourn AJ: Ulnar neuropathy. American Association of Electromyography and Electrodiagnosis, Rochester, Minnesota, Course A, 1985, pp 27.

152. Wongsam PE, Johnson EW, Weinerman JD: Carpal tunnel syndrome: Use of palmar stimulation of sensory fibers. Arch Phys Med Rehabil 64:16, 1983.

153. Wood WN: Thoracic outlet syndrome. West J Med 128:9, 1978.

154. Wu JS, Morris JD, Hogan GR: Ulnar neuropathy at the wrist: Case report and review of literature. Arch Phys Med Rehabil 66:785, 1985.

155. Yates SK, Hurst LN, Brown WF: Physiological observations in the median nerve during carpal tunnel surgery. Ann Neurol 10:227, 1981.

156. Yiannikas C, Shahani BT, Young RR: The investigation of traumatic lesions of the brachial plexus by electromyography and short latency somatosensory potentials evoked by stimulation of multiple peripheral nerves. J Neurol Neurosurg Psychiatry 46:1014, 1983.

157. Yiannikas C, Walsh JC: Somatosensory evoked responses in the diagnosis of thoracic outlet syndrome. J Neurol Neurosurg Psychiatry 46:234, 1983.

CHAPTER 5

Electrodiagnosis in Lower Extremity Nerve Compression

Robert G. Taylor, M.D.
James S. Lieberman, M.D.

Nerve compression syndromes are less common, or less frequently recognized, in the lower than in the upper extremity. As a result they are less well known. However, compartment syndromes are diagnosed more often in the lower than in the upper extremities.[35]

Compression Neuropathies

Lateral Femoral Cutaneous Nerve

This nerve is formed from the anterior primary divisions of the L 2 and L 3 mixed roots. The nerve cannot be stimulated for electrodiagnostic studies in the deep intra-abdominal portion of its course. However, it is accessible in the region of the inguinal ligament and the anterior superior iliac spine. Since this nerve has no motor component, the only electrodiagnostic tests available are sensory conduction studies.

Both antidromic[5] and orthodromic[44] sensory conduction techniques are described for the lateral femoral cutaneous nerve. In the antidromic method,[5] the nerve is stimulated using a needle electrode at the inguinal ligament near the anterior superior iliac spine, and the nerve action potential is recorded from the small branches of this nerve in its field on the anterolateral thigh. Special recording electrodes are required. In our experience, the orthodromic technique of Sarala, Nishihara, and Oh[40] is more likely to produce a detectable response. This is accomplished by recording from the nerve at or just proximal to the inguinal ligament and stimulating over the cutaneous area supplied by that nerve on the anterolateral thigh. Because of the relatively short distances available, it is not practical to stimulate at two sites, which would usually be necessary to calculate a velocity. However, an approximation of velocity can be obtained by dividing the distance from the stimulating electrode to the recording electrode (10-16 cm) by the latency. A side-to-side difference greater than 10 m/sec is considered abnormal. The other variables available are the latency and the amplitude of the evoked nerve action potential (N wave). N wave amplitudes are extremely variable, and may be very small in normal individuals. Amplitudes obtained by the orthodromic technique are usually larger than those obtained by the antidromic method.[4] A sensory latency more than 1 millisecond longer than the contralateral, asymptomatic side is considered abnormal.

A review of 17 cases in four separate studies[44,5,40,31] reveals that conduction was slow in four cases, absent in 12 cases, and one case had normal conduction. Unfortunately, the conduction studies of this nerve are technically very difficult, and Ma and Liveson suggest that no conclusions should be drawn if no response can be elicited.[32] With unilateral symptoms, both sides should be studied. An easily obtainable response on the asymptomatic side in combination with no response on the symptomatic side may be significant. When nerve conduction studies are not helpful, needle electromyography (EMG) should be performed to differentiate radiculopathy from peripheral nerve involvement.

Femoral Nerve

The femoral nerve originates from the lumbar plexus, and in its route to and through the pelvis follows or travels through the psoas muscle. In its proximal portion it is relatively immune to entrapment; however, its function is impaired in this region in diabetic patients, due to diabetic mononeuropathy or amyotrophy, or from bleeding into the psoas muscle or retroperitoneal space in patients on anticoagulant therapy or trauma victims.[24] It is theoretically possible for femoral nerve entrapment to occur as a result of soft tissue swelling pushing the nerve anteriorily against the inguinal ligament. This nerve also is occasionally injured during pelvic surgery or from prolonged immobilization in the lithotomy position.[24]

A technique to determine motor conduction velocity in the femoral nerve has been described[24] with recording from the vastus medialis and stimulation of the femoral nerve immediately proximal to the inguinal ligament, with a second stimulation site just distal to the inguinal ligament. However, the very small distances available may not be adequate to permit accurate calculation of velocities. It is also possible to record the latency to the vastus medialis,[14] with stimulation of the nerve at the inguinal ligament. The parameters that can be measured to assist in confirmation of diagnosis are the amplitude of the evoked muscle action potential (M wave) and the latency. Because of significant variations between patients, side-to-side (symptomatic versus asymptomatic) comparison is more reliable than comparison with "normal values." M wave amplitude 60 percent or less compared to the asymptomatic side, or a latency more than 1.5 milliseconds longer than the asymptomatic side, is considered an abnormal difference.

Sensory conduction studies are not available for study of the proximal femoral nerve. However, they are available for study of the saphenous nerve (see below). Needle EMG studies should be performed to differentiate radiculopathy from peripheral nerve dysfunction.

Saphenous Nerve

The saphenous nerve is the continuation of the femoral nerve into the leg. It is sensory only and provides a major articular branch to the knee then continues in the leg, just medial to the tibia, to the level of the ankle. It provides sensation to the skin of the anteromedial aspect of the leg. In its course through the thigh it must penetrate the fascia covering the adductor canal and the fascia lata in order to reach the subcutaneous layers. The saphenous nerve is vulnerable to entrapment or compression at the points where it penetrates these fasciae. Sensory nerve conduction study techniques have been developed for this nerve distal to the knee[42,48] but are not yet available for the regions across the area where the entrapment may occur. Somatosensory evoked potential techniques[45] can confirm that function is abnormal, but do not permit localization of the compression.

Obturator Nerve

This nerve is rarely evaluated for suspected entrapment neuropathy. It originates from the lower lumbar plexus and travels within the psoas muscle for a short distance before entering the pelvis. Potential for entrapment has been reported for this nerve as it exits the pelvis through the obturator canal and membrane. The obturator nerve is vulnerable to involvement from penetrating trauma, tumors, and surgical procedures. The sensory distribution for the obturator nerve is the posteromedial aspect of the thigh, and it innervates the adductor muscle group. No adequate techniques have been described for nerve conduction studies for this nerve. Therefore, needle EMG is the only electrodiagnostic technique available for study of the obturator nerve.

Sciatic Nerve

This nerve originates from the sacral plexus, levels L4, L5, S1, and S2, and as with the two previous nerves it is relatively immune to entrapment as it travels through the posterior pelvis. However, as with the other intrapelvic nerves, it can be injured by tumors, by direct trauma from penetrating wounds, by surgical procedures, or in individuals on anticoagulant therapy.[49] If sciatic nerve function is compromised within the pelvis, the involvement is usually moderate to severe as well as relatively acute. In these instances abnormalities can be readily detected by EMG two to three weeks after the event. Routine nerve conduction velocity studies are not available to evaluate intrapelvic abnormality; however, H reflex studies can be of assistance. The H reflex is a reflex response with the depolarization, from the stimulation, traveling up the sensory fibers to the spinal cord and then activating the anterior horn cells via the monosynaptic segmental reflex pathway. The H reflex response is obtained from the gastrocnemius muscle by stimulation of the sciatic nerve in the popliteal space. Nomograms with values for normal subjects that take into account the patient's age and leg length are available.[3] If symptoms are unilateral, the H reflex latencies are best compared to the asymptomatic side; the symptomatic to asymptomatic side difference greater than 1.5 milliseconds can be considered excessive. The H reflex cannot differentiate intrapelvic from peripheral nerve, plexus, or root level involvement; that can only be done by EMG, which can confirm whether the pattern of the involved muscles is in the distribution of the peripheral nerve or in a radicular or plexus distribution. The H reflex is usually obtainable only from the triceps surae muscle group with stimulation of the sciatic nerve and, with proper technique, can be found in most individuals. The F wave response is also a late response, but is not a reflex. It can be observed from most muscle groups. The F wave is a motor response and it cannot assess sensory dysfunction. In addition, a prolonged F wave latency does not localize the lesion to any particular site along the root, plexus or nerve. However, it has potential value for evaluating proximal sciatic function.[25] Finally, nerve root stimulation techniques for studying conduction through the lumbosacral plexus are described.[33] These are not generally available, however.

The sciatic nerve has potential for entrapment as it exits the pelvis via the sciatic notch or as it passes through the piriformis muscle. EMG is the best EDX procedure to evaluate this sciatic lesion. The abnormal findings would be limited to the muscles supplied by the divisions of the sciatic nerve, and not in a pattern to suggest plexus or root involvement, as the proximal muscles and the erector spinae muscles would be spared. Motor nerve conduction velocity techniques are available utilizing needle electrode stimulation of the sciatic nerve as it exits from the sciatic notch.[15,53] In addition, a sensory conduction technique is reported for the sciatic nerve.[4] These techniques are not in common use, however. As mentioned earlier, H reflex latency studies can also help to confirm abnormality but cannot differentiate between nerve, plexus, or root level of involvement. Somatosensory evoked potentials also may be of assistance in study of this nerve.

Tibial Nerve

The tibial nerve is one of the two major divisions of the sciatic nerve. It is a mixed nerve and carries sensation from the distal toes and plantar aspect of the foot (medial and lateral plantar nerves) and innervates the plantar flexor muscles in the calf and the intrinsic muscles of the foot, with the exception of the extensor digitorum brevis. When the tibial nerve is compressed in the popliteal space, if the nerve compression is moderately severe, the nerve conduction velocity for the tibial nerve will be slowed distal to the lesion and the M wave amplitude will be reduced.[22] In some individuals it may be possible to stimulate the tibial nerve at two levels in the popliteal space, proximal and distal to the site of compression. In this situation, a slowing of the nerve conduction velocity localized to the popliteal region might be identified.

At the ankle the tibial nerve branches into three divisions as it enters the tarsal tunnel: the medial and lateral plantar nerves and the calcaneal nerve. Electrodiagnostic tests are available for the plantar nerves, but no procedure is available for study of calcaneal nerve function.

Prior to the development of plantar nerve sensory conduction studies, the distal motor latency of the medial and lateral plantar nerves was the only nerve conduction technique available for tarsal tunnel diagnosis, and a number of early reports comment on its value,[10,17,23] while later studies concentrate on improving the techniques.[11,19] If the involvement is severe enough, the distal motor latency will be prolonged, and the M wave amplitude may be reduced if axonal loss has occurred. More recently Oh et al.[37] suggest that distal motor latency studies are abnormal in only 52 percent of the cases studied.

In recent years sensory nerve conduction studies have been developed for the medial and lateral plantar nerves.[2,18,20,36,37,39] One of the studies reports 90 percent accuracy using the sensory distal latency technique.[37] As in carpal tunnel syndrome, sensory conduction studies appear to be more sensitive than motor studies.

A recent review of tarsal tunnel syndrome[27] suggests that this syndrome is not analagous to carpal tunnel syndrome from an electrodiagnostic standpoint: Specifically, a number of reports suggest that distal motor latency may be normal in the presence of EMG abnormalities in the intrinsic muscles of the feet.[14,17,23,39] In this respect, tarsal tunnel syndrome seems more like an axonal neuropathy from trauma than a demyelinating neuropathy from compression.[27] In his recent review, Kraft[27] suggests that all patients being evaluated for possible tarsal tunnel syndrome undergo EMG of the back, leg, and intrinsic foot muscles. EMG of the intrinsic foot muscles is not routine in most EMG laboratories, because of patient discomfort and the frequent incidence of abnormal spontaneous activity (fibrillation and positive sharp wave potentials) in normal feet.[12]

Interdigital Neuropathy

Until recently no electrodiagnostic study was available for studying interdigital nerve conduction in the feet. Thus conditions such as Morton's neuroma could not be assessed by nerve conduction techniques. Recently a new technique has been reported[36] for studying sensory latencies from interdigital nerves. While not generally available, this technique shows promise.

Peroneal Nerve

The common peroneal nerve is the second of the major divisions of the sciatic nerve. This nerve must course in a lateral direction as it passes distally through the popliteal region. It then courses from posterior to anterior around the fibular neck where it divides into its superficial and deep branches. The common peroneal nerve can be compressed by expanding lesions in the popliteal space; however, compression neuropathy most commonly occurs as a result of compression of this nerve against the bony fibular head in crossed leg palsy.[26]

Nerve conduction studies of the peroneal nerve are the most useful test for peroneal nerve compression at the fibular head. Motor nerve conduction velocities can be obtained by recording from either the extensor digitorum brevis[7] or the tibialis anterior.[8] Most standard EMG textbooks suggest that slowing of motor nerve conduction across the fibular head is the most important finding in peroneal nerve compression at the knee.[16,25,30,47,50] However, one report[43] showed the diagnostic rate of motor conduction studies to be 36 percent, while sensory studies had a diagnostic rate of 82 percent.

Two of the most recent reports[38,51] suggest that the most useful electrodiagnostic finding in peroneal neuropathy is a drop in the amplitude of the evoked motor action potential ($>$20 percent) across the knee. This appears to be true when either the extensor digitorum brevis[38] or the tibialis anterior[51] is used for recording. Wilbourn also stresses that superficial peroneal nerve sensory conduction studies are of value in peroneal neuropathy.[51] However, the only value said to be of importance is the amplitude of the sensory nerve potential, since superficial peroneal nerve axons are more severely involved than motor axons in fibular head lesions.

Needle EMG in peroneal nerve lesions at the knee produces variable information. The proximal extent of the peroneal nerve involvement should be determined by EMG recording from the short head of the biceps femoris. In addition, peroneal neuropathy must be differentiated from radiculopathy.

The superficial branch of the peroneal nerve can be compromised by compression neuropathy in the distal portion of the leg as it exits the lateral compartment through its fascial covering to reach the subcutaneous layer. In this portion the nerve is purely sensory, with no motor component. Sensory nerve conduction studies are available for this nerve.[1,6,9,21,28,29,43] A side-to-side difference of greater than 10 m/sec velocity, or an impaired evoked potential amplitude are possible abnormal findings. As already noted, amplitude changes in a superficial peroneal nerve study may be caused by more proximal peroneal involvement of the nerve.

The deep peroneal nerve travels through the anterior compartment of the leg innervating the muscles of the anterior compartment as it passes through. It exits that compartment with the tendons at its inferior border. Entrapment or compression of this nerve is usually in its most distal segment where it is called the anterior tarsal tunnel syndrome.[34] At the present time there is no study available for sensory fibers of the deep peroneal nerve. Therefore, the electrodiagnostic findings seen in compression of this nerve are a prolonged distal motor latency to the extensor digitorum brevis muscle, with an impaired evoked muscle potential amplitude, normal conduction from knee to ankle, and EMG changes in the extensor digitorum brevis.[52]

Sural Nerve

The sural is a pure sensory nerve and provides sensation for the lateral aspect of the foot and the skin over the dorsum of the fifth metatarsal and toe. It is made up by small contributions from the tibial and the peroneal nerves, which meet in the posterior calf and exit the posterior compartment through the fascia covering that compartment to reach the subcutaneous level. It exits through the fascia slightly medial to the midline of the calf, at about the level of the musculotendonous junction of the gastrocnemius, and is vulnerable to entrapment in this fascia. Since this nerve has no motor component, only sensory nerve conduction studies are available, and these can be compared to normal values. The usual technique involves stimulation of the sural nerve over its trunk in the posterior calf and recording of the N wave from the nerve at the lateral malleolus.[1,41] Obviously this cannot identify the location of entrapment if it is within the fascia, as this technique studies the nerve after it has exited from the fascia. However, if the compromise is severe or has been present long enough the amplitude of the response will be decreased and the latency may be prolonged.

Compartment Syndromes

The decreased perfusion of tissues due to increased pressures in compartment syndromes can significantly compromise function of the nerves that traverse the involved compartment, as well as the muscle fibers themselves.[35,46] The compartment syndromes, in contrast to the other types of compression neuropathies, are more common in the lower than in the upper extremities.[35] The seven major compartments of the lower extremity, as described by Garfin[13] will be discussed in regard to the content likely to be involved and the electrodiagnostic studies appropriate for evaluation.

It is difficult clinically to determine if the impaired muscle function is due to reflex, inhibition of the muscles, pain, or to actual impairment of function of the nerve or the muscle from ischemic changes. As discussed in the introductory comments (Chapter 4) EMG and nerve conduction studies provide different information regarding what is occurring in the muscle or nerves in the involved compartment. Nerve conduction studies can help to confirm if nerve function has been impaired, and the EMG can help to confirm if muscle function is lost due to ischemic damage to the muscle fibers. Electrodiagnostic testing can be of significant assistance in monitoring recovery following treatment.

Gluteal Compartment Syndrome

The muscles contained in this compartment are the gluteus maximus, gluteus medius, and gluteus minimus. The major nerve traversing this compartment is the sciatic nerve. Monitoring function of the tibial or peroneal nerves is of little value during the period when information that would influence treatment is needed, as time is required for changes to occur in those distal areas. Even if many axons were lost due to the compression, in this proximal area it would take three to five days for the axons to degenerate far enough distally for reduction in the M wave amplitude to be observed, as the stimulus activating the nerve is delivered distal to the area of the compromise. EMG of the gluteus maximus and minimus can help monitor acute changes occurring in those muscles to confirm that muscle function is being lost. Other than EMG of the muscles of the gluteal compartment for acute changes, electrodiagnostic studies have little role in the evaluation of the gluteal compartment syndrome.

Iliacus Compartment

This compartment contains the iliacus and psoas major and minor muscles. The major nerve traversing this compartment is the femoral nerve. Since the contents of this compartment are on the inner surface of the pelvis it is relatively immune to minor trauma; however, it can be compromised by spontaneous hemorrhage into these tissues. Electrodiagnostic testing is of only very minor assistance in evaluating this condition. Only a small portion of the iliacus muscle is available for EMG study, and this portion of the muscle is distal to the compartment. Monitoring of function of the femoral nerve will show only late changes and is of little assistance in the early stage, as time is required for those changes to occur. As in all of the compartment syndromes, the electrodiagnostic studies can be of significant assistance to monitor recovery of function following treatment.

Thigh Anterior Compartment

The muscles contained in this compartment are the quadriceps muscles and the sartorius. The major nerve traversing this compartment is the femoral nerve. Monitoring of amplitude of the M wave from these muscles with stimulation of the femoral nerve at the inguinal ligament will show progressive reduction in amplitude and increase in latency as the condition worsens. In addition, EMG can also monitor acute changes occurring in the quadriceps muscles.

Thigh Posterior Compartment

The muscles contained in this compartment are the hamstrings and the adductor muscle groups. The major nerves traversing this compartment are the sciatic nerve and the obturator nerve. It is possible to stimulate the sciatic nerve at the level of the sciatic notch using a needle electrode placed close to the nerve.[15,53] Stimulation at this level with recording from muscles within or distal to this compartment allows monitoring of changes occurring in this nerve within the compartment. A progressive decline in the M wave amplitude on serial studies can confirm that nerve function is being compromised or lost because of the increased pressures within the compartment. EMG of the muscles within this compartment can help monitor acute changes occurring to those muscles, by confirming that muscle fibers are losing their ability to function or are being lost.

Leg Anterior Compartment

The anterior compartment syndrome is the best known and probably the most frequently diagnosed of the compartment syndromes.[35] The muscles contained in this compartment are the tibialis anterior, extensor hallucis longus and extensor digitorum longus. The major nerve traversing this compartment is the deep branch of the peroneal nerve. Motor or direct (mixed motor and sensory) nerve conduction studies for the peroneal nerve through this compartment will show slowing of the conduction velocity and reduction in the amplitude of the M wave evoked from the extensor digitorum brevis distal to the compartment. Serial EMG studies may document progressive reduction in ability to activate the muscles voluntarily and reduction in insertional activity suggests that the muscle fibers are losing the ability to maintain their resting membrane potential. This finding suggests that immediate monitoring of the compartment pressures is indicated as urgent decompression may be needed.

Leg Lateral Compartment

The muscles contained in this compartment are the peroneus longus and peroneus brevis. The major nerve traversing this compartment is the superficial branch of the peroneal nerve. Sensory nerve conduction study of the superficial peroneal nerve[1] evaluates the segment through the lateral compartment and can monitor change. EMG of these muscles can help to monitor acute changes occurring in these muscles. There are no muscles innervated by the superficial peroneal nerve distal to this compartment that can be used to monitor reduction in function of the nerve.

Leg Posterior Compartment

The posterior compartment of the leg is usually considered to be two separate compartments; a superficial and a deep compartment:

Superficial Compartment. The muscles contained in this compartment are the gastrocnemius, soleus, and plantaris muscles. The posterior tibial nerve provides muscular branches to innervate these muscles; however, the posterior tibial nerve does not traverse this compartment. The sural nerve is formed in this compartment; however, nerve conduction studies of this nerve would not show early changes, as the points for stimulation and recording are both distal to the compartment. EMG is the only useful study to assist in evaluation of acute changes occurring in the muscles in this compartment. As with the anterior compartment, evidence that the muscle fibers are losing their ability to maintain resting membrane potentials indicates that compartment pressure monitoring is urgently needed.

Deep Compartment. The muscles contained in this compartment are the flexor hallucis longus, tibialis posterior, and the flexor digitorum longus. The major nerve traversing this compartment is the posterior tibial nerve. Motor nerve conduction study with stimulation of the tibial nerve in the popliteal space and recording from the intrinsic muscles of the foot can monitor progressive loss or reduction of function of this nerve. The muscles of this compartment can be difficult to identify by EMG when voluntary function is limited by pain.

In summary, nerve conduction study techniques are of significantly greater value in localizing the level of a compressive (entrapment) neuropathy than the EMG. However, in compartment syndromes the relative value of these two techniques may be reversed. Nerve conduction study methods can confirm progressive reduction in amplitude of the evoked nerve action potential or the M wave with serial studies only if the nerve can be stimulated proximal to the site of compression or the involved compartment. EMG of the muscles within an involved compartment can confirm whether normal muscle function continues or is being lost as a result of the ischemic changes resulting from increased compartment pressures. In addition, if the insertional activity decreases or is lost, it suggests that the muscle fibers have been compromised by ischemia to the point that they are no longer able to maintain their resting membrane potential. In this event, if pressure monitoring studies have not already been initiated, they should be started as soon as possible as decompressive intervention may be essential to preserve muscle function.

References

1. Behse F, Buchthal F: Normal sensory conduction in the nerves of the leg in man. J Neurol Neurosurg Psychiatry 34:404, 1971.
2. Belen J: Orthodromic sensory nerve conduction of the medial and lateral plantar nerves. Am J Phys Med 64:17, 1985.
3. Braddom RL, Johnson EW: Standardization of H reflex and diagnostic use in S1 radiculopathy. Arch Phys Med Rehabil 55:161, 1974.
4. Buchthal F, Rosenfalck A: Evoked action potentials and conduction velocity in human sensory nerves. Brain Res 3:1, 1966.
5. Butler ET, Johnson EW, Kaye ZA: Normal conduction velocity in the lateral femoral cutaneous nerve. Arch Phys Med Rehabil 55:31, 1974.
6. Cape CA: Sensory nerve action potential of the peroneal, sural and tibial nerves. Am J Phys Med 50:220, 1971.
7. Checkels NS, Bailey JA, Johnson EW: Tape and caliper measurements in determination of peroneal nerve conduction velocity. Arch Phys Med Rehabil 50:214, 1969.
8. Devi S, Lovelace RE, Duarte N: Proximal peroneal nerve conduction velocity: Recording from anterior tibial and peroneus brevis muscles. Ann Neurol 2:116, 1977.
9. Di Benedetto M: Sensory nerve conduction in lower extremities. Arch Phys Med Rehabil 51:253, 1970.
10. Edwards WG, Lincoln CR, Bassett FH III, Goldner JL: The tarsal tunnel syndrome: Diagnosis and treatment. JAMA 207:716, 1969.
11. Fu R, DeLisa JA, Kraft BH: Motor nerve latencies through the tarsal tunnel in normal adult subjects: Standard determinations corrected for temperature and distance. Arch Phys Med Rehabil 61:243, 1980.
12. Gaetens PF, Saeed MH: Electromyographic findings in the intrinsic muscles of normal feet. Arch Phys Med Rehabil 63:317, 1982.

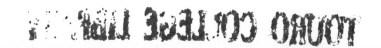

13. Garfin SR: Anatomy of the extremity compartments. *In* SJ Mubarak, AR Hargans (Eds): Compartments Syndromes and Volkman's Contracture. Philadelphia, W.B. Saunders Co., 1981, pp 17.
14. Gassel MM: A study of femoral nerve conduction time. Arch Neurol 9:607, 1963.
15. Gassel MM, Trojaborg W: Clinical and electrophysiological study of the pattern of conduction times in the distribution of the sciatic nerve. J Neurol Neurosurg Psychiatry 27:351, 1964.
16. Goodgold J, Eberstein A: Electrodiagnosis of Neuromuscular Diseases, 3rd ed. Baltimore, Williams and Wilkins, 1983.
17. Goodgold J, Kopell HP, Spielholz NI: The tarsal tunnel syndrome: Objective diagnostic criteria. N Engl J Med 273:742, 1965.
18. Guiloff RJ, Sherratt RM: Sensory conduction in medial plantar nerve: Normal values, clinical applications and a comparison with the sural and upper limb sensory nerve action potentials in peripheral neuropathies. J Neurol Neurosurg Psychiatry 40:1168, 1977.
19. Irani KD, Grabois M, Harvey SC: Standardized technique for diagnosis of tarsal tunnel syndrome. Am J Phys Med 61:26, 1982.
20. Iyer KS, Kaplan E, Goodgold J: Sensory action potentials of the medial and lateral plantar nerves. Arch Phys Med Rehabil 65:529, 1984.
21. Izzo KL, Sridhara CR, Rosenholtz H, Lemont H: Sensory conduction studies of the superficial peroneal nerve. Arch Phys Med Rehabil 62:24, 1981.
22. Jiminez J, Easton JK, Redford JB: Conduction studies of the anterior and posterior tibial nerves. Arch Phys Med Rehabil 51:164, 1970.
23. Johnson EW, Ortiz PR: Electrodiagnosis of tarsal tunnel syndrome. Arch Phys Med Rehabil 47:776, 1966.
24. Johnson EW, Wood PK, Power JJ: Femoral nerve conduction studies. Arch Phys Med Rehabil 49:528, 1968.
25. Kimura J: Electrodiagnosis in Diseases of Nerve and Muscle. Philadelphia, F.A. Davis, 1983.
26. Kopell HP, Thompson WAL: Peripheral Entrapment Neuropathies. Baltimore, Williams and Wilkins, 1963.
27. Kraft GH: Continuing Education Course E, American Association of Electromyography and Electrodiagnosis 13, 1986.
28. Lovelace RE, Meyers SJ, Zablow L: Sensory conduction in peroneal and posterior tibial nerves using averaging techniques. J Neurol Neurosurg Psychiatry 36:942, 1973.
29. Levin KH, Stevens JC, Daube JR: Superficial peroneal nerve conduction studies for electromyographic diagnosis. Muscle Nerve 9:322, 1986.
30. Ludin HP: Electromyography in Practice. New York, Thiene-Stratton, 1980.
31. Lysens R, Vandendriessch G, Von Mol Y, Roselle N: The sensory conduction velocity in the cutaneous femoris lateralis nerve in normal adults. Subjects and in patients with complaints suggesting meralgia paresthetica. Electromyogr Clin Neurophysiol 21:505, 1981.
32. Ma D, Liveson JA: Nerve Conduction Handbook. Philadelphia, F.A. Davis, 1983.
33. MacLean IC: Nerve root stimulation to evaluate conduction across the brachial and lumbo-sacral plexuses. Third Annual Continuing Education Course, American Association of Electromyography and Electrodiagnosis, 1980.
34. Marinacci AA: Neurological syndromes of the tarsal tunnels. Bull Los Angeles Neurol Soc 33:90, 1968.

35. Mubarak SJ, Hargans AR: Compartment Syndromes and Volkman Contracture. Philadelphia, W.B. Saunders Co., 1981.

36. Oh SJ, Kim HS, Ahmad BK: Electrophysiological diagnosis of interdigital neuropathy of the foot. Muscle Nerve 7:218, 1984.

37. Oh SH, Sarala PK, Kuba T, Elmore RS: Tarsal tunnel syndrome: Electrophysiological study. Ann Neurol 5:327, 1979.

38. Pickett JB: Localizing peroneal nerve lesions to the knee by motor conduction studies. Arch Neurol 41:192, 1984.

39. Saeed MA, Gatens PF: Compound nerve action potentials of the medial and lateral plantar nerves through the tarsal tunnel. Arch Phys Med Rehabil 63:304, 1982.

40. Sarala PK, Nishihara T, Oh SJ: Meralgia paresthetica—Electrophysiologic study. Arch Phys Med Rehabil 60:30, 1979.

41. Schuchmann JA: Sural nerve conduction: A standardized technique. Arch Phys Med Rehabil 58:166, 1977.

42. Senden R, Van Mulder J, Ghys R, Rosell N: Conduction velocity of the distal segment of the saphenous nerve in normal adult subjects. Electromyogr Clin Neurophysiol 21:3, 1981.

43. Singh N, Behse F, Buchthal F: Electrophysiological study of peroneal palsy. J Neurol Neurosurg Psychiatry 37:1202, 1974.

44. Stevens A, Roselle N: Sensory nerve conduction velocity of n. cutaneous femoris lateralis. Electromyogr 10:397, 1970.

45. Synek VM, Cowan JC: Saphenous nerve evoked potentials and the assessment of intraabdominal lesions of the femoral nerve. Muscle Nerve 6:453, 1983.

46. Szabo RM, Gelberman RH: Peripheral nerve compression: Etiology critical pressure threshold and clinical assessment. Orthopedics 7:1461, 1984.

47. Van der Most van Spijk D, Vingerhoets HM: Disorders of the lumbosacral roots and nerves. In SH Notermans (Ed): Current Practice of Clinical Electromyography. Amsterdam, Elsevier, 1984.

48. Wainaple SF, Kim DJ, Ebel A: Conduction studies of the saphenous nerve in healthy subjects. Arch Phys Med Rehabil 59:316, 1978.

49. Wallach HW, Oren ME: Sciatic nerve compression during anticoagulant therapy: Computerized tomography aids in diagnosis. Arch Neurol 36:448, 1979.

50. Weber R, Piero D: Entrapment syndromes. In EW Johnson (Ed): Practical Electromyography. Baltimore, Williams and Wilkins, 1980.

51. Wilbourn A: Common peroneal mononeuropathy at the fibular head. AAEE Case Report #12. Muscle Nerve 9:825, 1986.

52. Wilbourn A: Peroneal mononeuropathies. Course E, American Association of Electromyography and Electrodiagnosis 19, 1986.

53. Yap CB, Hirota T: Sciatic nerve motor conduction velocity study. J Neurol Neurosurg Psychiatry 30:233, 1967.

CHAPTER 6

Carpal Tunnel Syndrome

Robert M. Szabo, M.D.

"Carpal tunnel syndrome is the most common and the most important of all the nerve entrapment syndromes".[56]

The signs and symptoms resulting from median nerve compression at the wrist have previously been termed median neuritis, median neuropathy, and tardy median palsy, but since 1947 the condition has become known as the carpal tunnel syndrome.[10]

It is hard to believe that the carpal tunnel syndrome is probably the most commonly made diagnosis in a hand surgery practice, yet it is not too long ago that people complaining of numbness and discomfort in the fingers, particularly with night pain, were considered to have either thoracic outlet syndrome or hysteria. It is easy to see with statements like "The syndrome is characterized early by vague and fugitive complaints and occurs most frequently with middle-aged women who, may I add parenthetically, are possessed by other problems at that juncture" that the medical community took some time to adjust to this new entity.[63] A complete historical review of the carpal tunnel syndrome is provided by Dr. Paul Lipscomb earlier in this text.

Anatomy

The carpal tunnel is a narrow fibro-osseous canal. The floor of the canal is formed by a concave arch of carpal bones covered by the intrinsic and extrinsic palmar wrist ligaments. The roof of the canal is the transverse carpal ligament, which is firmly attached to the pisiform and hook of the hamate on its ulnar aspect and to the scaphoid tubercle and the crest of the trapezium on its radial aspect.[61]

The radial portion of the transverse carpal ligament divides into a superficial and a deep layer and forms a separate fibro-osseous tunnel for the flexor carpi radialis tendon. The distal palmar wrist crease represents the proximal border of the transverse carpal ligament, which then extends 3 to 4 cm distally from the crease. The ligament is 2½ to 3½ mm thick. The carpal tunnel contains the median nerve, the flexor pollicis longus tendon sheathed by the radial bursa, and four flexor digitorum superficialis tendons and four flexor digitorum profundus tendons, all of which are invested by the ulnar bursa. Proximally the ligament blends with the antebrachial fascia and distally with the palmar fascia.

The median nerve becomes superficial to the flexor digitorum superficialis muscle bellies about 5 cm proximal to the transverse carpal ligament. At about this level, the palmar cutaneous branch of the median nerve originates from its radial side and then runs parallel to the median nerve crossing the base of the thenar eminence over the scaphoid tubercle.[11] At the entrance to the tunnel, the median nerve consistently is radial to the flexor digitorum superficialis of the long and index fingers, and is ulnar to the flexor carpi radialis.

The median nerve is composed of 94 percent sensory fibers and 6 percent motor fibers at the level of the carpal tunnel. The motor branch, however, presents many anatomic variations of great significance to the surgeon who operates in the carpal tunnel. The normal position for the recurrent motor branch of the median nerve is extraligamentous just distal to the transverse carpal ligament. However, the branch can be subligamentous, or transligamentous. Other variations include high divisions of the median nerve in instances where the thenar branch leaves the median nerve proximal to the carpal tunnel. For a complete description of these variations, the reader is referred to the original work by Lanz.[44]

Etiology

The cause of compression in the carpal canal is a discrepancy between the volume of the contents of the canal and the size of the canal. Said another way, there is either too little space or too much substance within the carpal canal. The end result is increased pressure within the carpal tunnel causing median nerve compression.[69] Gelberman, using wick catheter techniques, has confirmed that the mean pressure within the intracarpal canal in patients with carpal tunnel syndrome is 32 mm Hg.[23] This compares to control subjects with a mean pressure of 2.5 mm Hg. This pressure is also dependent on wrist position as the pressure increases to 94 mm Hg with 90 degrees of wrist flexion in carpal tunnel patients and 110 mm Hg with wrist extension. In normal controls, the carpal tunnel pressure is 31 mm Hg in 90 degrees of wrist flexion and 30 mm Hg with wrist extension. Werner et al.[72] showed a relationship between the electrophysiologic abnormalities and pressure within the carpal canal that supports the view that raised pressure between the nerve and the ligament is an important factor for the nerve lesion in the carpal tunnel syndrome. The median nerve is compressed between extrinsic finger flexor tendons and the carpal bones during exertions of the hand. These rather high local intermittent pressures are most likely of great significance;[2,3] however, there are no experimental human or animal studies that shed light on the effect of intermittent compression of peripheral nerves.

The most common cause of increase in carpal canal contents is a nonspecific tenosynovial proliferation that occurs in otherwise healthy individuals.[18,47,56,57] Biopsy specimens of the flexor synovialis have demonstrated chronic fibrosis or thickening that seems to be associated with some kind of rheumatic process but frequently not rheumatoid arthritis.[74] The next most common group of patients with carpal tunnel syndrome, in fact, is patients with rheumatoid arthritis with accompanying rheumatoid tenosynovitis.[12,32] Other conditions that increase the volume of the contents of the carpal tunnel and tend to compress the median nerve include benign tumors (lypoma, hemangioma, and ganglia), deposits of calcium and gouty tophi, amyloidosis as seen in patients with multiple myoloma, myxedema[58] and fluid retention associated with pregnancy.[16] Congenital anomalies[19,45] with aberrant muscle bellies in the carpal canal have also been reported as a cause of median nerve compression.[7,42] Significant thickening of the transverse carpal ligament as found in acromegaly, pleonosteosis, and myxedema may be a contributing cause of median nerve compression.

We have seen schwannomas of the median nerve as well as lyphomas of the median nerve and aberrant median arteries[59] also cause compression of the median nerve in the carpal tunnel.

Factors that cause reduction of the capacity of the bony canal include first and foremost wrist arthritis. Other causes are malalignment or exuberant callus associated with distal radial fractures,[46] bony changes due to acromegaly, bony changes due to congenital abnormalities, or fracture dislocations leading to impingement from displaced carpal bones.[38,71]

As mentioned earlier, the position of the wrist is extremely important when considering pressure within the carpal canal and, thus, extremes of wrist position such as immobilization of a swollen wrist in flexion after a distal radius fracture may result in carpal tunnel syndrome.

One particular group of patients at risk for carpal tunnel syndrome are those on long-term hemodialysis.[5,64,70] Development of median nerve lesions during hemodialysis most likely is due to the increase of pressure within the carpal tunnel resulting from periodic increase of total body water in these patients. The development of carpal tunnel syndrome in hemodialysis patients is not influenced by age, sex, hand dominance, or mechanical or hormonal factors.[64]

Occupation as a contributor to carpal tunnel syndrome is a controversial issue.[29] Occupations or activities[36] that require highly repetitive finger or wrist flexion may predispose or aggravate a carpal tunnel syndrome, but it is not clear whether the occupational activities alone can be the cause of a carpal tunnel syndrome. Two studies[57,74] that had a combined group of 1000 patients had 50 percent of their patients working as housewives, an occupation not clearly associated with repetitive hand activities.

Poultry processing workers, butchers, meat wrappers, cashiers, and automotive assembly workers have been reported to have high rates of carpal tunnel syndrome. One study demonstrated nearly a 15 percent incidence of carpal tunnel disease in the meat-packing industry, which is higher than the usually reported 1 percent in the general population.[51] The cause has been attributed to highly repetitive motions involving extreme flexion and ulnar deviation while grasping of knives used in cutting meat. This study found that cost of days lost from work and compensation claims due to carpal tunnel syndrome in a small meat packing plant was in excess of one million dollars over five years. The implications are clear. As physicians we will be asked to perform pre-employment screening for workers at risk of developing carpal tunnel syndrome, and we will need to take an active role in suggesting modifications of job routine and redesign of tools to prevent carpal tunnel syndrome.

Pathogenesis

Relative roles of mechanical deformation and ischemia in production of nerve compression lesions are controversial and are discussed by Lundborg and Dahlin in Chapter 2. The pathologic basis and stages of median nerve compression in the carpal tunnel syndrome will be discussed here.

Using vital staining, Rydevick and Lundborg[62] have shown that pressures of 20-30 mm Hg applied to nerve will cause slowing of intraneural blood flow in venules. This venous congestion occurs at the same pressures that Gelberman found in patients with carpal tunnel syndrome in a very early stage of the lesion.[23] This might correspond to the first symptoms of pain that patients with carpal tunnel syndrome complain about. The immediate relief from pain following operative decompression indicates that this disturbance is rapidly reversible and suggests that the process is of vascular origin rather than involving morphologic changes.[21] If venous congestion persists from long-standing pressure, it will diminish the microvascular flow of nutrients to the fascicles, resulting in disturbances in nerve conduction. Vascular insufficiency will lead to anoxia and subsequent damage to the capillary endothelium, which results in leakage of proteins through the walls of the epineural venules, causing epineural edema. Early sensory and motor symptoms are found at this stage. If the pressure is relieved at this point, the edema will be resolved through the network of epineural lymphatics and capillaries. The swelling in this stage may be concealed within the epineurium or it may be great enough to cause physical enlargements like that seen in the median nerve above and below the edge of the flexor retinaculum while doing a carpal tunnel release. At this stage, symptoms from carpal tunnel syndrome are still reversible with decompression of the median nerve. The time it takes to progress from one stage to the next is not well established.

If compression persists, fibroblasts start to proliferate in the edema fluid, resulting in epineural fibrosis. The fibrosis leads to destruction of nerve fibers. Finally, nutrient vessels are obliterated, the funiculi atrophy, and with the increase of ischemia fibrosis becomes more marked. The affected nerve becomes somewhat thinned and as it converts into fibrous tissue, the lesion reaches the point of irreversibility, and decompression is without effect.[66]

There is a group of patients in whom less compression of the median nerve than usual in the carpal tunnel is required to produce symptoms. These patients have compression of the median nerve proximal to the carpal tunnel or compression at the cervical root level. This phenomenon is known as the "double crush syndrome." Similarly, the median nerve at the carpal tunnel may be more sensitive to lower levels of pressure in patients with diabetes mellitus, hypothyroidism, or other forms of systemic peripheral neuropathy.

Clinical Presentation

In a classic case of carpal tunnel syndrome there is a typical sequence of symptoms that often permits diagnosis.[34,48,73] The patient begins to complain of numbness and tingling in the median distribution of the hand; that is the thumb, the index, the middle, and the radial half of the ring fingers. Sometimes the symptoms are in only one finger, but more frequently the patient will complain of numbness in the whole hand. Careful questioning usually, but not always, eliminates the little finger as the site of any numbness or tingling. These symptoms are followed by numbness and pain, which is aggravated by persistent exertion. Frequently, the patient is awakened in the middle of the night by pain in the hand, which is relieved by hanging, shaking, massaging, or exercising the hand. Night pain is probably caused by persistent compression of the median nerve by the position assumed during sleep when it is not relieved by changes in posture, or it may be related to venous stasis. Patients often complain that their hands feel "swollen." Later on, symptoms appear related to the motor branch of the median nerve. With advancing atrophy of the thenar muscles, coordinated movements of the thumb and index finger become weak, stiff, and clumsy. This is usually noted in the morning hours and improves somewhat during the day. The motor disability becomes apparent during simple tasks such as buttoning clothes, sewing, and winding a watch.

Symptoms are frequently bilateral, with the dominant hand usually affected first and most severely. Interestingly, patients may only complain of unilateral symptoms, but when studied electrodiagnostically, bilaterality is often found. Repetitious acts such as gripping the steering wheel of a car, grasping and using a broom or a mop or a kitchen utensil, or any strenuous use of the hand almost always aggravates the symptoms. Symptoms can radiate to the elbow, shoulder, or along the forearm.

Acute carpal tunnel syndrome usually presents secondary to trauma.[4,52,71] A wrist fracture or dislocation may cause increased pressure in the carpal canal and actually jeopardize the viability of the median nerve. This often is difficult to differentiate from median nerve contusion. Intracarpal canal pressures are measured in order to differentiate between these two problems.

In obtaining the history relating to hand complaints, it is important to specifically seek out information about related systemic disease and conditions such as hypothyroidism, diabetes, rheumatoid arthritis, and pregnancy.

Physical Findings

Physical findings can be grouped into those related to decreased sensibility, response to provocative testing, or decreased strength. Pure objective sensory testing is not possible, as each test of sensibility depends on the patient's ability or inability to give an accurate assessment of the effect of the testing. Tests of sensibility include threshold tests (Semmes-Weinstein monofilaments, vibrometry, 256 cps vibration) and innervation density tests (two-point discrimination and moving two-point discrimination). Threshold tests evaluate a single nerve fiber innervating a receptor or group of receptor cells, whereas innervation density tests measure multiple overlapping peripheral receptor fields and the density of innervation in the region being tested. Innervation density tests are highly dependent on cortical integration of peripheral impulses and may remain apparently normal in a patient with nerve compression as long as a few fibers are conducting normally to their correct cortical end points. We have found in our laboratory, as well as in extensive clinical testing, that the most consistent and reliable way to evaluate sensibility in nerve compression is to use threshold testing.[25,67] We perform the von Frey pressure test using Semmes-Weinstein monofilaments (Fig. 6-1). The monofilament is applied perpendicularly to the palmar digital surface and pressure is increased until the monofilament begins to bend. Each probe is marked with the number that represents the logarithm of ten times the force (in milligrams) required to bow the monofilament. Light monofilaments (1.65 to 3.84) are bounced off the skin three times, whereas the heavier monofilaments (4.08 to 6.65) are applied in one motion. The response is considered positive when the patient, with eyes closed, can localize verbally which digit was receiving pressure. The test is performed on each digit and on both hands, and comparisons are made between the distribution of the affected median nerve, the ulnar nerve, and the contralateral median and ulnar nerves. Generally, a value of 2.83 or less is considered normal.

We also assess vibratory sensibility on each digit with a fixed frequency (120 hz) variable amplitude vibrometer (Fib. 6-2). The vibrating head is applied by the examiner and held in contact with the patient's fingertip while the intensity of the stimulus is gradually increased. The threshold is read as the voltage required to deliver one perceived stimulus. The voltage is then converted to micrometers of motion of the vibrating head using a calibration chart supplied with the instrument. While vibratory threshold data reflects the earliest clinical abnormalities, the Semmes-Weinstein monofilaments are only slightly less sensitive and are somewhat easier to use. We therefore reserve vibrometry testing for patients who we believe have very early carpal tunnel syndromes and test normally with the monofilaments. For a detailed description of this technique, the reader is

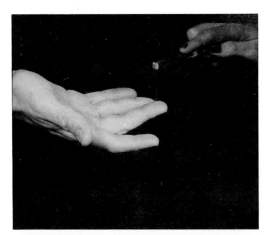

Figure 6-1. von Frey pressure test is performed using Semmes-Weinstein monofilaments. The monofilament is applied perpendicularly to the palmar digital surface, and the pressure is increased until the monofilament begins to bend. The response is considered positive when the patients, with eyes closed, can localize verbally which digit was receiving pressure.

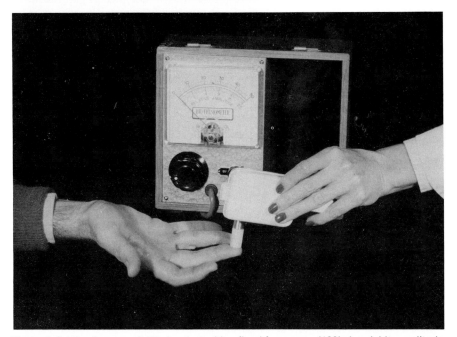

Figure 6-2. Vibratory sensibility is a test with a fixed frequency (120hz) variable amplitude vibrometer. The vibrating head is applied by the examiner and held in contact with the patient's finger tip while the intensity of the stimulus is gradually increased. The vibratory threshold is reported as the voltage required to deliver one perceived stimulus.

referred to the article, "Vibratory Sensory Testing in Acute Peripheral Nerve Compression".[68]

Weber two-point discrimination testing is performed and, if abnormal (more than 6 mm), advanced nerve compression is present (Fig. 6-3). In our series, abnormal vibratory thresholds were found in 87 percent, and abnormal determinations on Semmes-Weinstein monofilament testing in 83 percent of hands with carpal tunnel syndrome. Two-point discrimination

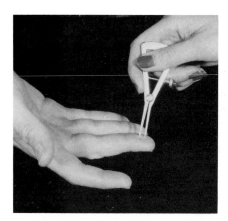

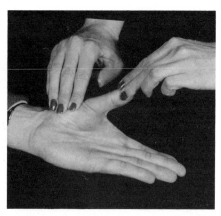

Figure 6-3. The Weber two-point discrimination test is performed using a blunt eye caliper or a paper clip. Pressure is applied in the longitudinal axis of the digit until the finger blanches. The distance between the two points perceived is then measured. Normal two-point discrimination is less than 6 mm.

Figure 6-4. The manual test of the abductor pollicis brevis is demonstrated. The thumb is placed in full palmar abduction and the patient is asked to maintain this position. The examiner palpates the abductor pollicis brevis with one hand and applies downward pressure with the other hand. The strength of the muscle is then graded.

was abnormal in only 22 percent. Moving two-point discrimination offered no advantage in the determination of sensory abnormalities in carpal tunnel syndrome.[67]

There are three provocative tests for carpal tunnel syndrome. These are the (1) wrist flexion (Phalen) test, (2) the median nerve percussion (Tinel) test, and (3) the tourniquet test. The wrist flexion test is performed by actively placing the wrist in complete, but unforced flexion. If numbness or tingling is produced or exaggerated in the median nerve distribution within 60 seconds, the test is considered positive. The median nerve percussion test is performed by the examiner who gently taps the area over the median nerve at the wrist. The test is positive if this produces tingling in the fingers. The tourniquet test is performed by placing a pneumatic blood pressure cuff proximal to the elbow and inflating it to a pressure higher than the patient's systolic blood pressure. If the patient experiences paresthesia or numbness in the distribution of the median nerve within 60 seconds of inflation, the test is considered positive. We found that these tests are positive in approximately 60 to 70 percent of patients with carpal tunnel syndrome; however, Gellman demonstrated that the wrist flexion test is the most sensitive and most useful of the three provocative tests.[26] The percussion test was least sensitive, but the most specific, with only a 6 percent false positive rate. A very important finding was that the tourniquet test presented a 40 percent false positive rate and, thus, cannot be considered very useful.

An evaluation of the motor branch in the median nerve includes observation for thenar atrophy and specific muscle testing of the abductor pollicis brevis and opponens pollicis brevis (Fig. 6-4).

Recently, an additional provocative test has been described designed to reproduce the patient's symptoms.[55] The test, called the "median nerve compression test," is performed by applying gentle, sustained firm pressure with one's thumbs to the median nerve at its entrance to the carpal tunnel. If the patient's symptoms are reproduced within 15 seconds to two minutes, the test is considered positive. The second phase of the test is to remove the pressure and question the patient as to the relief of his symptoms. More data are needed to evaluate the sensitivity and specificity of this test.

Diagnostic Studies

Carpal tunnel syndrome is generally a clinical diagnosis; however, several conditions may mimic the chief characteristics of pain, numbness, and paresthesias in the hand. Basic laboratory studies should routinely be included in the workup. These include screening for collagen vascular disease, renal and thyroid disease, and diabetes mellitus. One study revealed a 14 percent incidence of associated diabetes mellitus in a group of carpal tunnel syndrome patients.[17]

Anteroposterior and lateral roentgenograms of the wrist should be performed, even though in most cases they are normal. In some patients they may demonstrate recent or old fractures resulting in encroachment of bone into the carpal tunnel, foreign bodies, tumors, or other lesions that may cause secondary compression of the median nerve. If some abnormality is seen on plain x-rays, then it is sometimes useful to obtain a carpal tunnel projection view of the wrist. Computerized tomography of the carpal tunnel may become more useful.[35]

The most sensitive and objective test used to diagnose carpal tunnel syndrome is electrodiagnosis.[13,28,31,33,40,50] Electrical abnormalities are often found early and correlate with clinical findings in greater than 90 percent of patients.[39] While normal electrodiagnostic studies do not exclude the diagnosis of carpal tunnel syndrome, the median nerve is rarely significantly compressed in the face of a negative exam performed by an experienced electromyographer. In a patient with carpal tunnel syndrome, the distal latency is prolonged and the conduction velocity is delayed of either the sensory or motor or both components of the median nerve when compared with normal values or uninvolved nerves elsewhere in the patient. Electrodiagnostic standards vary with given investigators; however, in general distal motor latencies of more than 4.5 milliseconds and distal sensory latencies of more than 3.5 milliseconds are considered abnormal. Asymmetry of conduction between both hands of more than one millisecond for motor conduction or 0.5 milliseconds for sensory conduction time is also considered abnormal. Complete nerve conduction studies including measurements of velocity, amplitude, and latency, in addition to electromyographic studies of the thenar muscles, can help quantitate the severity of nerve compression. I obtain electrodiagnostic studies in all patients who I suspect to have carpal tunnel syndrome in order to confirm the clinical diagnosis and, equally as important, eliminate other diagnoses.

For further discussion of electrodiagnostic studies and nerve compression, the reader should refer to Chapters 4 and 5 in this text.

Treatment

There are three basic treatment modalities: medical, steroid injections, and surgical.

Medical

Conservative therapy is offered to mildly symptomatic patients with normal clinical and electromyographic studies. Treatment typically consists of splinting the wrist in neutral position; oral anti-inflammatory medications to reduce synovitis; diuretics to reduce edema; and management of underlying systemic diseases, such as hypothyroidism and diabetes mellitus.

Recently there has been a great interest in treating carpal tunnel syndrome with pyridoxine (vitamin B_6). Ellis[15] has claimed that carpal tunnel syndrome is a primary deficiency of vitamin B_6, based on determination of the specific activities and percentage deficiencies of the glutamic-oxaloacetic transaminase of erythrocytes. This claim has been challenged by Byers et al.,[8] who have reminded us that for many years B complex vitamins have been used to treat peripheral neuropathies. They pointed out that the patients treated by Ellis were not studied electrodiagnostically, and many of these patients had signs and symptoms that were also compatible with peripheral neuropathy. A more recent study was performed on 19 consecutive patients with documented carpal tunnel syndrome. Treatment of these patients with pyridoxine did not appear to modify the natural history of their disease.[1]

I can only conclude at this time that patients with isolated distal median nerve compression at the wrist probably do not benefit from treatment with vitamin B_6.

Steroid Injections

Over 80 percent of patients will obtain transient relief from injection of steroids[27,28] into the carpal canal; however, only 22 percent will be symptom-free 12 months after the injection.[22] Gelberman identified patients likely to benefit the most from steroid injections to have symptoms of less than one year duration, numbness that was diffuse and intermittent, normal two-point discrimination without evidence of weakness or atrophy, one to two millisecond prolongations of distal motor and sensory latencies, and no denervation potentials on needle examination of the thenar muscles.[22] Forty percent of this group with mild symptoms and clinical findings were found to be symptom-free for longer than 12 months. Carpal tunnel injection and splinting were not effective in patients with severe symptoms of more than 12 months duration who had atrophy and weakness or marked abnormalities on nerve conduction velocity testing.

Steroid injection of the carpal tunnel also serves a diagnostic purpose. Green has demonstrated a strong correlation between the results of injections and subsequent operations, in that a patient who obtained a good response from a steroid injection will have a high probability of responding to surgical management.[30] However, poor relief from injection did not necessarily mean that the patient was a poor candidate for surgery.

The injection into the carpal tunnel is made with a 22-gauge needle one centimeter proximal to the distal wrist flexion crease between the palmaris longus and flexor carpi radialis tendons. The needle is angled 45 degrees distally and dorsally and advanced until touching the floor of the carpal canal. It is then withdrawn 0.5 centimeters. A solution of 1 ml (8 milligrams) of dexamethasone acetate and 2 ml of 1 percent lidocaine is injected slowly into the carpal canal. If median paresthesias are elicited, the needle is withdrawn and redirected. Techniques vary and some authors prefer to place their needle just ulnar to the palmaris longus tendon. In any case, a temporary median nerve block should result from the local anesthetic and confirm proper placement of the medication into the carpal canal. I prefer to splint the wrist continuously for three weeks after steroid injection.

Patients are warned that they may experience increased pain in their wrist and actually have exacerbations of their symptoms for 24 to 48 hours after steroid injection, but this discomfort usually subsides.

Surgery

Patients with moderate to severe symptoms; symptoms of more than one year duration, atrophy or weakness of thenar muscles; abnormalities on electromyographic studies of the thenar muscles; or severely prolonged distal motor and sensory latencies, should undergo carpal tunnel release without delay. A steroid injection may be used as a temporary therapeutic or a diagnostic modality. However, patients should be warned that even if symptoms are relieved their nerve is in jeopardy and surgery is indicated.

Operative Technique.

Surgery is performed using Loupe magnification. The carpal tunnel is approached through a curved longitudinal incision, paralleling the thenar crease and crosses the wrist crease obliquely in an ulnar direction at a point in line with the long axis of the ring finger (Fig. 6-5). The transverse incision is no longer popular because it does not provide adequate exposure and is associated with a high rate of incomplete division of the transverse carpal ligament. The transverse carpal ligament is divided on the ulnar side of the median nerve in order to avoid injury to the palmar cutaneous branch of the median nerve and the recurrent motor branch of the median nerve. In addition, the antebrachial fascia is divided for about 3 centimeters proximal to the distal flexion wrist crease. The contents and the floor of the carpal canal are always inspected for any space-occupying lesion. The procedure is performed under local or regional anesthesia with the aid of a tourniquet (Fig. 6-6).

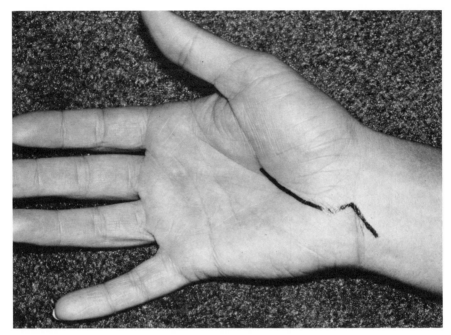

Figure 6-5. Surgery on the carpal tunnel is approached through a curved longitudinal incision, paralleling the thenar crease and crossing the wrist crease obliquely in an ulnar direction at a point in line with the long axis of the ring finger.

Routine tenosynovectomy is not performed. This procedure increases postoperative morbidity and, at times, may decrease excursion of the flexor tendons. It is indicated, however, when the synovium is extremely proliferative, such as in a very active rheumatoid patient.

The need for internal neurolysis is often debated in the literature[20,60] (Fig. 6-7). Proponents cite atrophy of the thenar muscles, loss of two-point discrimination, or both as indications for neurolysis. Those opposed to neurolysis claim the extra dissection of the nerve results in increased scarring about the nerve and further nerve damage. In attempts to answer this question, we studied our own patients and at first found that while internal neurolysis did no further harm to the median nerve if used according to the criteria already stated[60] neither did it improve the results when compared to sectioning of the transverse carpal ligament alone.[24] At this point, we can not predict which patients would benefit from internal neurolysis.

A significant percentage of patients with carpal tunnel syndrome also have signs and symptoms of ulnar nerve compression at the wrist. Most of these patient's symptoms will improve with carpal tunnel release alone, and it is rarely necessary to explore and release Guyon's canal.[65]

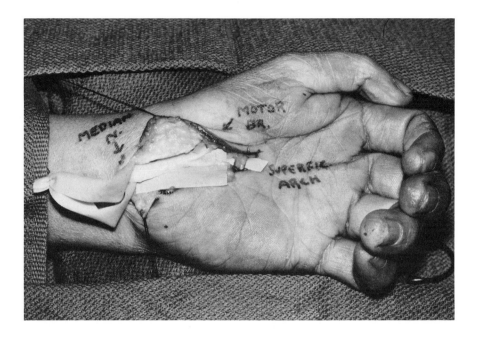

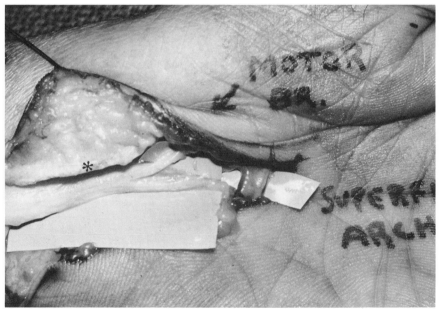

Figure 6-6. *A,* An operative case demonstrating the release of the transverse carpal ligament and the anatomy of the median nerve as it courses through the carpal canal. *B,* Close up view. Note the radial edge of the thick transverse carpal ligament (*). Also note the radial position of the motor branch of the median nerve and the proximity of the superficial arch at the distal edge of the transverse carpal ligament.

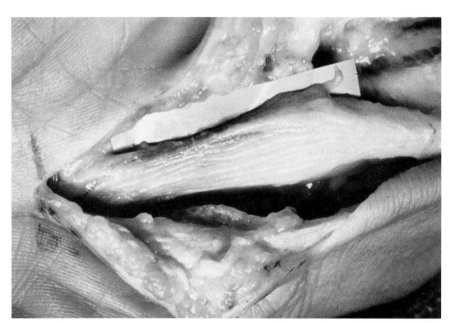

Figure 6-7. Surgical case demonstrating an internal neurolysis. Individual fascicles can be seen dissected on the palmar two-thirds of the median nerve.

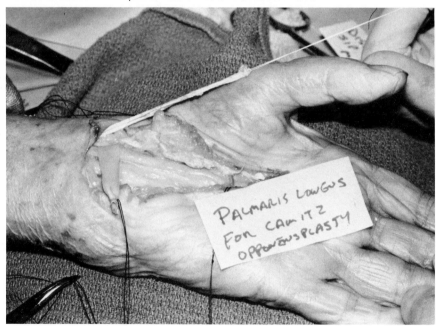

Figure 6-8. This is an 85-year-old female with a long-standing median nerve compression secondary to a malunited Colles' fracture, which occurred 50 years previous to her present operation. A tag is placed on the median nerve, which was then decompressed in the carpal tunnel. The palmaris longus tendon was then isolated with a strip of palmar fascia and subsequently inserted into the abductor pollicis brevis tendon.

Tendon Transfer for
Restoration of Thumb Opposition

Patients with severe thenar atrophy and weakness are good candidates for opponensplasty at the time of carpal tunnel release. An ideal procedure is to use the palmaris longus tendon as described by Camitz[6,9] (Fig. 6-8). This transfer attempts to duplicate abductor brevis function, is properly phased for pinch activity, and requires minimal retraining. If the palmaris longus tendon is not available, my preference is to perform an opponensplasty using either the flexor digitorum superficialis tendon of the ring finger or the extensor indicis proprius; however, I do not do this at the same time as the carpal tunnel release for fear of scarring.

Postoperative care of the wrist and hand is important. A bulky compression dressing is applied until suture removal, maintaining the wrist in neutral position. Each patient is then fitted with a palmar wrist splint, and the wrist is continuously immobilized in the neutral position for a total of three weeks. Digital motion is encouraged from the onset. Splinting should not be discontinued early because the flexor tendons may bowstring when the wrist is flexed and get caught up in the healing process of the transverse carpal ligament.

After splint removal, full range of motion of the wrist is allowed, but strenuous activity is avoided for a minimum of six weeks. The incision may remain tender, and the grip may feel noticeably weak for several months after surgery. Full recovery actually does not occur for six to twelve months. A person who needs to return to manual labor will have a significantly longer recovery time than the elderly rheumatoid patient. Physicians must be sensitive to the different demands a patient will place upon his or her hands and not be too fast to label a person a malingerer.

Complications

Phalen stated, "There are few operations that are as successful and rewarding as the operation for carpal tunnel syndrome."[57] Complications of surgical release for carpal tunnel syndrome have become more appreciated.[14,37] Failure to release the transverse carpal ligament adequately has been thought to be the most frequent complication leading to suboptimal results after carpal tunnel release. Incomplete release was much more common with the transverse incision, which is no longer recommended. Recent information has confirmed that poor results after carpal tunnel release are more commonly associated with the presence of either local or systemic conditions or what has become known as the "double crush" syndrome. A thorough investigation of proximal areas of nerve compression will often demonstrate cervical arthritis with associated C5-6 or C6-7 disc space narrowing. The combination of neck pain and carpal tunnel syndrome should alert the physician to the possibility of a "double crush syndrome."[54]

Other complications following carpal tunnel syndrome include recurrent median nerve compression secondary to either tenosynovitis or a fibrous proliferation within the carpal canal.[41,43,49] Iatrogenic injury to the palmar cutaneous branch of the median nerve can occur from incisions radial to the thenar crease. The neuroma that forms in this branch subsequent to its injury can cause exquisite tenderness and pain in the palm, which interferes with normal hand use. Similarly, the recurrent motor branch can be sectioned if the incision of the carpal ligament is performed on the anterior or radial side of the median nerve.

Bow-stringing of the flexor tendons or pinching of the median nerve in the healing process of the flexor retinaculum can occur if splinting is discontinued and the wrist falls into flexion too early in the postoperative course.

Damage to the superficial palmar arch or even to the ulnar nerve or artery can occur during carpal tunnel release if the surgeon does not appreciate the exact position of these anatomic structures.

Adhesion of the flexor tendons and stiffness may result from tenosynovectomy if digital motion is delayed.

Reflex sympathetic dystrophy occasionally occurs, and has no correlation to the severity of the initial disease. Its incidence is increased when carpal tunnel release is performed simultaneously with excision of Dupuytren's contracture.[53]

Many patients have persistent pain at the wrist at the entrance to the carpal tunnel after carpal tunnel release. This pain is not associated with neuroma and is poorly described in the literature. Sometimes referred to as "pillar pain," the etiology is unclear. Some people feel that this may represent a periostitis caused by an altered mechanics after carpal tunnel release. Others claim it may be due to very small nerve fibers that are sectioned in this area. Still others consider this to be a form of sensitive scar. This pain eventually goes away, but often may take six months to a year to completely resolve.

References

1. Amadio PC: Pyridoxine as an Adjunct in the Treatment of Carpal Tunnel Syndrome. J Hand Surg 10:237-241, 1985.
2. Armstrong TJ, Castelli WA, Evans FG, Diaz-Perez RJ: Some histological changes in carpal tunnel contents and their biomechanical implications. J Occup Med 26(3):197-201, 1984.
3. Armstrong TJ, Chaffin DB: Some Biomechanical Aspects of the Carpal Tunnel. J Biomechanics 12:567-570, 1979.
4. Bauman TD, Gelberman RH, Mubarak SJ, Garfin SR: The acute carpal tunnel syndrome. CORR 156:151-156, 1981.
5. Blodgett RC, Lipscomb PR, Hill RW: Incidence of hematologic disease in patients with carpal tunnel syndrome. JAMA 182:814-815, 1962.
6. Braun RM: Palmaris longus tendon transfer for augmentation of the thenar musculature in low median palsy. J Hand Surg 3(5):488-491, 1978.

7. Butler B, Bigley EC: Aberrant index (first) lumbrical tendinous origin associated with carpal tunnel syndrome. J Bone Joint Surg 53A(1):160-162, 1971.

8. Byers CM, DeLisa JA, Frankel DL, Kraft GH: Pyridoxine metabolism in carpal tunnel syndrome with and without peripheral neuropathy. Arch Phys Med Rehabil 65:712-716, 1984.

9. Camitz H: Surgical treatment of paralysis of opponens muscles of thumbs. Acta Chir Scand 65:77-81, 1929.

10. Cannon BW, Love JG: Tardy median palsy; Median neuritis; Median thenar neuritis amenable to surgery. Presented at the Third Annual Meeting of the Central Surgical Association, Chicago, Illinois, Feb. 22-23, 1946.

11. Carroll RE, Green DP: The significance of the palmar cutaneous nerve at the wrist. CORR 83:24-28, 1972.

12. Chamberlain MA, Corbett M: Carpal Tunnel Syndrome in Early Rheumatoid Arthritis. Ann Rheum Dis 29:149-152, 1970.

13. Cseuz KA, Thomas JE, Lambert EH, Love JG, Lipscomb PR: Long-term results of operation from carpal tunnel syndrome. Mayo Clin Proc 41:232-241, 1966.

14. Eason SY, Belsole RJ, Greene TL: Carpal Tunnel Release: Analysis of Suboptimal Results. J Hand Surg 10B(3):365-369, 1985.

15. Ellis JM, Folkers K, Levy M, Shizukuishi S, Lewandowski J, Nishii S, Schubert HA, Ulrich R: Response of Vitamin B-6 Deficiency and the Carpal Tunnel Syndrome to Pyridoxine. Proc Natl Acad Sci USA 79:7494-7498, 1982.

16. Entin MA: Carpal tunnel syndrome and its variants. Surg Clin North Am 48(5):1097-1112, 1968.

17. Eversmann WW, Colonel L, Ritsick JA: Intraoperative Changes in Motor Nerve Conduction Latency in Carpal Tunnel Syndrome. J Hand Surg 3(1):77-81, 1978.

18. Faithfull DK, Moir DH, Ireland J: The Micropathology of the Typical Carpal Tunnel Syndrome. J Hand Surg 11B(1):131-132, 1986.

19. Feingold MH, Hidvegi E, Horwitz SJ: Bilateral carpal tunnel syndrome in an adolescent. Am J Dis Child 134:394-396, 1980.

20. Fissette J, Onkelinx A: Treatment of carpal tunnel syndrome: Comparative study with and without epineurolysis. Hand 11(2):206-210, 1979.

21. Fullerton PM: The effect of ischaemia on nerve conduction in the carpal tunnel syndrome. J Neurol Neurosurg Psychiatry 26:385-397, 1963.

22. Gelberman RH, Aronson D, Weisman MH: Carpal tunnel syndrome: Results of a prospective trial of steroid injection and splinting. J Bone Joint Surg 62A(7):1181-1184, 1980.

23. Gelberman RH, Hergenroeder PT, Hargens AR, Lundborg GN, Akeson WH: The carpal tunnel syndrome: A study of carpal canal pressures. J Bone Joint Surg 63A(3):380-383, 1981.

24. Gelberman RH, Pfeffer GB, Galbraith RT, Szabo RM, Rydevik B, Dimick M: Results of treatment of severe carpal tunnel syndrome without internal neurolysis of the median nerve. J Bone Joint Surg (in press).

25. Gelberman RH, Szabo RM, Williamson RV, Dimick MP: Sensibility testing in peripheral nerve compression syndromes: An experimental study in humans. J Bone Joint Surg 65A(5):632-638, 1983.

26. Gellman H, Gelberman RH, Tan AM, Botte MJ: Carpal tunnel syndrome: An evaluation of the provocative diagnostic tests. J Bone Joint Surg 68A(5):735-737, 1986.

27. Goodman HV, Foster JB: Effect of local corticosteroid injection on median nerve conduction in carpal tunnel syndrome. Ann Phys Med 6(7):287-294, 1962.

28. Goodwill CJ: The carpal tunnel syndrome: Long-term follow-up showing relation of latency measurements to response to treatment. Ann Phys Med 8(1):12-21, 1965.

29. Graham RA: Carpal tunnel syndrome: A statistical analysis of 214 cases. Orthopedics 6(10):1283-1287, 1983.

30. Green DP: Diagnostic and Therapeutic Value of Carpal Tunnel Injection. J Hand Surg 9:850-854, 1984.

31. Harris CM, Tanner E, Goldstein MN, Pettee DS: The surgical treatment of the carpal-tunnel syndrome correlated with preoperative nerve-conduction studies. J Bone Joint Surg 61A(1):93-98, 1979.

32. Herbison GJ, Teng C, Martin JH, Ditunno JF: Carpal tunnel syndrome in rheumatoid arthritis: A preliminary study. Am J Phys Med 52(2):68-74, 1973.

33. Hongell A, Mattsson HS: Neurographic studies before, after, and during operation for median nerve compression in the carpal tunnel. Scand J Plast Reconstr Surg 5:103-109, 1971.

34. Inglis AE, Straub LR, Williams CS: Median nerve neuropathy at the wrist. C.O.R.R., No. 83:48-54, 1972.

35. John V, Nau HE, Nahser HC, Reinhardt V, Venjakob K: CT of carpal tunnel syndrome. AJNR 4:770-772, 1983.

36. Kellner WS, Felsenthal G, Anderson JM, Hilton EB, Mondell DL: Carpal tunnel syndrome in the nonparetic hands of hemiplegics: Stress-induced by ambulatory assistive devices. Orthop Rev 15(9):87-90, 1986.

37. Kessler FB: Complications of the Management of Carpal Tunnel Syndrome. Hand Clin 2(2):401-406, 1986.

38. Kinley DL, Evarts CM: Carpal tunnel syndrome due to a small displaced fragment of bone. Cleve Clin Qu 35:215-221, 1968.

39. Kopell HP, Goodgold J: Clinical and electrodiagnostic features of carpal tunnel syndrome. Arch Phys Med Rehabil pp. 371-375, July 1968.

40. Kraft GH, Halvorson GA: Median nerve residual latency: Normal value and use in diagnosis of carpal tunnel syndrome. Arch Phys Med Rehabil 64:221-226, 1983.

41. Kulick MI, Gordillo G, Javidi T, Kilgore ES: Long-term analysis of patients having surgical treatment for carpal tunnel syndrome. J Hand Surg 11:59-66, 1986.

42. Lakey MD, Aulicino PL: Anomalous muscles associated with compression neuropathies. Orthop Rev 15(4):19-28, 1986.

43. Langloh ND, Linscheid RL: Recurrent and unrelieved carpal tunnel syndrome. C.O.R.R. 83:41-47, 1972.

44. Lanz U: Anatomical variations of the median nerve in the carpal tunnel. J Hand Surg 2:44-53, 1977.

45. Leslie BM, Ruby LK: Congenital carpal tunnel syndrome: A case report. Orthopedics 8(9):1165-1167, 1985.

46. Lewis MH: Median nerve decompression after Colles's fracture. J Bone Joint Surg 60B(2):195-196, 1978.

47. Lipscomb PR: Carpal tunnel syndrome: Guide to office diagnosis. J Musculoskeletal Med Aug. 1984.

48. Lipscomb PR: Tenosynovitis of the hand and the wrist: Carpal tunnel syndrome, de Quervain's disease, trigger digit. Clin Orthop 13:164-181, 1959.

49. MacDonald RI, Lichtman DM, Hanlon JJ, Wilson JN: Complications of surgical release for carpal tunnel syndrome. J Hand Surg 3(1):70-76, 1978.

50. Marin EL, Vernick S, Friedman LW: Carpal tunnel syndrome: Median nerve stress test. Arch Phys Med Rehabil 64:206-208, 1983.
51. Maesear VR, Hayes JM, Hyde AG: An Industrial Cause of Carpal Tunnel Syndrome. J Hand Surg 11A(2):222-227, 1986.
52. McClain EJ, Wissinger HA: The acute carpal tunnel syndrome: Nine case reports. J Trauma 16(1):75-78, 1976.
53. Nissenbaum M: Treatment consideration in carpal tunnel syndrome with coexistent Dupuytren's disease. J Hand Surg 5:544-547, 1980.
54. Osterman AL: Causes of failure in carpal tunnel surgery. Fifty-third Annual Meetinng of the American Academy of Orthopaedic Surgery, 1986.
55. Paley D, McMurtry RY: Median nerve compression test in carpal tunnel syndrome diagnosis: Reproduces signs and symptoms in affected wrist. Orthop Rev 14(7):41-45, 1985.
56. Phalen GS: The carpal tunnel syndrome: Clinical evaluation of 598 hands. C.O.R.R. 83:29-40, 1972.
57. Phalen GS: The carpal tunnel syndrome: Seventeen years' experience in diagnosis and treatment of six hundred fifty-four hands. J Bone Joint Surg 48A(2):211-228, 1966.
58. Purnell DC, Daly DD, Lipscomb PR: Carpal Tunnel Syndrome Associated with Myxedema. Arch Intern Med 108:751-756, 1961.
59. Rayan GM: Persistent median artery and compression neuropathy. Orthop Rev 15(4):89-92, 1986.
60. Rhoades CE, Gelberman RH, Szabo RM, Botte M: The results of carpal tunnel release with and without internal neurolysis of the median nerve for severe carpal tunnel syndrome. Orthop Trans 10:206, 1986.
61. Robbins H: Anatomical study of the median nerve in the carpal tunnel and etiologies of the carpal tunnel syndrome. J Bone Joint Surg 45A(5):953-966, 1963.
62. Rydevick B, Lundborg GN: The effects of graded compression on intraneural blood flow: An in vivo study on rabbit tibial nerve. J Hand Surg 6:3-12, 1981.
63. Schlesinger EB, Liss HR: Fundamentals, fads and fallacies in the carpal tunnel syndrome. Am J Surg 97:466-470, 1959.
64. Schwarz A, Keller F, Seyfert S, Poll W, Molzahn M, Distler A: Carpal tunnel syndrome: A major complications in long-term hemodialysis patients. Clin Nephrol 22(3):133-137, 1984.
65. Silver MA, Gelberman RH, Gellman H, Rhoades CE: Carpal tunnel syndrome: Associated abnormalities in ulnar nerve function and the effect of carpal tunnel release on these abnormalities. J Hand Surg 10A(5):710-713, 1985.
66. Sunderland S: The nerve lesion in the carpal tunnel syndrome. J Neurol Neurosurg Psychiatry 39:615-626, 1976.
67. Szabo RM, Gelberman RH, Dimick MP: Sensibility testing in patients with carpal tunnel syndrome. J Bone Joint Surg 66A(1):60-64, 1984.
68. Szabo RM, et al.: Vibratory sensory testing in acute peripheral nerve compression. J Hand Surg 9:104-109, 1984.
69. Tanzer RC: The carpal tunnel syndrome: A clinical and anatomical study. J Bone Joint Surg 41A(4):626-634, 1959.
70. Teitz CC, DeLisa JA, Halter SK: Results of carpal tunnel release in renal hemodialysis patients. C.O.R.R. 198:197-200, 1985.
71. Weiland AJ, Lister GD, Villarreal-Rios A: Volar fracture dislocations of the second and third carpometacarpal joints associated with acute carpal tunnel syndrome. J Trauma 16(8):672-675, 1976.

72. Werner C, Elmqvist D, Ohlin Per. Pressure and nerve lesion in the carpal tunnel. Acta Orthop Scand 54:312-316, 1983.
73. Wertsch JJ, Melvin J: Median nerve anatomy and entrapment syndromes: A review. Arch Phys Med Rehabil 63:623-627, 1982.
74. Yamaguchi DM, Lipscomb PR, Soule EH: Carpal Tunnel Syndrome. Minn Med 48:22-33, 1965.

CHAPTER 7

Ulnar Nerve Compression at the Wrist

Michael J. Botte, M.D.
and Richard H. Gelberman, M.D.

The anatomic space of Guyon was described in 1861.[24] Fifty years later, compression of the ulnar nerve within this space was reported.[29] The term "ulnar tunnel syndrome" was introduced by Dupont in 1965 and subsequently became the accepted term to describe this condition.[13,37] The characteristic features include pain in the wrist with numbness, tingling, burning, or pain radiating to the ring and little fingers. The pain and numbness are intensified at night and accentuated by tapping over the ulnar nerve at the wrist or by sustained hyperflexion or hyperextension of the wrist. Intrinsic weakness occurs with possible wasting of the ulnar innervated intrinsic muscles of the hand. Multiple causes of compression, both intrinsic and extrinsic to the space of Guyon, have been reported. This chapter will review the pertinent anatomy, etiology of compression, clinical symptoms, prediction of site of compression, and the methods of management of ulnar nerve compression at the wrist.

Anatomy

Anatomic studies of this region provide an explanation for the predisposition of the ulnar nerve to compression and provide a basis for understanding the various manifestations of the syndrome.[11,16,17,23,27,30,38,42,43] The distal ulnar tunnel is approximately four centimeters long. It originates at the proximal edge of the palmar carpal ligament and extends to the fibrous arch of the hypothenar muscles[23] (Fig. 7-1). The boundaries change from proximal to distal, and four distinct walls are not present throughout the entire course. The roof of the tunnel is composed of the palmar carpal ligament, the palmaris brevis, and hypothenar fat and fibrous tissue. The floor consists of tendons of the flexor digitorum profundus, the transverse carpal ligament, the pisohamate and pisometacarpal ligaments, and the

Figure 7-1. Artist's drawing of the distal ulnar tunnel showing anatomic landmarks. 1 = ulnar nerve, 2 = superficial branch of the ulnar nerve, 3 = hamulus, 4 = fibrous arch of the hypothenar muscles, 5 = pisiform, 6 = transverse carpal ligament, 7 = palmaris brevis, and 8 = palmar carpal ligament. (With permission, Gross MS, Gelberman RH: Anatomy of the distal ulnar tunnel. Clin Orthop 196:238, 1985.)

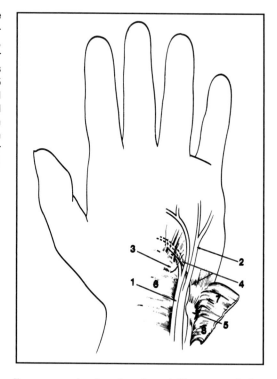

opponens digiti minimi. The flexor carpi ulnaris, the pisiform, and the abductor digiti minimi constitute the medial wall. The tendons of the extrinsic flexors, the transverse carpal ligament, and the hook of the hamate constitute the lateral wall.[23]

The distal ulnar tunnel has been divided in three zones based on topography of the nerve and its relationship to the surrounding structures[23] (Fig. 7-2). An understanding of the anatomic aspects of each zone allows possible prediction or diagnosis of specific sites or types of compression lesions involving the nerve based on presenting clinical symptoms. Zone I consists of the portion of the tunnel proximal to the bifurcation of the nerve. Zone II encompasses the deep motor branch of the nerve and surrounding structures. Zone III includes the superficial branch and adjacent distal and lateral tissues.

Zone I

Zone I extends approximately three centimeters from the proximal edge of the palmar carpal ligament to the bifurcation of the ulnar nerve. The palmar carpal ligament is a thickening of the superficial forearm fascia and becomes distinct approximately two centimeters proximal to the pisiform. The ligament arises ulnarly from the tendon of the flexor carpi ulnaris, and inserts radially on the palmaris longus tendon and the transverse carpal ligament, forming the roof (palmar surface) of the proximal part of Zone I. The ulnar nerve, along with the ulnar artery,

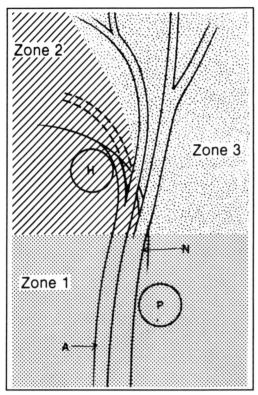

Figure 7-2. Schematic drawing of the distal ulnar tunnel showing the location of the three zones. Zone 1 (coarse stippling), zone 2 (lines), zone 3 (fine stippling). P = pisiform, H = hamulus, A = ulnar artery, N = ulnar nerve. (With permission, Gross MS, Gelberman RH: Anatomy of the distal ulnar tunnel. Clin Orthop 196:238, 1985.)

passes under the palmar carpal ligament to enter the ulnar tunnel. The artery is located slightly superficial and radial to the nerve at this level. The floor (dorsal surface) of Zone I is composed of tendons of the flexor digitorum profundus and the ulnar portion of the transverse carpal ligament. The lateral wall is formed by the most distal fibers of the palmar carpal ligament, which curve radially and posteriorly to wrap around the neurovascular bundle and merge with the fibers of the transverse carpal ligament (Fig. 7-3). The pisiform and tendon of the flexor carpi ulnaris constitute the medial wall of the tunnel at this level.

Distal to the palmar carpal ligament, the roof of the tunnel is comprised of the palmaris brevis muscle. This muscle originates from the distal palmar aspect of the pisiform and the hypothenar muscle fascia and inserts on the ulnar margin of the palmar aponeurosis and the transverse carpal ligament. The length of the palmaris brevis from the proximal to distal border is approximately 2.5 centimeters.

Deep to the palmaris brevis, approximately one centimeter distal to the proximal edge of the pisiform, the ulnar nerve bifurcates into the deep motor branch and the superficial branch of the ulnar nerve. Three to seven millimeters beyond the bifurcation of the nerve, the ulnar artery divides into two branches. The larger of the arterial branches accompanies the

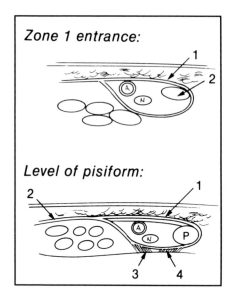

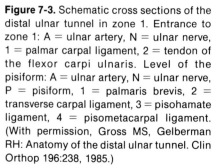

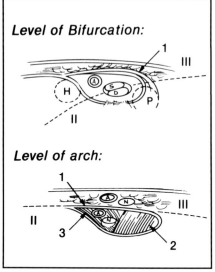

Figure 7-3. Schematic cross sections of the distal ulnar tunnel in zone 1. Entrance to zone 1: A = ulnar artery, N = ulnar nerve, 1 = palmar carpal ligament, 2 = tendon of the flexor carpi ulnaris. Level of the pisiform: A = ulnar artery, N = ulnar nerve, P = pisiform, 1 = palmaris brevis, 2 = transverse carpal ligament, 3 = pisohamate ligament, 4 = pisometacarpal ligament. (With permission, Gross MS, Gelberman RH: Anatomy of the distal ulnar tunnel. Clin Orthop 196:238, 1985.)

Figure 7-4. Schematic cross sections of the distal ulnar tunnel at the proximal and distal ulnar boundaries of zones 2 and 3. Level of the bifurcation of the ulnar nerve: A = ulnar artery, S = superficial branch of the ulnar nerve, D = deep branch of the ulnar nerve, P = pisiform, H = hamulus, II = zone 2, III = zone 3. Level of the fibrous arch of the hypothenar muscles: 1 = fibrous arch of the hypothenar muscles, 2 = abductor digiti minimi, 3 = flexor digiti minimi. In zone II: A = deep branch of the ulnar artery, N = deep branch of the ulnar nerve. In zone III: A = superficial branch of the ulnar artery forming the superficial arch, N = superficial branch of the ulnar nerve. (With permission, Gross MS, Gelberman RH: Anatomy of the distal ulnar tunnel. Clin Orthop 196:238, 1985.)

superficial branch of the nerve and becomes the superficial palmar arch. The smaller arterial branch continues with the motor branch into the deep space of the palm and terminates in the deep palmar arch. Both arteries remain superficial and radial to the nerves they accompany.[23]

The distal extent of Zone I terminates at the level of the bifurcation of the nerve. At this level, the roof of the tunnel is formed by the palmaris brevis and the floor formed by the pisohamate and pisometacarpal ligaments (Fig. 7-4). The pisohamate ligament arises from the distal, radial, and dorsal aspect of the pisiform and inserts on the proximal, ulnar, and palmar aspect of the hook of the hamate. Ulnar to the pisohamate ligament, the pisometacarpal ligament arises from the distal aspect of the pisiform and inserts on the palmar radial aspect of the base of the fifth metacarpal. The divergence of these ligaments leaves an opening in the floor of the tunnel that is filled with fibrofatty tissue overlying the capsule of the triquetro-hamate joint.[23]

In Zone I, the nerve has both motor and sensory fibers. Therefore, a lesion in Zone I will have a high likelihood of producing both motor and sensory deficits. The nerve fibers are arranged in two distinct groups of fascicles. The palmar-radial fibers contain the fascicles that become the superficial branch of the ulnar nerve, while the dorsal-ulnar fibers become the deep motor branch. Thus, in Zone I, the ulnar nerve is actually two nerves contained within a common epineural sheath.[23,31]

Zone II

Zone II surrounds the deep motor branch of the ulnar nerve in the dorsal radial portion of the tunnel (Fig. 7-2). On the palmar medial aspect, this zone is bordered by the palmaris brevis and superficial branch of the nerve (Zone III). Laterally, the transverse carpal ligament forms a wall that merges with the floor of the tunnel. The floor consists of the pisohamate and pisometacarpal ligaments. At the distal extent of Zone II, the fibrous arch of the hypothenar muscles lies palmar to the nerve, the opponens digiti minimi lies posterior, the hook of the hamate and flexor digiti minimi are located laterally, and the abductor digiti minimi lies on the medial aspect. The deep branch passes under the fibrous arch and between the abductor digiti minimi and flexor digiti minimi muscles. It innervates these muscles as it exits the tunnel. The nerve to the abductor digiti minimi is usually given off just proximal to its entrance into these muscles. The motor branch innervates the opponens digiti minimi as it continues radially and posteriorly around the hook of the hamate. The nerve then extends across the palm.[23]

The ulnar artery enters Zone II radially and palmarly, just distal to the level of nerve bifurcation. The artery follows the nerve, lying palmar and slightly radially. Both structures continue distally and pass under the arch of the origin of the hypothenar muscles.

The deep branch of the ulnar nerve in Zone II is purely motor in composition, thus lesions restricted to this zone produce only motor deficits.

Zone III

Zone III originates just distal to the bifurcation of the ulnar nerve (Fig. 7-2). This zone encompasses the superficial branch of the nerve. At the entrance to Zone III, the boundaries are comprised of the palmaris brevis palmarly, the abductor digiti minimi medially, the pisometacarpal ligament and capsule of the triquetro-hamate joint dorsally, and the border of Zone II laterally and dorsally.

As the superficial nerve continues distally, it gives off two small motor branches that innervate the palmaris brevis. Distal to this point, the nerve is purely sensory. It emerges from Zone III by passing over the fibrous arch of the hypothenar muscles. The ulnar artery accompanies the nerve throughout Zone III and remains superficial and radial to it. At the distal extent of the zone, the nerve lies between the hypothenar fascia posteriorly and the artery and a fibrofatty layer deep to the subcutaneous tissues palmarly.

The superficial branch in Zone III contains mostly sensory fibers along with motor fibers to the hypothenar muscles. Lesions in this zone will produce primarily sensory deficits with possible motor weakness of the hypothenar muscles.

The dorsal branch of the ulnar nerve is not a component of Guyon's canal; however, an awareness of the location and path of this nerve is important in distinguishing ulnar nerve compression that may occur proximal to Guyon's canal. The dorsal branch of the ulnar nerve arises from the main trunk of the ulnar nerve beneath the flexor carpi ulnaris in the distal third of the forearm. It carries only sensory fibers and diverges from the ulnar nerve as the two run distally. A few centimeters proximal to the wrist, the dorsal branch courses medially and dorsally, passing beneath the flexor carpi ulnaris to emerge onto the dorsum of the hand. It pierces the deep fascia and divides into two or three digital branches to supply sensation to the dorsal ulnar aspect of the hand, the dorsal proximal aspect of the ring finger, and the dorsal aspect of the little finger.[47] Since this nerve exits the main trunk of the ulnar nerve proximal to the wrist, lesions within Guyon's canal will spare sensation to the dorsal aspect of the ring and little fingers. If sensibility in this distribution is impaired as well, a lesion proximal to Guyon's canal should be suspected.

Etiology of Compression

Multiple causes of ulnar nerve compression in the region of Guyon's canal have been described (Table I). These causes include tumors,[3,5,41,42,44,50,51,53,57,61,70,72] anatomic abnormalities,[8,16,18,21,22,33,40,46,55,56,60,64,66,68] sequelae of rheumatoid or osteoarthritis,[10,35,47,62] vascular lesions,[9,32,36,45,63] and ulnar neuropathy associated with carpal tunnel syndrome.[59] Single reported cases of unusual etiologies of nerve compression include edema secondary to infection,[39] and iatrogenic nerve compression by a malpositioned tendon transfer.[73]

Tumors

Tumors causing ulnar neuropathy in the region of Guyon's canal include ganglia, lipomas, benign giant cell tumors, and desmoid tumors[3,5,34,41,42,44,50,51,53,57,61,70,72] (Table I).

Ganglia are the most common and account for 29 to 45 percent of reported causes of ulnar tunnel syndrome.[5,23,41,44,51,57,58] The onset of symptoms may be insidious, allowing for advanced neuropathy before the patient seeks medical help. Most ganglia arise from the palmar aspect of the carpus and present in Zones I or II.[23,50] The ganglion may arise from the carpal tunnel and subsequently erode or encroach into the space of

Table 7-1. Common Causes of Ulnar Nerve Compression at the Wrist*

Cause	Number
Tumors	
Ganglion	46
Lipoma	3
Giant Cell Tumor	2
Desmoid Tumor	1
Anatomic Abnormalities	
Anomolous Muscles	22
Thickened Ligaments	4
Anomalous Hamulus	3
Trauma	
Fractures	19
Repetitive Trauma	8
Edema Following Burns	10
Other	3
Vascular Pathology	9
Arthritis	
Rheumatoid	4
Degenerative	1
	——
	135

*Based on 135 reported cases. (Refs. 1, 2, 8, 10, 13, 15, 17, 18, 19, 20, 21, 22, 23, 25, 27, 28, 29, 32, 33, 36, 37, 39, 41, 42, 44, 46, 53, 54, 55, 56, 57, 60, 61, 62, 65, 66, 67, 69, 70, 74, 76)

Guyon. The cystic mass may not be palpable, but can often be visualized by CAT or MRI scan.

Lipomas and benign giant cell tumors causing ulnar neuropathy are rare, accounting for 2 and 1 percent, respectively, of reported cases of ulnar tunnel syndrome.[27,44,72] These tumors present as solitary masses in the proximal ulnar palm in conjunction with signs and symptoms consistent with ulnar neuropathy. The giant cell tumor may cause erosions of the hook of the hamate. These erosions can be visualized by carpal tunnel view roentgenograms.[44]

A rare case of an extra-abdominal desmoid tumor of the hand producing an ulnar tunnel syndrome has also been reported.[53]

Anatomic Abnormalities

Anatomic abnormalities causing ulnar nerve compression at the wrist include anomalous muscle bellies,[16,18,21,33,40,46,55,56,60,64,66,68] anomalous or thickened ligaments,[23] and congenital or developmental carpal bone abnormalities[18,22] (Table I). Anomalous muscle bellies are the most common of these abnormalities, accounting for approximately 16 percent of reported cases of ulnar tunnel syndrome. The anomalous muscles consist either of muscles that are normally present but are abnormal in size, shape, or location, or anomalous accessory muscles that are not normally present.[21,56] In both cases, spatial encroachment occurs on the ulnar nerve, from either intrinsic or extrinsic compression. Anomalous muscles causing compression include: the palmaris longus (with an anomalous extension into Guyon's canal),[64] accessory flexor digiti minimi,[55,60] and an accessory abductor digiti minimi.[33,68]

Thickening of the pisohamate ligament may compress the ulnar nerve.[23] This ligamentous band runs from the pisiform to the hook of the hamate anterior to the deep branch of the ulnar nerve in Zone II. The deep branch of the ulnar nerve carries only motor fibers and is vulnerable to compression as it passes under the pisohamate ligament. These lesions present with motor deficits only.

Abnormalities of the size or shape of the hamate have been associated with ulnar tunnel syndrome. The presence of a bipartite hamulus has also been associated with ulnar tunnel syndrome.[18,22]

Trauma

Ulnar tunnel syndrome may occur following fractures or dislocations of the distal forearm or carpus,[1,12,26,28,48,67,69,76] repetitive occupational trauma,[2,25,29,54] thermal burns of the hand and wrist,[19,20] or sustained hyperextension of the wrist[15,47] (Table I).

Fractures or dislocations of the distal radius, ulna, or carpus may result in acute ulnar neuropathy either by direct compression or traction of the nerve from fracture displacement, or by resulting soft tissue swelling and edema. These acute lesions tend to occur in young adults following high-energy trauma with severe, dorsally displaced fractures.[67] A previously intact nerve may be subject to an iatrogenic ulnar tunnel syndrome following fracture reduction from interposition of the nerve between fracture fragments or soft tissue.

Cyclic occupational trauma to the extremity that involves repetitive blows or severe vibratory insults to the extremity (such as with jackhammers or pneumatic drills) may precipitate an ulnar tunnel syndrome[2,25,29,54,74] (Table I). These are more likely to occur if the wrist is used predominantly in a extended position. There may be underlying pathology or predisposing factors that should be investigated before this diagnosis is made. Since many of these types of ulnar neuropathy respond by nonsurgical methods, the actual incidence of this condition is probably higher than that reported.

Thermal burns to the region of the wrist may precipitate soft tissue swelling and edema that result in ulnar tunnel syndrome. The diagnosis may be difficult because of the overlying pain and muscle weakness from the burns. A high index of suspicion and electromyographic studies will aid in the correct diagnosis[19,20] (Table I).

Prolonged dorsiflexion of the wrist in long distance bicycle riders may produce symptoms of ulnar tunnel syndrome.[15,47]

A rare cause of ulnar tunnel syndrome has been reported that was precipitated by multiple insect bites to the hand. Secondary infection led to soft tissue swelling and resulted in an ulnar nerve compression.[39]

Iatrogenic ulnar tunnel syndrome has occurred following opponensplasty. The flexor digitorum superficialis tendon, transferred subcutaneously through the palm to the thumb, pierced and compressed the ulnar nerve. An anomalous muscle within Guyon's canal was also encountered.[73]

Vascular Pathology

Thrombosis, aneurysm, or false aneurysm of the ulnar artery within Guyon's canal can compress the adjacent ulnar nerve.[9,32,36,63] These account for approximately 9 percent of reported cases of ulnar tunnel syndrome.

Arthritis

Patients with rheumatoid arthritis are at risk for ulnar tunnel syndrome from compression by edema, excess tenosynovium, synovial cysts, and carpal deformity. These account for approximately 3 percent of the reported cases of ulnar tunnel syndrome. Tenosynovitis of the flexor carpi ulnaris and the flexor digitorum superficialis can cause ulnar tunnel syndrome.[10,62] Rheumatoid synovial cysts arising from the proximal edge of Guyon's canal can compress the ulnar nerve.[10] Osteoarthritis of the pisiform-triquetral joint may cause ulnar neuropathy.[35]

Associated and Carpal Tunnel Syndrome

Signs or symptoms consistent with ulnar nerve compression at the wrist have been shown to occur in 34 percent of patients with concommitant carpal tunnel syndrome.[59] These findings may be caused by (1) an antomic abnormality in osseous or soft tissue structures that simultaneously causes narrowing of both canals, (2) the possibility that a significant proportion of these patients have an underlying subclinical neuropathy that predisposes them to entrapment neuropathies, or (3) the existence of a hereditary susceptibility to peripheral nerve pressure palsies.

Clinical Symptoms and Prediction of Site of Compression

Clinical symptoms and signs associated with ulnar nerve compression at the wrist region include pain at the wrist that radiates to the little and ring fingers; numbness, burning and tingling of the little and ring fingers (palmar aspect); and weakness and possible wasting of the ulnar innervated intrinsic muscles of the hand (hypothenar muscles, palmar and dorsal interosseus, lumbricals to the ring and little fingers, and the adductor pollicis). The symptoms are usually worse at night and exacerbated with placement of the wrist in marked dorsiflexion or palmar flexion. Longstanding compression may lead to clawing of the digits (hyperextension of the metacarpophalangeal joints and flexion of the proximal interphalangeal joints) due to loss of intrinsic muscle function. Weakness of the adductor pollicis will be evident by a positive Froment's sign (flexion of the interphalangeal joint of the thumb on attempt to key pinch as the flexor pollicis longus muscle substitutes for the weak adductor).

Depending on the specific site of nerve compression, differences in clinical presentation may occur. These subtleties in presentation will give evidence to the location of nerve compression and may allow preoperative prediction of the involved zone. The following sites of nerve compression may exist:

Proximal to the dorsal sensory branch: A patient who presents with numbness or paresthesias on the *dorsum* of the ring and little fingers along with palmar numbness and paresthesias of these digits and intrinsic muscle weakness may have nerve compression at or proximal to the point of exit of the dorsal sensory branch in the forearm (assuming two separate lesions are not present).

Distal to the dorsal sensory branch or within Zone I: These patients will usually present with numbness and paresthesias on the palmar aspect of the ring and little fingers along with weakness of the ulnar innervated intrinsic muscles. In Zone I the nerve contains both motor and sensory fibers. However, the motor fibers are located posteriorly within the nerve and the sensory fibers located in the palmar aspect. Early or mild compression lesions in this area that arise from the dorsal surface of the tunnel may compress only the motor fibers, while superficial lesions may initially compress only the sensory fibers. Usually, however, lesions in this area will present with both motor and sensory impairment (Table II).

Zone II: In Zone II, which is distal to the bifurcation of the ulnar nerve, the nerve contains only motor fibers. Patients with lesions restricted to this zone present with motor impairment only (Table II). A compression

Table 7-2. Distribution of Cases by Zone and Deficit

Zone	Deficit			Total
	M/S	M	S	
1	39	1	7	47
2		36		36
3			10	
Total (complete data)	39	37	17	93
Incomplete data				49
Total				142

M/S = both motor and sensory deficits. M = motor deficit only. S = sensory deficit only.

(By permission, Gross, M.S., Gelberman, R.H.: Anatomy of the Distal Ulnar Tunnel. Clin. Orthop. 196:238-247, 1985)

lesion at the most distal aspect of Zone II, however, may spare the hypothenar muscles because their innervation arises proximal to the most distal aspect of this zone.

Zone III: In Zone III, which is distal to the bifurcation of the ulnar nerve, the nerve contains predominantly sensory fibers (with the exception of the motor fibers to the palmaris brevis muscle). Patients with lesions in this zone will present with sensory impairment to the palmar aspect of the little and ulnar half of the ring finger. Motor function will be preserved (Table II).

Patient Evaluation

A thorough patient history should investigate past occurrences of trauma, repetitive or occupational related activities, and past diagnoses of inflammatory conditions such as rheumatoid arthritis or osteoarthritis. The nature, extent, location, pattern of involvement, and exacerbating factors of the symptoms are important. Associated carpal tunnel syndrome should be noted. A past history of medical illness that can lead to peripheral neuropathy may require further investigation.

Physical examination includes investigation for areas of tenderness, presence and nature of masses, soft tissue swelling, bruits, pulsitile lesions, evidence of previous trauma (puncture wound scars), or wrist deformity. Motor and sensory investigation includes manual muscle testing of the intrinsic muscles, and Semmes-Weinstein monofilament and two-point sensory discrimination. Nerve percussion and Phalen's tests should be performed. Patency of the ulnar artery can be assessed with the Allen's test. The cubital tunnel regions should be examined to rule out tenderness, masses, positive nerve percussion sign, or deformity indicative of a more proximal lesion.

Laboratory investigation includes screening tests to rule out inflammatory conditions or metabolic causes of neuropathy.

Radiographs should include standard anteroposterior, lateral, and oblique views as well as the carpal tunnel view. The carpal tunnel view is useful for identification of erosions, fractures, or congenital pathology of the hook of the hamate. Computerized axial tomography and magnetic resonance imaging of the wrist are useful in identification and evaluation of tumors, fractures, congenital abnormalities, or vascular pathology.

Electromyography and nerve conduction velocity studies will confirm the diagnosis.[14] Sparing of only sensory or only motor fibers may aid in locating the site of compression within Guyon's canal (Zone II or III, respectively).

Treatment

The method of treatment depends on the etiology and duration of the neuropathy. Most chronic or mild cases may be approached with an initial trial of conservative treatment (cessation of any implicated activity, administration of anti-inflammatory medication, and short-term immobilization of the wrist). Severe or refractory cases require surgical decompression and correction or removal of the offending cause.[6,17,65,67,68]

When a tumor or mass is responsible for nerve compression, the treatment is decompression of Guyon's canal and excision of the tumor. In most cases, a ganglion will be found to be responsible. Giant cell tumors or lipomas should be similarly excised.

Nerve compression by anomalous muscles or hypertrophied ligaments require decompression of Guyon's canal and excision of offending muscle or ligament. The diagnosis is often delayed until surgical exploration is carried out.

In chronic cases where repetitive trauma or occupational factors appear responsible, a trial of conservative management is indicated. This includes removal or adjustment of the implicated activity, splinting of the wrist in a neutral position, oral nonsteroidal anti-inflammatory medication, and possible steroid injection into Guyon's canal. Surgical decompression of Guyon's canal is indicated for refractory cases or those who show initial severe neural compromise (those with intrinsic muscle wasting or those with severe electromyographic changes).

Acute ulnar nerve compression following fractures requires prompt fracture reduction and stabilization. Restrictive bandages should be avoided. If nerve function does not improve within a few hours following fracture reduction, surgical decompression of Guyon's canal is indicated. If the function of a previously intact nerve deteriorates following fracture or reduction, nerve interposition into the fracture may have occurred, and prompt surgical exploration should be carried out.

Neuropathy caused by edema from infection or burns requires surgical decompression and proper wound and infection care.

In patients with rheumatoid arthritis, ulnar neuropathy caused by soft tissue swelling, synovitis, or tenosynovitis may be initially treated conservatively. Refractory or severe cases should be treated with decompression and synovectomy or tenosynovectomy.

Osteophytes protruding into Guyon's canal from osteoarthritis may require excision if refractory to conservative care.

Vascular lesions associated with ulnar nerve compression require excision of the aneurysm or thrombosis and possible repair with vein grafting. Assessment of collateral flow through the radial artery should be made preoperatively.

Ulnar nerve compression at the wrist associated with carpal tunnel syndrome often resolves following carpal tunnel release.[59] The routine release of Guyon's canal in these patients is probably not warranted.

Technique of decompression of the ulnar nerve at the wrist: The hook of the hamate, pisiform, and distal aspect of the flexor carpi ulnaris provide palpable landmarks for placement of the incision over Guyon's canal. A six centimeter zig zag incision is placed over the canal, extending one centimeter into the forearm and five centimeters into the ulnar aspect of the palm. The incision should avoid crossing the wrist crease at right angles.

The tendon of the flexor carpi ulnaris is retracted ulnarly to expose the ulnar nerve and artery. The artery will be located slightly radial to the nerve (Fig. 7-1). The nerve and artery are traced distally to where they enter Guyon's canal under the palmar carpal ligament. The palmar carpal ligament, the palmaris brevis muscle, and hypothenar fat and fibrous tissue are incised to decompress the nerve along the course of the canal. An exploration of the floor, walls, and contents of the canal should be performed to identify any offending masses, muscles, ligaments, osteophytes, protruding fracture or nonunited fragments, or excess tenosynovium. The ulnar artery is examined for vascular pathology. The palmar carpal ligament is not repaired. The skin is closed and a bulky hand dressing applied.

The results following surgery are related to the time and severity of compression. In most cases, pain is resolved a few weeks following surgery, and sensibility and motor function improve over a four- to twelve-month period.[10,13,47,55,67] Severe long-standing compression may result in permanent neuropathy. Reconstruction of intrinsic function can be performed using tendon transfers; however, these are rarely required or indicated following compression lesions in the ulnar tunnel.[4,6,7,49,52,71,75] In many cases of occupation-related symptoms, the symptoms resolve following adjustment of activity.

Proper management of ulnar nerve compression at the wrist is dependent on a knowledge of the anatomic aspects of the region, thorough physical and laboratory assessment of the presenting signs and symptoms, and a treatment regimen based on severity, duration, and probable etiology of the compression.

References

1. Baird DB, Predenberg ZB: Delayed ulnar nerve palsy following a fracture of the hamate. J Bone Joint Surg (Am) 50:570, 1968.
2. Bakke JL, Wolff HG: Occupational pressure neuritis of the deep palmar branch of the ulnar nerve. Arch Neurol Psychiatry 60:549, 1948.
3. Bayer WL, Shea JD, Curiel DC et al.: Excision of a pseudocyst of the hand in a hemophiliac (PTC-deficiency). Use of a plasma thromboplastin component concentrate. J Bone Joint Surg 51:1423, 1969.
4. Brand RW: Tendon transfers for median and ulnar nerve paralysis. Orthop Clin North Am 2:447, 1973.
5. Brooks DM: Nerve compression by simple ganglia. J Bone Joint Surg (Br) 34:391, 1952.
6. Brown PW: Reconstruction for pinch in ulnar intrinsic palsy. Orthop Clin North Am 2:323, 1974.
7. Bunnell S: Tendon transfers in the hand and forearm. *In* JW Edwards (Ed): American Academy of Orthopaedic Surgeons, Instructional Course Lecturers, vol. 6. Ann Arbor, MI, 1949.
8. Comtet JJ, Quicot L, Moyen B: Compression of the deep palmar branch of the ulnar nerve by the arch of the adductor pollicis. Hand 10:176, 1978.
9. Costigan DG, Riley JM, Coy FE: Thrombofibrosis of the ulnar artery in the palm. J Bone Joint Surg (Am) 41:702, 1959.

10. Dell PC: Compression of the ulnar nerve at the wrist secondary to a rheumatoid synovial cyst: case report and review of the literature. J Hand Surg 4:468, 1979.
11. Denman EE: The anatomy of the space of Guyon. Hand 10:69, 1978.
12. Dunn WA: Fractures and dislocations of the carpus. Surg Clin North Am 52:1513, 1972.
13. Dupont C, Cloutier GE, Prevost Y et al.: Ulnar-tunnel syndrome at the wrist. J Bone Joint Surg (Am) 42:757, 1965.
14. Ebeling P, Gilliatt RW, Thomas DK: A clinical and electrical study of ulnar nerve lesions in the hand. J Neurol Neurosurg Psychiatry 23:1, 1960.
15. Eckman PB, Perstein G, Altrocchi PH: Ulnar neuropathy in bicycle riders. Arch Neurol 32:130, 1975.
16. Fahrer M: The proximal end of the palmar aponeurosis. Hand 12:33, 1980.
17. Fahrer M, Millroy PJ: Ulnar compression neuropathy due to an anomalous abductor digiti minimi: clinical and anatomic study. J Hand Surg 6:266, 1981.
18. Fennay JB: Deep ulnar nerve paralysis resulting from an anatomical abnormality. J Bone Joint Surg (Am) 47:1381, 1965.
19. Fissette J, Onkelinx A, Fandi N: Carpal and Guyon tunnel syndrome in burns at the wrist. J Hand Surg 6:13, 1981.
20. Frank DH, Robson MD: Unusual occurrence of chronic nerve compression syndromes at the wrists of thermally injured patients. Orthop Rev 8:180, 1979.
21. Gloobe H, Pecket P: An anomalous muscle in the canal of Guyon. Anat Anz 133:477, 1973.
22. Greene MH, Hadied AM: Bipartite hamulus with ulnar tunnel syndrome—case report and literature review. J Hand Surg 6:605, 1981.
23. Gross MS, Gelberman RH: The anatomy of the distal ulnar tunnel. Clin Orthop 196:238, 1985.
24. Guyon F: Note sur une disposition anatomique propre a la face anterieure de la region du poignet et non encore decrite par le docteur. Bull Soc Anat Paris 6:184, 1861.
25. Harris W: Occupational pressure neuritis of the deep palmar branch of the ulnar nerve. Br Med J 1:98, 1921.
26. Hart UL: Two unusual injuries of the wrist. J Bone Joint Surg 23:948, 1941.
27. Hayes JR, Mulholland RC, O'Connor BT: Compression of the deep palmar branch of the ulnar nerve. J Bone Joint Surg (Br) 51:469, 1969.
28. Howard FM: Ulnar nerve palsy in wrist fractures. J Bone Joint Surg (Am) 43:1197, 1961.
29. Hunt JR: Occupational neuritis of the deep palmar branch of the ulnar nerve. J Nerv Ment Dis 35:676, 1908.
30. Hunt JR: Thenar and hypothenar types of neural atrophy of the hand. Br Med J 2:642, 1930.
31. Jabaley ME, Wallace WH, Heckler FR: Internal topography of major nerves of the forearm and hand: a current view. J Hand Surg 5:1, 1980.
32. Jackson JP: Traumatic thrombosis of the ulnar artery in the palm. J Bone Joint Surg (Br) 36:438, 1954.
33. Jeffery AK: Compression of the deep palmar branch of the ulnar nerve by an anomalous muscle. J Bone Joint Surg (Br) 53:718, 1971.
34. Jenkins SA: Solitary tumors of peripheral nerve trunks. J Bone Joint Surg (Br) 34:401, 1952.
35. Jenkins SA: Osteoarthritis of the pisiform-triquetral joint. J Bone Joint Surg (Br) 33:532, 1957.

36. Kalisman M, Laborde K, Wolff TW: Ulnar nerve compression secondary to ulnar artery false aneurysm at the Guyon's canal. J Hand Surg 7:137, 1982.

37. Kleinert HE, Hayes JW: Ulnar tunnel syndrome. Plast Reconstr Surg.47:21, 1971.

38. Lassa R, Shrewsbury MM: A variation of the path of the deep branch of the ulnar nerve at the wrist. J Bone Joint Surg 57A:990, 1975.

39. Leslie IJ: Compression of the deep branch of the ulnar nerve due to edema of the hand. Hand 12:271, 1980.

40. Lipscomb PR: Duplication of hypothenar muscles simulating soft tissue tumor of the hand. Report of a case. J Bone Joint Surg 42:1058, 1960.

41. Mallet BL, Zilkha KJ: Compression of the ulnar nerve at the wrist by a ganglion. Lancet 268:8901, 1955.

42. McFarland GB, Hoffer MM: Paralysis of the intrinsic muscles of the hand secondary to lipoma in Guyon's tunnel. J Bone Joint Surg 53:375, 1971.

43. McFarland RM, Mayer JR, Hugill JV: Further observations on the anatomy of the ulnar nerve at the wrist. Hand 8:115, 1976.

44. Milberg P, Kleinert HE: Giant cell tumor compression of the deep branch of the ulnar nerve. Ann Plast Surg 4:426, 1980.

45. Millender LH, Nalebuff E, Kasdon E: Aneurysms and thromboses of the ulnar artery in the hand. Arch Surg 105:686, 1972.

46. Muller LH: Anatomical abnormalities at the wrist joint causing neurological symptoms in the hand. J Bone Joint Surg (Br) 45:431, 1963.

47. Nakano KK: The entrapment neuropathies. Muscle Nerve 1:264, 1978.

48. Nisenfield FG, Neviaser RJ: Fracture of the hook of the hamate: a diagnosis easily missed. J Trauma 14:612, 1974.

49. Omer GE Jr: Tendon transfers in combined nerve lesions. Orthop Clin North Am 2:377, 1974.

50. Packer NP, Fisk GR: Compression of the distal ulnar nerve with clawing of the index finger. HJand 14:38, 1982.

51. Richmond DA: Carpal ganglion with ulnar nerve compression. J Bone Joint Surg (Br) 45:513, 1963.

52. Riordan DC: Tendon transplantations in median nerve and ulnar nerve paralysis. J Bone Joint Surg (Am) 35:312, 1953.

53. Ritter MA, Marshall JL, Straub LR: Extra-abdominal desmoid of the hand. A case report. J Bone Joint Surg 51:1641, 1969.

54. Russell WR, Whitty CWM: Traumatic neuritis of the deep palmar branch of the ulnar nerve. Lancet 1:828, 1947.

55. Salgeback S: Ulnar tunnel syndrome caused by anomalous muscles. A case report. Scand J Plast Reconstr Surg 11:255, 1977.

56. Schjelderup H: Aberrant muscle in the hand causing ulnar nerve compression. J Bone Joint Surg (Br) 46:361, 1964.

57. Seddon HJ: Carpal ganglion as a cause of paralysis of the deep branch of the ulnar nerve. J Bone Joint Surg (Br) 34:386, 1952.

58. Shea JD, McClain EJ: Ulnar nerve compression syndromes at and below the wrist. J Bone Joint Surg (Am) 51:1095, 1969.

59. Silver MA, Gelberman RH, Gellman H et al.: Carpal tunnel syndromme: associated abnormalities in ulnar nerve function and the effect of carpal tunnel release on these abnormmalities. J Hand Surg 10A:710, 1985.

60. Swanson AB, Biddulph SL, Baughman FA et al.: Ulnar nerve compression due to an anomalous muscle in the canal of Guyon. Clin Orthop 83:64, 1972.

61. Tashima Y, Kimata Y: A case of ganglion causing paralysis of intrinsic muscles innervated by the ulnar nerve. J Bone Joint Surg (Br) 43:153, 1961.
62. Taylor AR: Ulnar nerve compression at the wrist in rheumatoid arthritis. J Bone Joint Surg (Br) 56:142, 1974.
63. Teece LG: Thrombosis of the ulnar artery. Aust NZ J Surg 19:156, 1949.
64. Thomas CG: Clinical manifestations of an accessory palmaris muscle. J Bone Joint Surg (Am) 40:929, 1958.
65. Thomsen PB: Compression neuritis of the ulnar nerve treated with simple decompression. Acta Orthop Scand 48:164, 1977.
66. Turner MS, Caird DM: Anomalous muscles and ulnar nerve compression at the wrist. Hand 9:140, 1977.
67. Vance RM, Gelberman RH: Acute ulnar neuropathy with fractures at the wrist. J Bone Joint Surg (Am) 60:692, 1978.
68. Vanderpool DW, Chalmers J, Whiston TB: Peripheral compression lesions of the ulnar nerve. J Bone Joint Surg.
69. Watson-Jones R: Carpal semilunar dislocations and other wrist dislocations with associated nerve lesions. Proc R Soc Med 22:1071, 1929.
70. White NB: Neurilemomas of the extremities. J Bone Joint Surg (Am) 49:1605, 1967.
71. White WL: Restoration of function and balance of the wrist and hand by tendon transfer. Surg Clin North Am 40:427, 1960.
72. White WL, Hauna DC: Troublesome lipomata of the upper extremity. J Bone Joint Surg (Am) 44:1353, 1962.
73. Wood VE: Nerve compression following opponensplasty as a result of wrist anomalies: report of a case. J Hand Surg 5:279, 1980.
74. Worster-Drought C: Pressure neuritis of the deep palmar branch of the ulnar nerve. Br Med J 1:247, 1929.
75. Zancolli EA: Claw hand caused by paralysis of the intrinsic muscles: a simple surgical procedure for its correction. J Bone Joint Surg (Am) 39:1076, 1957.
76. Zoega H: Fracture of the lower end of the radius with ulnar nerve palsy. J Bone Joint Surg (Br) 48:514, 1966.

CHAPTER 8

Median Nerve Compression In The Forearm: The Pronator Tunnel Syndrome

Richard K. Johnson, M.D.
and Morton Spinner, M.D.

Complaints of paresthesia and numbness in the thumb, index, and middle fingers can arise from any of five levels in the upper extremity. These most commonly are in the neck, thoracic outlet, upper arm, pronator tunnel, and carpal tunnel levels. Of these, the most commonly overlooked is the pronator tunnel.

In 1977, the authors presented their results of 54 operative cases of median nerve compression at the pronator tunnel level. Since that time, Johnson has added 34 operative decompressions at that level and Spinner has added 15, a total of 103 cases. Further observations on the clinical presentation of median nerve compression in the forearm and operative findings have been collected, and perhaps a clearer picture can be derived at this time in order to differentiate the entity from other compression neuropathies.[1,3,5,7-12,16,17,19,20-25]

Observations

Since our initial study, the same clinical pattern has been observed with female patients predominating in a ratio of roughly 4:1. The mean age is between 40 and 45 years.

The clinical pattern is that generally associated with compression of the median nerve, including paresthesias and numbness in the thumb, index, middle, and radial one-half of the ring fingers; pain and a feeling of fullness in the proximal forearm on the palmar surface, which is increased by

Continued page 140

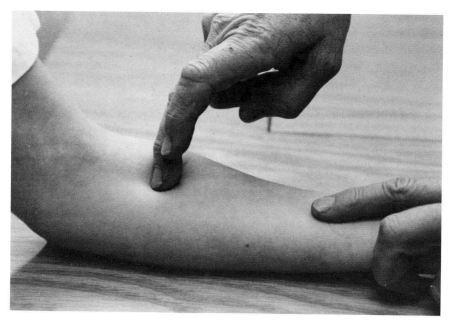

Figure 8-1. Percussion over pronator teres muscle for tinel sign.

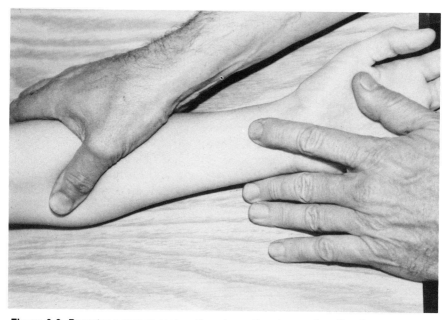

Figure 8-2. Pronator pressure test — Examiners thumb pressing directly over pronator teres muscle and median nerve.

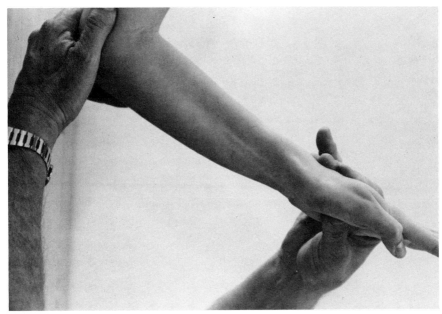

Figure 8-3A. Pronator stress test — patient is pronating forcefully as examiner attempts to supinate the forearm.

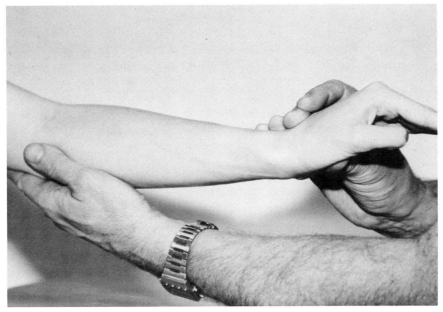

Figure 8-3B. Pronator stress test — continuated pronation against resistance as elbow is extended.

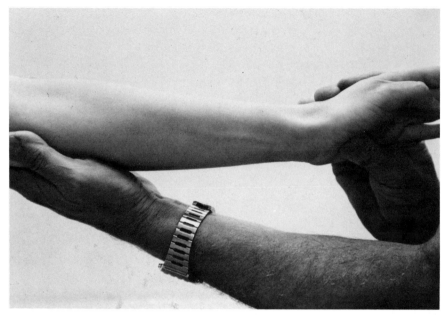

Figure 8-3C. Pronator stress test — continued pronation against resistance and elbow now fully extended.

resistance to pronation; occasional radiation of pain into the axilla, neck, and subscapular region; and frequently, a subjective feeling of weakness of grip in the affected forearm and hand.

Physical findings are varied, and while few of the patients have had all of the following findings, establishment of the diagnosis has been based on having a clear majority present. These generally are as follows:

1. Tenderness, firmness, and sometimes measurable fusiform enlargement of the pronator teres muscle.
2. Tingling and parasthesias reproduced on percussion in the region of the pronator tunnel over the distal margin of the pronator teres muscle (Fig. 8-1).
3. *No* weakness of the median nerve innervated intrinsic or extrinsic muscles.
4. Marked increase in paresthesia in the radial three and one-half fingers of the hand after mild compression of the proximal muscle mass of the pronator teres (Fig. 8-2).
5. Increase in paresthesias or reproduction of paresthesias in the affected digits after pronation of the flexed forearm against resistance, and further increase in paresthesia and discomfort in the forearm when the elbow is gradually extended (Fig. 8-3).
6. Reproduction of paresthesias by flexion of the elbow with supination of the forearm against resistance to test specifically for encroachment by the lacertus fibrosis (Fig. 8-4).

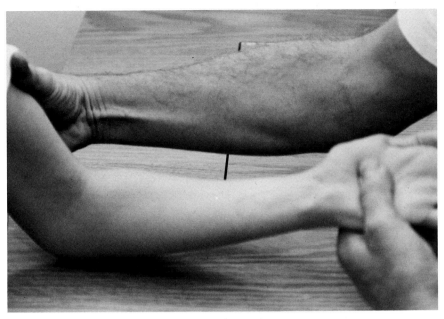

Figure 8-4. Lacertus test — Elbow flexed and patient supinating against resistance of examiner.

7. Reproduction or increase in paresthesias in the radial three and one-half fingers with independent flexion of the flexor superficialis of the middle finger or ring finger, which is an indication of a localized area of compression at the fibrous arcade of the flexor superficialis.

8. Reproduction of symptoms by placement of a tourniquet on the upper arm inflated to above diastolic pressure and with reproduction of numbness and tingling.

9. Rare conduction defect in the median nerve by electrodiagnostic studies when specifically tested in the area of the pronator, but occasionally seen in the superficialis muscles when specifically tested by electromyographic means.[2,4,14,15,19]

10. An absence of night symptoms in the arm proximal to the site of compression by the pronator teres muscle.

11. Severe muscle cramping and muscle spasms in the forearm, which are associated with repetitious pinching maneuvers, such as writing and, not infrequently, reported by the patient to be "writer's cramp."

Anatomic Relationships

The median nerve passes from the upper arm to the forearm beneath the lacertus fibrosus and then traverses the interval between the humeral and ulnar heads of the pronator teres. The nerve then passes distal beneath the cover of the flexor superficialis musculature. Anatomic variations in this area have been thoroughly described in the past.[6,13,18,24] At the time of our initial study, 40 preserved cadaver specimens were dissected and, in 50 percent of the dissections, there was a structurally distinct but variable fibrous band generally arising from the superficial head of the pronator teres overlying the median nerve. Forty percent of the dissections demonstrated a fibrous band dorsal to the nerve. The fibrous band encountered in these dissections were occasionally a component of the deep ulnar head of the pronator teres muscle when the latter was present, or when the deep head was absent, a separate fibrous structure was occasionally present, which was attached to the coronoid process of the ulna proximally. Only 20 percent of the dissections showed fibrous bands involving the superficial and deep heads of the muscle. In these instances, a definite fibrous arcade was formed which surrounded most of the median nerve in its passage through the muscle. Furthermore, in one-half of the dissections, there was an intramuscular fibrous element within the humeral head of the pronator teres that did not overlie the median nerve, but rather contacted it directly as the nerve passed beneath it.

In 30 percent of the dissections a fibrous acrade was observed at the proximal margin of the flexor superficialis muscle to the middle finger. Twenty percent of the total showed a strong fibrous band belonging to the flexor carpi radialis. Both sets of bands were seen in conjunction with the presence of fibrous elements for both the pronator teres and the flexor superficialis. When viewed together, all three components united proximally and appeared as an intramuscular septum that either surrounded or covered the median nerve in the region. In 25 percent of our observations there were no fibrous bands relating to the passage of the median nerve through the cubital region.

In approximately 90 percent of the dissections, the anterior interosseous nerve separated from the median nerve distal to its passage through the pronator teres muscle. The anterior interosseous nerve accompanied the median nerve through the pronator muscle on the posterior radial aspect of the median nerve and both nerves were sheathed together by epineurium through the pronator tunnel. Branching of the anterior interosseous nerve from the median nerve usually occurred 3 to 10 mm distal to the pronator teres muscle and, in only 10 percent was the anterior interosseous nerve seen to separate from the median nerve within the pronator tunnel. In no instances was there a separation of the two nerves proximal to the pronator teres muscle.

Treatment (Fig. 8-5)

Using the previously stated criteria for diagnosis, attempts were made in all patients with a diagnosis of a pronator tunnel syndrome to effectively treat the condition conservatively. This treatment consisted of anti-inflammatory medication, guarded and graded activity, and immobilization prior to consideration of surgical treatment. In approximately half the treated cases, surgical intervention was not necessary.

Continued page 148

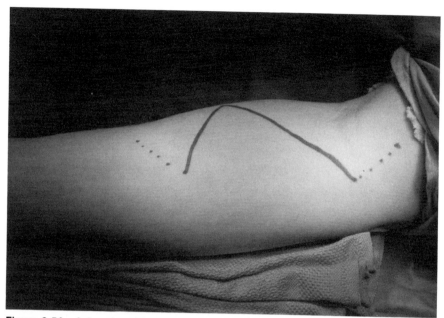

Figure 8-5A—J A series showing operative decompression of the median nerve in the proximal forearm. A) Essential skin incision in solid line and dotted line proximal and distal indicate extensions if necessary.

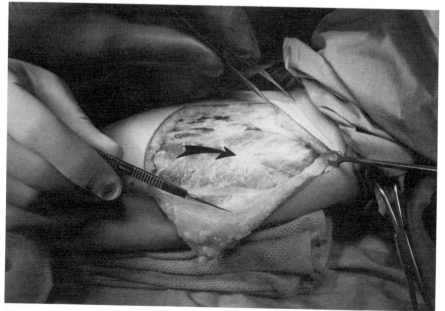

Figure 8-5B. Skin reflected exposing fascia and terminal fibers of laceratus fibrosis. Arrow indicates internal between pronator teres and flexor garpi radialis.

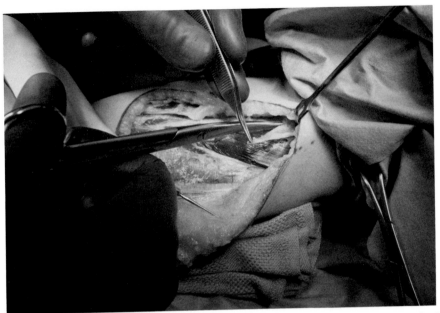

Figure 8-5C. Fascia incised between pronator teres and flexor carpi radialis and terminal portion of Lacertus Fibrosis (in forceps) being resected.

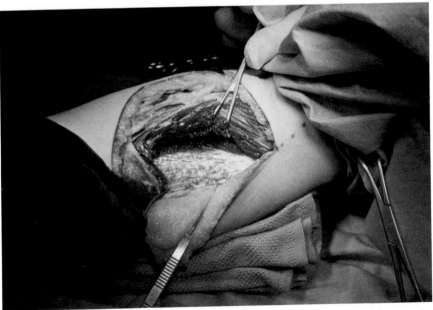

Figure 8-5D. Pronator teres muscle being elevated from facial septum between pronator teres and flexor carpi radialis.

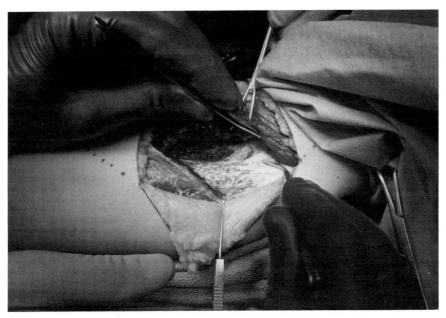

Figure 8-5E. Pronator teres muscle elevated from intermuscular fascia and median nerve (tip of angled probe).

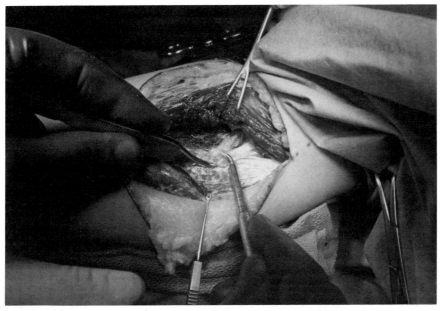

Figure 8-5F. Angled probe beneath abnormal fascial band which arises from intermuscular fascia passes around median nerve and insert into coronoid process of ulna.

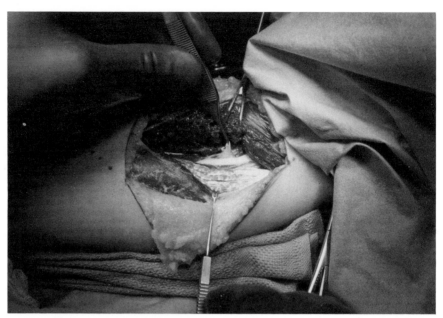

Figure 8-5G. Abnormal band detached from fascia and elevated from median nerve. Note slight irregularity in contour of nerve beneath the band.

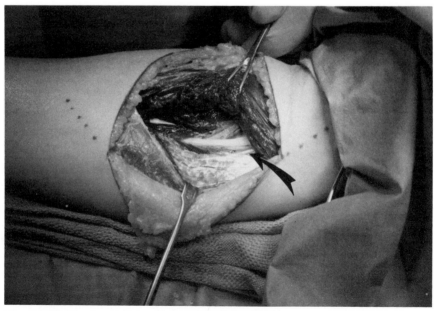

Figure 8-5H. Band resected and nerve free from distal pronator tunnel through superficialis arcade. Note branch to flexor carpi radialis (arrow).

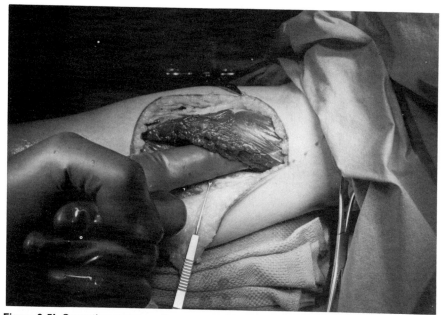

Figure 8-5I. Operating surgeons finger passed through pronator tunnel to complete nerve decompression and to palpate for abnormal intramuscular bands within the pronator teres.

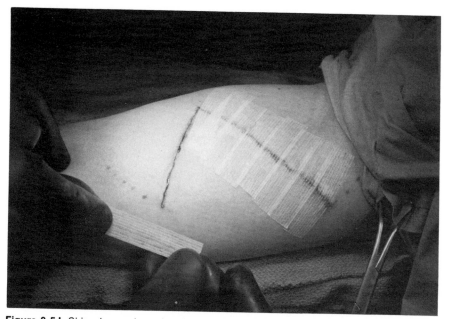

Figure 8-5J. Skin closure by subcuticular suture and steri-tape reinforcement. This has provided most satisfactory post-operative appearance to date.

The median nerve has been explored and decompressed in 103 cases. An incision is made from just proximal to the medial aspect of the antecubital crease, extending distally and radially to the junction of the proximal and middle one-thirds of the forearm. It is then turned ulnarly and distally across the forearm. The flap is elevated from the antebrachial fascia. The medial and lateral cutaneous nerves of the forearm can be exposed and protected in soft tissue slings, or not exposed and left protected in soft tissue. The lacertus fibrosus is easily visualized; its distal insertion into the antebrachial fascia is near the junction of the pronator teres and flexor carpi radialis muscle bellies. After sectioning of the antebrachial fascia and removal of a portion of the lacertus fibrosus distally, the fascial intervals between the pronator teres and flexor carpi radialis can readily be seen. By careful sharp dissection, the muscle belly of the pronator teres is then separated from the fascial plane between the two muscles and, using a careful blunt retracting technique, the pronator teres is then separated from the fascia, preserving the total musculature and readily visualizing the median nerve and the one or more of its branches to the flexor carpi radialis. While several different areas of compression of the nerve had been observed in the region, the most common in the last 40 cases has been a variable size band extending from the fascial interval between the pronator teres and the flexor carpi radialis, which passes about the nerve on the radial side and turns proximally and attaches to the coronoid process of the ulna. In previous dissections in the prior series of operative cases, this is the band that was felt to be arising from the dorsal portion of the pronator teres. Its origin has now been seen clearly to be from the fascial interval between the pronator teres and the flexor carpi radialis. The other sources of nerve compression have been variable, with only two cases accounted for by lacertus fibrosus, three instances of an accessory origin of the flexor carpi radialis from the ulna, and varying degrees of hypertrophy of the pronator teres muscle and vascular anomalies in the area about the median nerve in the region of the pronator teres muscle. Few instances have been seen in recent times with fibrous bands within the muscle mass of the pronator teres. All apparent fibrous bands encountered should be released and, if possible, removed. The pronator tunnel is always enlarged enough to allow the passage of the surgeon's finger proximally through the tunnel to the level of the antecubital space.

Results

Total follow-up time has been from one to thirty years. All patients who have had decompression of the median nerve in the proximal forearm for sensory complaints only have reported relief of the symptoms. The preoperative pain is usually improved immediately following decompression of the nerve, with maximum relief varying from one day to six weeks after the surgery. Physical findings from the original diagnostic criteria were generally absent by the time the sutures were removed.

The resultant scar of this surgical decompression is generally unattractive. Attempts at serpentine incisions or variable types of angular incisions have all produced a cosmetically poor scar, whether they are closed with subcuticular sutures and then bridged with Steri-strip or merely closed in a routine fashion. Probably our best cosmetic results have been in those which were done in an angular fashion and closed with subcuticular sutures and Steri-stripped, leaving the Steri-strips intact for two to three weeks. Postoperative splinting is done long-arm with the elbow at 90° and the wrist in neutral and held for two to three weeks. It must be emphasized that a transverse or longitudinal incision will not provide adequate visualization of the nerve and the associated areas of pathology.

Discussion

Median nerve compression syndrome in the proximal forearm is the least frequently diagnosed median nerve compression neuropathy in the upper extremity. It must carefully be excluded from carpal tunnel syndrome, thoracic outlet syndrome, and cervical radiculopathy. It should be stressed that the syndrome is a condition that almost uniformly occurs while the patient is awake. It is associated with physical activity, especially stressful activity of the forearm and hand. Generally, by careful history and physical examination, it can easily be distinguished from the other three entities. The condition can occur in conjunction with any of the other three and has frequently been seen as a two-level entrapment neuropathy by both the authors. To relieve the patient's complaint it is vital to identify if nerve compression is present at multiple levels: more than one level may then be relieved with one surgery. It is not unusual for us to operate for a pronator tunnel syndrome and carpal tunnel syndrome. Electrical conduction findings and clinical findings localize the double lesion levels. Thoracic outlet and cervical radiculopathy associated with pronator tunnel entrapment often improve with release only of the pronator tunnel entrapment.

Multiple neural entrapments of several peripheral nerves can coexist in the same extremity at one time, or can appear sequentially over several years. These cases have been identified and documented by the authors, and it is felt that in these cases there is probably some underlying predisposition for these multiple neural compression problems. A common pathologic mechanism may be the occurrence of increased intraneural vesicular pressure in these cases from possible multiple etiologies, such as hereditary problems, enzymatic or metabolic irregularities and toxic exposures.

As a solitary entity, median nerve compression in the proximal forearm is generally caused by the presence of fibrous bands and occurs at three distinct levels in the proximal forearm: the pronator teres, the flexor superficialis arch, and the lacertus fibrosus. Along with the clinical findings and the historical pattern, three resistive tests have been found to be helpful in making the diagnosis. These are as follows:

1. Pronation of the forearm against resistance with the elbow flexed and then gradually extended, with pain or paresthesias following, thus localizing the lesion to the pronator teres.
2. Independent flexion of the flexor superficialis of the long finger or ring finger, with reproduction of or increase in pain and paresthesia in the proximal forearm and median nerve supplied area of the hand, indicative of entrapment at the flexor superficialis arcade.
3. Flexion and supination of the elbow against resistance, indicative of entrapment and compression by the lacertus fibrosus.

Finally, it must be constantly borne in mind that the pronator tunnel syndrome is a daytime syndrome, aggravated by increased activity in the forearm and relieved by rest of the forearm and hand.

References

1. Bayerl W, Fischer K: The pronator teres syndrome. Clinical aspects, pathogenesis and therapy of a non-traumatic median nerve compression syndrome in the space of the elbow joint. Handchirurgie, 11(2):91, 1979.
2. Benson YR, de Bissschop G, Lavaivre M, Claparede P, Decaillet JM, Commandre F, Doumoulin J: Diagnostic and therapeutic problems in atypical carpal tunnel syndrome. Electrodiagnostic Therapy 18(2):37, 1981.
3. Bouche P, Travers MA, Saillant G, Laplane D, Cathala HP: The anterior interosseous nerve syndrome. A rare lesion of the median nerve branch in the forearm. A case. Presse Med 12:14(1):31, 1985.
4. Cornwall MW, Nelson C: Median nerve F-wave conduction in healthy subjects. Phys Ther 64(11):1679, 1984.
5. Crotti FM, Manisasalli EP, Rampini P: Supracondyloid process and anomalous insertion of pronator teres as sources of median nerve neuralgia. J Neurosurg Sci 25(1):41, 1981.
6. Crutchfield CA, Gutmann L: Hereditary aspects of median-ulnar nerve communications. J Neurol Neurosurg, Psyuchiatry 43(1):53, 1980.
7. Farrell WF: Pain and the pronator teres syndrome. Bull Hosp Joint Dis 37(1):59, 1976.
8. Flory PJ, Berser A: The accessory brachial tendon—A cause of pronator teres syndrome. Handchir Mikrochir Plast Chir 17(5):270, 1985.
9. Gressini L, Jandolo B, Pietranseli A, Bove L: The Seyffarth syndrome (round pronator syndrome), Considerations on 19 cases. Chir Organi Mov 66(4):481, 1980.
10. Hartz CR, Linschied RL, Gramse RR, Daube JR: The pronator teres syndrome: Compressive neuropathy of the median nerve. J Bone Joint Surg 63A(6):885, 1981.
11. Haussmann P, Kendel K: Olisofascicular median nerve compression syndrome. Handchirurgie 13(3-4):268, 1981.
12. Hill NA, Howard FM, Huffer BR: The incomplete anterior interosseous nerve syndrome. J Hand Surg 31(1):123, 1985.
13. Jabaley ME, Wallace WH, Heckler FR: Internal topography of major nerves of the forearm and hand: A current view. J Hand Surg 5(1):1, 1980.
14. Kimura I, Ayyar DR: The hand neural communication between the ulnar and median nerves: Electrophysiological detection. Electromyosurg Clin Neurophysiol 24(5):409, 1984.

15. Kimura I, Ayyar DR, Lippmann SM: Electrophysiological verification of the ulnar to median nerve communications in the hand and forearm. Tohoku J Exp Med 141(3):269, 1983.
16. Kutz JE, Singer R, Lindsay M: Chronic exertional compartment syndrome of the forearm: A case report. J Hand Surg 10(2):302, 1985.
17. Martinelli P, Gabellini AS, Foppi M, Gasassi R, Pozzati E: Pronator syndrome due to thickened bicipital aponeurosis. Neurol, Neurosurg, Psychiatry 45(2):131, 1982.
18. Matini K: Abnormal distribution of the median nerve at the wrist and forearm. Plast Reconst Surg 71:711, 1983.
19. Morris HH, Peters BH: Pronator syndrome: Clinical and electrophysiological features in seven cases. J Neurol, Neurosurg, Psychiatry 39(5):461, 1976.
20. Morsan RF, Terranova W, Nichter LS, Edserton MT: Entrapment Neuropathies of the upper extremity. Am Fam Physician 31(1):123, 1985.
21. Stern MB: The anterior interosseous nerve syndrome (Kiloh-Nevin syndrome): Report and follow-up of three cases. Clin Orthop (137):223, 1984.
22. Tirrins S, Sommer J: Pronator teres syndrome. Compression of the median nerve in the proximal forearm. Useskr laeser 28:142(18):1152, 1980.
23. Torres J: The clinical significance of the processur supratrochlearis. Handchirurgie 3(1):15, 1971.
24. Wertsch JJ, Melvin J: Median nerve anatomy and entrapment syndrome: A review. Arch Phys Med Rehabil 63(12):623, 1982.
25. Wissins CE: Pronator syndrome. South Med J 75(2):240, 1982.

CHAPTER 9

Anterior Interosseous Nerve Palsy

Larry K. Chidgey, M.D.
Robert M. Szabo, M.D.

Isolated palsy of the anterior interosseous nerve is uncommon, comprising less than 1 percent of all upper extremity peripheral nerve palsies.[28] Paresis or paralysis of the muscles innervated by the anterior interosseous nerve—the flexor pollicis longus, the radial portion of the flexor digitorum profundus, and the pronator quadratus—results in a characteristic pinch deformity with the thumb interphalangeal joint and the index distal interphalangeal joint collapsing into extension (Fig. 9-1).

One of the earliest descriptions of anterior interosseous nerve palsy can be attributed to Parsonage and Turner[31] in 1948. In their review of 136 cases of acute brachial neuritis (neuralgic amyotrophy) they described five patients with weakness of the long flexors of the thumb and index finger occurring in addition to shoulder-girdle weakness. They also described one case of isolated thumb and index finger involvement. It is interesting to note that they felt this isolated case must represent an anterior-horn-cell lesion and not a peripheral nerve lesion. They provided no followup of the case. Kiloh and Nevin,[15] in 1952, first reported isolated involvement of the anterior interosseous nerve with a description of two cases. Both cases were treated conservatively with some recovery beginning after one year but neither recovered fully by the end of followup. They attributed the pathology to "isolated neuritis" of the anterior interosseous nerve. Fearn and Goodfellow[9] were the first to suggest the etiology of mechanical compression that could be treated surgically. They documented a case in which surgical exploration revealed a fibrous band that when cut provided decompression and complete recovery from the paralysis in a relatively short time. Since their report, most authors have regarded spontaneous anterior interosseous nerve palsy as one of the peripheral nerve entrapment syndromes.[34]

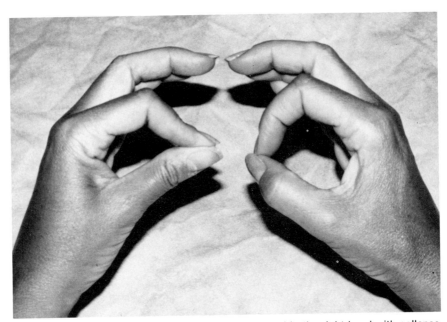

Figure 9-1. Characteristic pinch deformity demonstrated in the right hand with collapse of the thumb interphalangeal and the index distal interphalangeal joints into extension.

Figure 9-2. Anatomy of the anterior interosseous nerve.

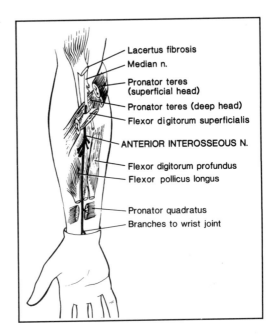

Lacertus fibrosis

Median n.

Pronator teres (superficial head)

Pronator teres (deep head)

Flexor digitorum superficialis

ANTERIOR INTEROSSEOUS N.

Flexor digitorum profundus

Flexor pollicus longus

Pronator quadratus

Branches to wrist joint

Anatomy (Fig. 9-2)

The anterior interosseous nerve arises from the posterior radial surface of the median nerve 2 cm to 8 cm (average 5 cm) below the level of the medial epicondyle.[19,42] This point of origin is usually immediately distal to the proximal border of the superficial head of the pronator teres. The funiculi that form the anterior interosseous nerve can be isolated as a separate bundle within the median nerve for at least 2.4 cm before the bifurcation site.[39] The median and anterior interosseous nerves most commonly course through the two heads of the pronator teres but this is variable; these nerves pass between the superficial and deep heads in 82 percent of cases, beneath the superficial head with an absent deep head in 9 percent of cases, beneath both heads in 7 percent of cases, and through the superficial head in 2 percent of cases.[1] After exiting the pronator teres, the anterior interosseous nerve continues to accompany the median nerve beneath the arcade of the flexor digitorum superficialis origin. About 4 cm distal to its bifurcation from the median nerve, the anterior interosseous nerve gives off a motor branch to the flexor pollicis longus.[34] This motor branch may be single but more commonly divides into two to six branches, which enter the muscle proximally and medially close to the radius.[42] At about the same level from one to six branches arise to supply the radial portion of the flexor digitorum profundus.[42] The flexor digitorum profundus to the index finger is exclusively innervated by the anterior interosseous nerve, but exclusive innervation of the flexor digitorum profundus of the long finger is present only 50 percent of the time.[40,41] In the remaining 50 percent the flexor digitorum profundus of the long finger is at least partially supplied by the ulnar nerve. In rare cases the flexor digitorum profundus may be completely innervated by the anterior interosseous nerve.[35] Sunderland has found a 30 percent incidence of a branch from the anterior interosseous nerve supplying a portion of the flexor digitorum superficialis.[40,41]

After supplying these motor branches the anterior interosseous nerve continues distally between the flexor digitorum profundus and the flexor pollicis longus to accompany the anterior interosseous artery distally on the interosseous membrane. The larger of the two terminal branches supplies the pronator quadratus while the smaller branch continues deep to the pronator quadratus as sensory innervation to the palmer aspect of the radio-carpal and intercarpal joints. The anterior interosseous nerve has no cutaneous sensory component.

Connection between the median and ulnar nerves in the forearm, in the form of a Martin-Gruber anastomosis, can be found in 15 percent of limbs.[43] In 50 percent of the cases the communicating branch from the median nerve originates from the anterior interosseous nerve. Median nerve fibers may therefore supply some of the intrinsic muscles with the first, second, and third dorsal interosseous, the adductor pollicis, and the abductor digiti minimi being the most common ones receiving median nerve innervation.[23,34]

Clinical Presentation

In approximately a third of the cases the patient will present with a history of the insidious onset of proximal forearm pain followed in several hours by the onset of paresis or paralysis of the affected muscles. The pain may radiate distally or proximally to the elbow. The pain may present as isolated elbow pain.[32] In the remaining two-thirds of cases, a careful history will reveal an inciting cause including strenuous or repetitive activity, prolonged pressure on the forearm, or acute trauma.[8,11,16,18,21,32,34,35,37,45] The paresis or paralysis may not be obvious even to the patient unless specifically looked for. There have been reports of patients presenting with a deterioration in their handwriting as their only complaint.[38]

On physical examination there is weakness or absence of flexion of the thumb interphalangeal and index distal interphalangeal joint, with the long finger distal interphalangeal joint variably affected. A characteristic pinch deformity results (Fig. 9-1). Spinner and Schrieber[36] have stated "the attitude in pinch position is as constant as any of the other classical peripheral nerve injuries. It should be kept in mind as representative of a distinct entity." To test the pronator quadratus, Spinner[35] has suggested eliminating the rotary action of the pronator teres on the forearm by fully flexing the elbow. Since the pronator teres usually has two heads, the humeral head can be made ineffective by flexing the elbow so that only about 25 percent of the muscle's pronating strength from the ulnar head remains. In this position, if there is a paralyzed pronator quadratus, there will be very weak resistance to forced supination of the forearm. If the pronator quadratus is intact then resistance to supination will be normal with the elbow either flexed or extended.

Innervation anomalies will add variability to the classic examination findings.[23,34,40,41] There may be some weakness in the flexor digitorum superficialis or some of the intrinsic muscles. These findings may be compatible with an isolated anterior interosseous nerve palsy.

Other findings on physical examination are a positive Tinel's sign over the proximal forearm with radiation distally into the area of the pronator quadratus.[32] Pain may be reproduced with the modified Mills' test.[32] The wrist and fingers are flexed with the forearm hyperpronated. As the elbow is brought from a flexed to an extended position, pain will be reproduced in the proximal forearm.

There are no cutaneous sensory deficits related to anterior interosseous nerve palsy, but the terminal sensory fibers to the palmer wrist joint have been implicated as a source of wrist pain.[6] The cases reported have been related to a hyperextension injury to the wrist causing a traction injury to the nerve.

Electromyographic studies are positive for denervation of the affected muscles in the majority of cases if care is taken to evaluate the individual muscles. Nerve conduction studies are not affected.

The flexor pollicis longus and the flexor digitorum profundus to the index finger are innervated exclusively by the anterior interosseous nerve, so in a complete palsy these muscles are always affected. There has been one reported exception by Sunderland in a rare case where the ulnar nerve supplied the entire flexor digitorum profundus.[41] There have been reported cases presenting with paralysis of only the flexor pollicis longus or the flexor digitorum profundus to the index finger.[13] These cases represent incomplete anterior interosseous nerve palsy.

There are a number of conditions that must be ruled out in a patient presenting with the inability to flex the terminal phalanx of the thumb or the index finger. Isolated rupture of the flexor pollicis longus or, less commonly, rupture of the index flexor digitorum profundus may occur secondary to attritional changes in the tendon related to rheumatoid arthritis, osteoarthritis, gout, scaphoid nonunion or Kienbock's disease.[10,14,22,24] In the case of rheumatoid arthritis, osteophytes on the distal pole of the scaphoid may often be seen roentgenographically with a carpal tunnel view as described by Mannerfelt.[24] On physical examination the differential between a tendon rupture and nerve palsy may be made by looking for a tenodesis effect with alternating wrist flexion and extension or by simply squeezing on the forearm over the muscle bellies of the flexor pollicis longus and index flexor digitorum profundus. If the tendon is intact, then the interphalangeal joint will flex down. These tests may not be as reliable in patients with subluxation of the wrist related to rheumatoid arthritis or deforming wrist pathology because the force is not transmitted as well. Electromyographic studies are imperative with this differential to look for any denervation of the involved muscles. Brachial plexus neuritis and neurologic amyotrophy will usually present with accompanying shoulder pain, and the muscles about the shoulder will be involved.[21,31] Electromyography is helpful in this differential as well. Spinner has described a case of congenital absence of the flexor pollicis longus and all of the flexor digitorum profundus.[35] To help with the differential in this case there may be absent muscles elsewhere, such as in the legs, and electrical studies will also be helpful. The median nerve is formed by contributing fibers from the medial and lateral cords of the brachial plexus. Sunderland has documented that the funiculi making up the anterior interosseous nerve pass through both medial and lateral cords, so any lesion affecting either of these cords in the axilla may present with findings similar to an anterior interosseous nerve palsy.[41] Anomalous perforation of the lateral cord or the median nerve itself by the posterior humeral circumflex artery may occur, resulting in symptoms simulating anterior interosseous nerve palsy.[25,35] The reported cases have been associated with shoulder pain.

Etiology

Anterior interosseous nerve palsy will arise spontaneously in approximately one-third of cases.[3,8,13,17,29,34,47] In the majority of the reported cases of spontaneous anterior interosseous nerve palsy that went on to surgical exploration a compressing structure was found.[8,9,13,16,18,21,28,32,34,35,37,45] The compressing structure most commonly found has been a fibrous band originating from the deep head of the pronator teres, which blends with the brachialis fascia.[9,13,34,35] Other fibrous structures found to be causing compression have included a fibrous band from the superficial head of the pronator teres inserting into the brachialis fascia, the tendinous origin of the deep head of the pronator teres, and a fibrous band from the superficialis arcade.[5,13,34,35] Several accessory and variant muscles have been noted as compressing structures. These have included Gantzer's muscle, which is an accessory head of the flexor pollicis longus, the palmaris profundus, and the flexor carpi radialis brevis.[34,35] The anterior interosseous nerve is crossed by the ulnar collateral vessels and may be crossed by an aberrant radial artery. Thrombosis of these may be a source of compression.[35] Other compressing structures have included an enlarged bicipital bursa and fibrosis of necrotic muscle secondary to Volkmann's ischemic contracture.[35]

Traumatic causes of anterior interosseous nerve palsy have included supracondylar fractures in both children and adults,[4,8,20,21,35,36] forearm fractures,[7,34,46] penetrating injuries of the proximal forearm,[34,35] iatrogenic injury related to plating radius fractures[12] and flexor-pronator slide procedures,[30] blunt trauma or external compression to the proximal forearm by plaster casts, lying on the forearm, carrying a heavy purse, or a single direct blow to the forearm.[8,11,27,34,45] Pure anterior interosseous nerve palsy related to supracondylar fractures is a result of traction on the less mobile anterior interosseous nerve while the median nerve, which is more mobile in the proximal forearm, is spared.[4] This is in contrast to direct trauma to the anterior interosseous component of the median nerve at the level of the fracture. The posterior portion of the median nerve in the supracondylar region, in addition to fibers of the anterior interosseous nerve, also contain motor fibers to the pronator teres and the flexor digitorum superficialis as well as sensory fibers to the forearm.[39] Therefore direct involvement of the median nerve at the fracture site would present with findings more than isolated anterior interosseous nerve palsy.

Neuritis related to several of the immune complex disorders has also been implicated.[2]

Treatment

The management of anterior interosseous nerve palsy is related to the specific etiology. With spontaneous nerve palsy initial treatment should be conservative. Many will show signs of return within two to three months.[5,34,35] Numerous conservative measures have been tried but their effectiveness has not been documented. These include avoidance of strenuous use of the forearm, particularly supination and pronation, plaster immobilization, steroid injections and anti-inflammatory medications. During this initial waiting period baseline electromyography should be obtained after three weeks from the time of onset. Some authors have recommended continued nonsurgical treatment for prolonged periods of time, as there are some documented cases of return even up to 18 months after onset.[11,14,15,26,33] The return with such expectant treatment has been less predictable than surgical intervention, and recovery often is incomplete. Surgical decompression has lead to a more rapid recovery in the majority of cases. Therefore, if there are no signs of clinical or electromyographic improvement in 8 to 12 weeks, surgical exploration should be undertaken. Anterior interosseous nerve palsy associated with supracondylar humerus fractures in children may be an exception to early exploration, as long term followup in this group of lesions suggests that function returns in all cases.[44] Anterior interosseous nerve palsy associated with penetratinng wounds in the proximal forearm and about the elbow should be explored primarily. Neurorrhaphy or nerve grafting should be carried out at the time of exploration or as soon as the wound conditions permit.

Technique:

Exploration of the anterior interosseous nerve should start by identifying the median nerve proximal to the elbow and tracing it distally. Only in this way may an adequate appreciation of the many anatomic variations of the median and anterior interosseous nerves be attained. The incision starts 5 cm above the level of the medial epicondyle over the palpable medial border of the biceps muscle belly (Fig. 9-3). The incision curves distally along the margin of the biceps to the antecubital crease just medial to the biceps tendon where it then zig-zags back in a medial direction. The incision continues distal over the medial flexor muscle mass. In the proximal extent of the incision the median nerve is identified medial to the brachial artery. The median nerve is traced distally and the lacertus fibrosus divided. The nerve is followed to the proximal extent of the superficial head of the pronator teres. Retracting the superficial head distally will assist in defining any variation of the nerve's course in relation to

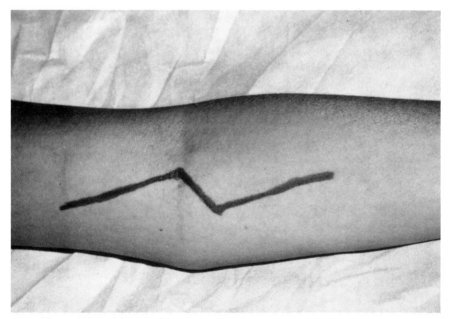

Figure 9-3. Incision used for exploration of the anterior interosseous nerve.

the two heads of the pronator teres. In the majority of cases the median and anterior interosseous nerves pass between the superficial and deep heads of the pronator teres. If this is the case, then the insertion of the superficial head should be divided from the radius and reflected proximally from the deep head to expose the median and anterior interosseous nerves. In the majority of cases this will provide adequate exposure to identify the anterior interosseous nerve and its compressing structure. If one of the less common variants is encountered, such as the anterior interosseous and median nerves passing under both heads of the pronator teres, further exposure may be obtained by detaching the insertion of the deep head of the pronator teres and reflecting it proximally and ulnarly to fully expose the superficialis arcade. If still further exposure is needed the radial origin of the superficialis may be released. Once the offending structure has been identified and released or, in the case of a penetrating wound, the nerve has been repaired, the tourniquet should be deflated and strict hemostasis achieved. The pronator teres is sutured back to its insertion site and the wound closed.

Postoperatively, a bulky dressing incorporating splints is applied, maintaining the elbow at 90 degrees of flexion and the forearm in 45 degrees of pronation. At 10 days the dressing is changed and the sutures removed. Immobilization is continued for an additional two weeks maintaining the same position and then all immobilization discontinued.

If the function of the anterior interosseous nerve fails to return following decompression or repair, or if the nerve is irreparable, appropriate tendon transfers should be considered.[34,35] Patients find the inability to flex the terminal joints of the thumb and index fingers annoying and disabling and will usually request reconstructive surgery. To restore thumb interphalangeal joint flexion one can transfer the flexor digitorum superficialis of the ring finger to the flexor pollicis longus tendon. Alternative motors to the flexor pollicis longus tendon are the brachioradialis or the flexor carpi radialis. To provide flexion of the index distal interphalangeal joint the index flexor digitorum profundus tendon is transferred to the long or ring flexor digitorum profundus tendon at the distal forearm.

Summary

Anterior interosseous nerve palsy presents with a characteristic pinch deformity with the thumb interphalangeal joint and the index distal interphalangeal joint collapsing into extension and should be looked for in any patient with a suggestive history or predisposing injury. With spontaneous nerve palsy, if there are no signs of recovery by 12 weeks the nerve should be explored. A mechanical cause of compression will be found in the majority of these cases.

References

1. Beaton LE, Anson BJ: The relation of the median nerve to the pronator teres muscle. Anat Rec 75:23, 1939.

2. Belsole RJ, Lister GD, Kleinert HE: Polyarteritis: A cause of nerve palsy in the extremity. J Hand Surg 3:320, 1978.

3. Bucher TPJ: Anterior interosseous nerve syndrome. J Bone Joint Surg 54B:555, 1972.

4. Collins DN, Weber ER: Anterior interosseous nerve avulsion. Clin Orthop 181:175, 1983.

5. Collins DN, Weber ER: Anterior interosseous nerve syndrome. South Med J 76:1533, 1983.

6. Dellon AL, MacKinnon SE, Daneshvar A: Terminal branch of anterior interosseous nerve as source of wrist pain. J Hand Surg 9B:316, 1984.

7. Engber WD, Keene JS: Anterior interosseous nerve palsy associated with a Monteggia fracture. A case report. Clin Orthop 174:133, 1983.

8. Farber JS, Bryan RS: The anterior interosseous nerve syndrome. J Bone Joint Surg 50A:521, 1968.

9. Fearn CBA, Goodfellow JW: Anterior interosseous nerve palsy. J Bone Joint Surg 47B:91, 1965.

10. Folmar RC, Nelson CL, Phalen GS: Ruptures of the flexor tendons in hands of non-rheumatoid patients. J Bone Joint Surg 54A:579, 1972.

11. Gardner-Thorpe C: Anterior interosseous nerve palsy: Spontaneous recovery in two patients. J Neurol Neurosurg Psychiatry 37:1146, 1974.

12. Griffiths JC: Nerve injuries after plating of forearm bones. Br Med J 2:277, 1966.

13. Hill NA, Howard FM, Huffer BR: The incomplete anterior interosseous nerve syndrome. J Hand Surg 10A:4, 1985.

14. Huffmann G and Leven B: Interosseous anterior syndrome. Bericht uber 4 Eigene und 49 Falle aus der Literatur. J Neurol 213:317, 1976.

15. Kiloh LG, Nevin S: Isolated neuritis of the anterior interosseous nerve. Br Med J 1:850, 1952.

16. Knight CR, Kozub P: Anterior interosseous syndrome. Ann Plast Surg 3:72, 1979.

17. Krag C: Isolated paralysis of the flexor pollicis longus muscle. An unusual variation of the anterior interosseous nerve syndrome. A case report. Scand J Plast Reconstr Surg 8:250, 1974.

18. Lake PA: Anterior interosseous nerve syndrome. J Neurosurg 41:306, 1974.

19. Linell EA: The distribution of nerves in the upper limb, with reference to variabilities and their clinical significance. J Anat 55:79, 1921.

20. Lipscomb PR, Burleson RJ: Vascular and neural complications in supracondylar fractures in children. J Bone Joint Surg 37A:487, 1955.

21. Maeda L, Miura T, Komada T, Chiba AA: Anterior interosseous nerve paralysis. Report of 13 cases and review of Japanese literatures. Hand 9:165, 1977.

22. Mahring M, Semple C, Gray ICM: Attritional flexor tendon rupture due to a scaphoid non-union imitating an anterior interosseous nerve syndrome: A case report. J Hand Surg 10B62, 1985.

23. Mannerfelt L: Studies on the hand in ulnar nerve paralysis. A clinical-experimental investigation in normal and anomalous innervation. Acta Orthop Scand Supplementum 87, 1966.

24. Mannerfelt L, Norman O: Attrition ruptures of flexor tendons in rheumatoid arthritis caused by bony spurs in the carpal tunnel. J Bone Joint Surg 51B:270, 1969.

25. Miller R: Observations upon the arrangement of the axillary artery and brachial plexus. Am J Anat 64:143, 1939.

26. Nakano KK, Lundergan C, Okihiro MM: Anterior interosseous nerve syndromes. Diagnostic methods and alternative treatments. Arch Neurol 34:477, 1977.
27. Neundorfer B, Kroger M: The anterior interosseous nerve syndrome. J Neurol 213:347, 1976.
28. Nigst H, Dick W: Syndromes of compression of the median nerve in the proximal forearm (pronator teres syndrome; anterior interosseous nerve syndrome). Arch Orthop Trauma Surg 93:307, 1979.
29. O'Brien MD, Upton ARM: Anterior interosseous nerve syndrome. A case report with neurophysiological investigation. J Neurol Neurosurg Psychiatry 35:531, 1972.
30. Page CM: An operation for the relief of flexion-contracture in the forearm. J Bone Joint Surg 5:233, 1923.
31. Parsonage MJ, Turner JWA: Neuralgic amyotrophy. The shoulder-girdle syndrome. Lancet 1:973, 1948.
32. Rask MR: Anterior interosseous nerve entrapment: (Kiloh-Nevin syndrome). Report of seven cases. Clin Orthop 142:176, 1979.
33. Smith BH, Herbst BA: Anterior interosseous nerve palsy. Arch Neurol 30:330, 1974.
34. Spinner M: The anterior interosseous nerve syndrome. With special attention to its variations. J Bone Joint Surg 52A:84, 1970.
35. Spinner M: Injuries to the Major Branches of Peripheral Nerves of the Forearm, 2nd Ed. Philadelphia, W.B. Saunders Co., 1978.
36. Spinner M, Schrieber SN: The anterior interosseous nerve paralysis as a complication of supracondylar fractures in children. J Bone Joint Surg 51A:1584, 1969.
37. Stern MB, Rosner LJ, Blinderman EE: Kiloh-Nevin syndrome. Report of a case and review of the literature. Clin Orthop 53:95, 1967.
38. Stern PJ, Kutz JE: An unusual variant of the anterior interosseous nerve syndrome: A case report and review of the literature. J Hand Surg 5:32, 1980.
39. Sunderland S: The intraneural topography of the radial, median and ulnar nerves. Brain 68:243, 1945.
40. Sunderland S: The innervation of the flexor digitorum profundus and lumbrical muscles. Anat Rec 93:317, 1945.
41. Sunderland S: Nerves and Nerve Injuries. Baltimore, Williams & Wilkins Co., 1978.
42. Sunderland S, Ray LJ: Metrical and non-metrical features of the muscular branches of the median nerve. J Comp Neurol 85:191, 1946.
43. Thomson A: Third annual report on the Committee of Collective Investigation of the Anatomical Society of Great Britain and Ireland for the year 1891—1892. J Anat Physiol 27:183, 1893.
44. Vahvanen V, Aalto K: Supracondylar fracture of the humerus in children: A long-term follow-up of 107 cases. Acta Orthop Scand 49:225, 1978.
45. Vichare NA: Spontaneous paralysis of the anterior interosseous nerve. J Bone Joint Surg 50B:806, 1968.
46. Warren JD: Anterior interosseous nerve palsy as a complication of forearm fractures. J Bone Joint Surg 45B:511, 1963.
47. Weins E, Lau SCK: The anterior interosseous nerve syndrome. Can J Surg 21:354, 1978.

CHAPTER 10

The Cubital Tunnel Syndrome

George E. Omer, M.D., M.S., F.A.C.S.

The cubital tunnel syndrome, or "tardy ulnar palsy", was defined in 1958 by Feindel and Stratford[14,15] although the ability of the anatomic structures near the elbow joint to produce external pressure on the ulnar nerve was known more than a century ago.[49] It is the most common entrapment of the ulnar nerve.[33]

Anatomy

The ulnar nerve arises as the extension of the medial cord of the brachial plexus and lies medial to the brachial artery as far as the middle third of the arm. The ulnar nerve then pierces the medial intermuscular septum and descends subfascially on the medial side of the triceps muscle. At the elbow, the ulnar nerve is accompanied by the superior ulnar collateral artery[14,49] as the nerve passes through the cubital tunnel during its course from the arm to the forearm.

The ulnar nerve can be compressed by the arcade of Struthers or the ligament of Struthers in the distal portion of the arm.[43] The arcade of Struthers is formed by fascial attachments between the internal brachial ligament, the medial head of the triceps muscle, and the medial intermuscular septum (Fig. 10-1). In an anatomic study, Spinner[43] found the arcade of Struthers to be present in 14 of 20 upper extremities. The ligament of Struthers arises from a supracondylar process and attaches to the junction of the medial epicondyle and the humeral metaphysis. The ligament of Struthers is found in only 1 percent of all upper extremities.[43]

The cubital tunnel begins at the condylar groove between the medial epicondyle of the humerus and the olecranon of the ulna. In this area a condensation of connective tissue has been reported to extend from the nerve to the subcutaneous fascia and skin.[22,43] The floor of the cubital tunnel is the medial collateral ligament (ulnar lateral ligament) of the elbow joint, and the sides are formed by the two heads of the flexor carpi ulnaris muscle.

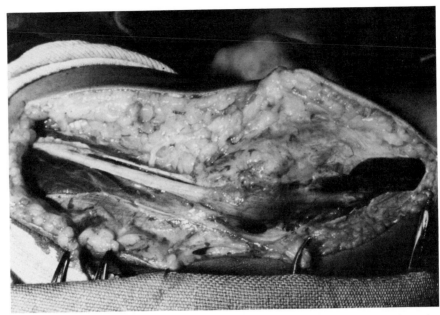

Figure 10-1. The medial intermuscular septum is a taut fibrotic ridge just anterior (superior in this view) to the ulnar nerve proximal to the medial epicondyle. The nerve is fixed in fibrous tissue in the condylar groove. (After Omer GE Jr: The ulnar nerve at the elbow. In JW Strickland, JB Steichen (Eds): Difficult Problems in Hand Surgery. St. Louis, C.V. Mosby Co., 1982.)

The roof is formed by the triangular arcuate ligament (aponeurotic band) that bridges from the medial epicondyle of the humerus to the medial aspect of the olecranon.[2,38,43,48] In the cubital tunnel the ulnar nerve can be palpated in its course behind and beneath the humeral medial epicondyle until the nerve passes between the two heads of the flexor carpi ulnaris muscle.

The capacity of the cubital tunnel is greatest when the elbow is in extension, because the triangular arcuate ligament (aponeurotic band) is slack. Measurements in cadaveric material demonstrate that the distance between the humeral and ulnar attachments of the triangular arcuate ligament lengthens 5 mm for each 45 degrees of flexion.[47] During flexion the medial head of the triceps pushes the ulnar nerve anteromedially 0.73 centimeters.[43] At 90 degrees of elbow flexion, the proximal edge of the triangular arcuate ligament is rigidly taut. In addition, the floor of the tunnel is elevated during flexion by the bulging medial collateral ligament.[25]

After the ulnar nerve passes through the cubital tunnel, it remains in the interval between the humeral and ulnar heads of the flexor carpi ulnaris muscle. Fibrous bands have been described that compress the ulnar nerve distal to the cubital tunnel.[22]

Pathophysiology

Pressure may be applied to the ulnar nerve in three ways: compression, stretch, and friction.[43] Low pressure applied to a nerve trunk initially affects the endoneural microcirculation. The nocturnal paresthesias seen in the first phases of compression are based upon edema within the nerve secondary to a nocturnal increase in tissue pressure in the cubital tunnel. A critical pressure level has been reported to be 30 mm Hg within the tunnel.[29] Functional loss due to acute compression is due to ischemia and not to mechanical deformation.[29] Pechan and Julis[40] have measured intraneural pressure in the ulnar nerve at the cubital tunnel in cadaver experiments: the pressure was 7 mm Hg with full elbow extension and 11 to 24 mm Hg at 90 degrees of flexion. Experimental studies[30] have demonstrated a progressive thickening of the external and internal epineurium as well as thickening of the perineurium. A progressive thinning of the myelin in large myelinated fibers was noted. This change was more pronounced in the peripheral than in the central fascicles of the nerve. This suggests a basis for the patient who presents with marked symptoms but normal electrodiagnostic studies. The abnormal morphometric findings in the worst fascicles account for the symptoms, while the normal myelinated fibers in the best fascicles account for the normal electrodiagnostic findings. Persistent paresthesias are related to chronic alterations in the blood flow due to intraneural fibrosis.[29,30] The muscle wasting and loss of two-point discrimination found in advanced nerve compression are related to loss of nerve fiber function.

Etiology

Wadsworth[48,49] classifies the cubital tunnel syndrome on an etiologic basis: (I) acute and subacute external compression, and (II) chronic internal compression caused by space-occupying lesions or lateral shift of the ulna (injury of the capitular epiphyses in childhood). Acute ulnar compression neuropathy can follow a single episode of blunt trauma such as fracture or dislocation of the elbow. Tardy ulnar palsy present in the adult as a consequence of injury about the elbow joint in childhood has been well documented.[17,21] However, tardy ulnar palsy in the child is an infrequent occurrence.[21] Congenital cubitus valgus deformity will result in chronic compression and dysfunction.[4] Childress[7] studied 2000 ulnar nerves in 1000 normal subjects and found an incidence of 16 percent with subluxation of the ulnar nerve from the humeral epicondylar groove during elbow flexion. Childress defined two types of subluxation: (A) the nerve moves onto the tip of the epicondyle when the elbow is flexed to or beyond 90 degrees; and (B) the nerve passes completely across and anterior to the epicondyle when the elbow is completely flexed. Approximately 75 percent of ulnar nerves with recurring subluxation are type A. Excursion of the ulnar nerve across the epicondyle makes it more accessible to trauma from direct pressure.[27]

Compression of the ulnar nerve can result from fascial bands or from lesions within the cubital tunnel, such as arthritic spurs,[20] rheumatoid synovitis, muscle anomalies,[42,43] ganglia, lipomata, and other soft tissue tumors.

Cubital tunnel syndrome has followed elective surgery or confinement to bed for a variety of reasons.[48] Certain extremity positions, such as marked elbow flexion, put the ulnar nerve within the cubital tunnel at risk during operations. A prolonged period of extreme elbow flexion should be avoided in all chair-bound or bedridden patients. During a surgical procedure, the nerve should be protected by appropriate positioning of soft pads. Sleep position may account for some cases where the patient observes that symptoms are present when the elbow is acutely flexed during sleep, but relieved by extending the elbow.

Diabetes, chronic alcoholism, and renal disease may increase the sensitivity of the ulnar nerve to compression. Hansen's disease should be considered if there is obvious thickening of the nerve.[33]

Diagnosis

The first symptoms of compression of the ulnar nerve near the elbow joint is sharp or aching pain on the medial side of the proximal forearm.[12,13] The pain may radiate proximally or distally and may be accompanied by paresthesias, dysesthesias, or anesthesia in the ring and little fingers. The exact distribution of sensory loss should be determined, because involvement of the dorsal cutaneous branch of the ulnar nerve establishes the lesion proximal to the wrist. The numbness, tingling, or "falling asleep" is related often to repetitive exercises or work involving the elbow. Severe pain in the hand is not as common as in carpal tunnel syndrome.[16] Localizing physical findings are a positive percussion test over the ulnar nerve at the elbow, abnormal mobility of the ulnar nerve over the medial epicondyle of the humerus, or a positive elbow flexion test of Wadsworth[48] (Fig. 10-2).

Patients complain of weakness and loss of dexterity for handling objects. A more recognizable clinical feature is atrophy of the intrinsic muscles with clawing of the ring and little fingers. When weakness of the extrinsic flexor carpi ulnaris muscle and the flexor digitorum profundus muscle to the little finger is demonstrated, the ulnar neuropathy can be localized at the elbow. Sunderland's studies[46] of the intraneural topography of the ulnar nerve show that the sensory axons and the intrinsic motor axons lie in a more vulnerable superficial position within the ulnar nerve at the elbow, while the motor axons to the flexor carpi ulnaris and flexor digitorum profundus muscles are deep within the nerve and relatively protected from pressure (Fig. 10-3).

A nerve conduction velocity study is usually expressed in meters per second.[18,39] The loss of the evoked sensory potential is a very sensitive indicator of altered conduction.[1] Reduced velocities of less than 25 percent are probably not significant, but greater than 33 percent are always significant.[12,13] Electromyographic studies may show denervation potentials in the ulnar innervated muscles and are consistent with cubital tunnel

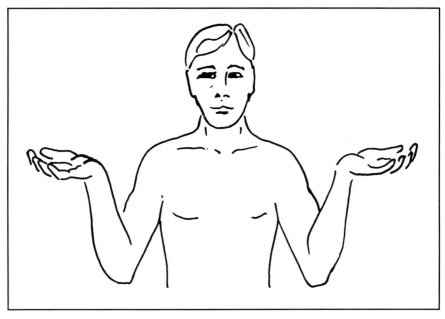

Figure 10-2. The elbow flexion test, which increases pressure within the cubital canal similar to the wrist flexion test of Phalen. Note that the wrists are held in extension.

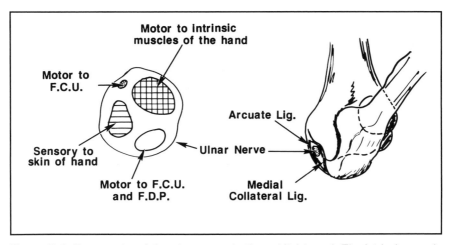

Figure 10-3. Topography of the ulnar nerve in the cubital tunnel. The intrinsic muscle fibers and cutaneous sensory fibers lie superficially under the arcuate ligament and are very vulnerable to external compressive force.

syndrome when nerve conduction velocity is less than 41 mm per second or the conduction latency across the elbow is greater than 9 or 10 mm per second.[11] It is important to remember that a peripheral nerve can be entrapped simultaneously at two levels.[36,37] Degenerative disc disease, with C8 root radiculopathy, is more likely to involve the radial aspect of the ring finger than more distal lesions at the elbow.[6] Roentgenographic studies should be done to determine the degree of cubitus valgus or evaluate bony lesions compromising the cubital tunnel. Wadsworth[48] described a cubital tunnel view: a slightly oblique anteroposterior view with the elbow in full flexion and the arm externally rotated about 20 degrees.

McGowan[34] developed a clinical classification of ulnar neuropathy: Grade I has no detectable motor weakness in the hand; Grade II has weakness of the interosseoi and the ulnar-innervated lumbricals, and Grade III demonstrates paralysis of one or more of the ulnar intrinsic muscles.

Treatment

Conservative Treatment

In the early case, management includes education of the patient regarding sleep positions and protection of the nerves from the edges of furniture and other potentially sharp objects. One should avoid repetitive flexion and extension of the elbow, such as occurs when a carpenter uses a hammer. In hospitalized patients with instructions for strict bed rest, lamb's wool elbow pads are useful, and the overhead "monkey bar" should be used to move about the bed.[25] The arms should be extended during the recovery period as well as during an operation. Local heat and ultrasound may be applied, while anti-inflammatory agents could be prescribed.[10,33] Once an ulnar nerve becomes symptomatic, either spontaneously or secondary to identified trauma, the symptoms persist. The accepted treatment of an established cubital tunnel syndrome is surgical.

Nerve Decompression

The surgical approach is a posteromedial longitudinal incision that is a series of 60 degree "steps" or turns (Fig. 10-4A). The incision should extend 8 to 10 cm proximal to the medial epicondyle and an equal distal distance to the flexor carpi ulnaris muscle. The purpose of this procedure is to decompress the nerve, but also to retain the vincula-like deep attachments that contain the segmental blood supply to the nerve. The nerve should not sublux from the humeral epicondylar groove when the elbow is flexed.

In every case the ulnar nerve must be released from tight fibrous bands. Proximal to the medial epicondyle, the medial intermuscular septum forms a taut fibrous ridge. A section of this fascial septum must be excised to prevent kinking of the nerve.[27] The ulnar nerve should be freed for at least 8 cm proximal to the medial epicondyle to determine if the nerve is entrapped in the arcade of Struthers[44,45] or entrapped on the medial intermuscular septum. Failure to release the nerve proximally will lead to continued ulnar neuropathy (Fig. 10-4B).

The aponeurotic roof of the cubital tunnel should be incised and the area inspected. An hourglass compression of the ulnar nerve at the proximal edge of the aponeurotic roof suggests an epineurotomy or an internal

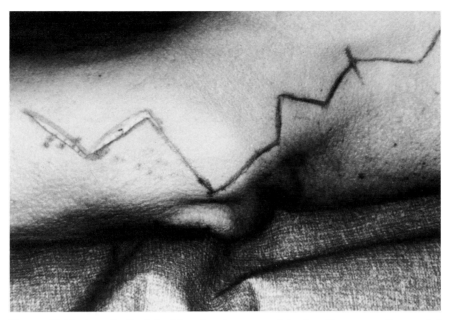

Figure 10-4A. Longitudinal incision in zig-zag or "step" pattern over the medial epicondylar area.

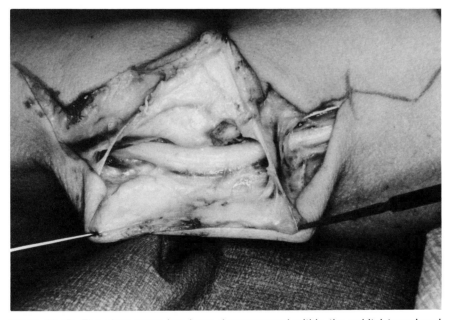

Figure 10-4B. The ulnar nerve has been decompressed within the cubital tunnel and from the medial intermuscular septum.

neurolysis. My experience has been that epineurotomy is useful in restoring a circulatory blush across a compressed segment, but there is no direct relationship between intraneural neurolysis and improved sensory or motor function of the ulnar nerve. A saline neurolysis is never indicated. A more reliable prognostic indicator is the duration of clinical symptoms, and a McGowan[34] Grade III lesion does not recover function following intraneural neurolysis.

Fixation of the ulnar nerve at the level of the medial epicondylar groove can result in traction neuritis.[2,22,50] Condensation of connective tissue and aponeurotic bands should be released. Bone fragments must be removed. The groove should be carefully inspected, because friction neuritis can develop with repeated movement of the ulnar nerve against osteophytes or bony spurs of the distal aspect of the humerus. The aponeurotic roof of the cubital tunnel may be utilized as a fasciodermal sling[10] or excised. The superior ulnar collateral artery, which accompanies the ulnar nerve in the condylar groove, should not be injured.

I prefer to leave the ulnar nerve attached to the soft tissue in the depth of the groove and within the cubital tunnel, provided this vincula-like tissue is elastic and not fibrotic. The fibrous arcade over the flexor carpi ulnaris is incised, and the ulnar nerve should be explored to the midportion of the proximal third of the forearm. The ulnar nerve is not disturbed in its bed. After the nerve is decompressed, the elbow should be extended and flexed to observe the excursion of the nerve trunk. If the nerve is compressed against the posterior aspect of the medial epicondyle, but is not subluxing across the medial epicondyle, an epicondylectomy is indicated (Fig. 10-4C).

Epicondylectomy

Removal of the medial epicondyle permits the ulnar nerve to be under minimal tension during extension and flexion of the elbow.[8,16,23,24,35] The ulnar nerve is decompressed without releasing it from the condylar groove, as previously described. The humeral medial epicondyle is exposed by sharp subperiosteal dissection, reflecting the common origin of the flexor-pronator muscles. After the medial epicondyle and the adjacent supracondylar ridge are exposed, both are removed with a bone saw or osteotomes (Fig. 10-4D). The ulnar nerve is protected with a broad-blade retractor. The medial collateral ligament and its bony attachments must remain intact. Bony spurs are removed with a rongeur. The flexor-pronator muscle flap is reattached to the redundant periosteal flaps, leaving a smooth buttress for the ulnar nerve, which should not be compressed by the remaining medial epicondyle during flexion. I deflate the tourniquet and ensure hemostasis before subcutaneous and skin closure (Fig. 40-4E).

Subcutaneous Transposition

If there is subluxation of the ulnar nerve across the medial epicondyle with flexion of the elbow after decompression, anterior subcutaneous transposition is indicated. Curtis is reported[3,10] to have described in 1898 a technique for subcutaneous anterior transposition of the ulnar nerve, and

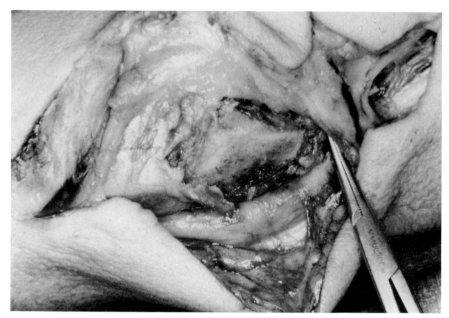

Figure 10-4C. The ulnar nerve is decompressed more with an epicondylectomy. The flexor-pronator origin has been released and the bone partially removed.

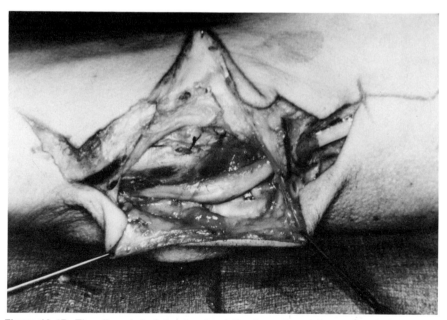

Figure 10-4D. The elbow is in full extension following epicondylectomy and ulnar nerve decompression. (After Omer GE Jr: The ulnar nerve at the elbow. In JW Strickland, JB Steichen (Eds): Difficult Problems in Hand Surgery. St. Louis, C.V. Mosby Co., 1982.)

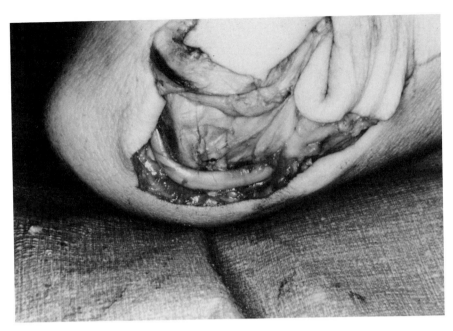

Figure 10-4E. The elbow is in full flexion following epicondylectomy and ulnar nerve decompression. The nerve is not subluxed onto the tip of the condyle, and is free of pressure. (After Omer GE Jr: The ulnar nerve at the elbow. In JW Strickland, JB Steichen (Eds): Difficult Problems in Hand Surgery. St. Louis, C.V. Mosby Co., 1982.)

the procedure was standardized by Platt.[41] After the ulnar nerve is exposed from at least 8 cm above the medial epicondyle to between the heads of the flexor carpi ulnaris muscle in the proximal forearm, the nerve is mobilized as a neurovascular bundle that includes both the arteries and veins that accompany the nerve. The neurovascular bundle is transposed anteriorly beneath the elevated skin flap. Eaton, Crowe, and Parkes[10] have described a fasciodermal sling to support the transposed ulnar nerve. A flap of antebrachial fascia 1 cm wide and 1 cm long, based on the medial epicondyle, is raised and reflected medially. The fascial flap is passed posterior to the transposed ulnar nerve and is sutured to the subcutaneous tissue anterior to the medial epicondyle, preventing the ulnar nerve from returning to its original position. Subcutaneous slings have been reported to result in constriction or kinking of the ulnar nerve[3,28] and these procedures are not indicated unless there has been symptomatic subluxation prior to surgery.

Submuscular Transposition

Submuscular transposition of the ulnar nerve is indicated for a Childress[7] type B subluxation, where the nerve passes completely across and anterior to the medial epicondyle when the elbow is flexed. In addition, submuscular transposition should be considered in cases with severe hypertrophic osteoarthritis.[47]

Learmonth[26] decompresses the ulnar nerve from the point where it penetrates the medial intermuscular septum to beyond the cubital tunnel. The flexor-pronator muscle mass is detached from the medial epicondyle and turned distally and radially to expose the median nerve. The ulnar nerve is transposed to lie alongside the median nerve on the brachialis muscle. The flexor-pronator muscle origin is then reattached to the medial epicondyle. This procedure permits arthrotomy of the elbow joint and inspection of the medial collateral ligament.[9] The technique has been modified by performing an osteotomy of the medial epicondyle with the attached flexor-pronator muscles and then reattaching the epicondyle with screw fixation.[27,32] Fibrous constriction of the ulnar nerve has been observed following submuscular transposition.[16] Campbell, Morantz, and Post[5] have recommended encasing the ulnar nerve in a silastic sleeve to halt progressive fibrosis.

Postoperative Care

A bulky soft dressing is used for 24 to 48 hours after nerve decompression. If an epicondylectomy has been done, the soft dressing is replaced with a posterior plaster splint with the elbow in 90 degrees of flexion for two weeks. If the nerve has been transposed, the elbow is immobilized in 90 degrees of flexion and the forearm fully pronated. The initial bulky dressing is replaced by a long arm plaster dressing for three weeks. Active range of motion exercises are then initiated with emphasis on regaining full extension at the elbow.

Results

Treatment by in-situ decompression, anterior subcutaneous transposition, and submuscular transposition have all been reported to produce satisfactory results.[1,27,34,47] Pain is usually relieved, and other sensory symptoms show consistent improvement. Improvement of the evoked sensory potential correlates well with improvement in clinical symptoms.[1] However, weakness tends to persist, and intrinsic muscular atrophy is the least likely to improve.[1,16,19,31] There is little prognostic difference between successful surgical procedures, but a guarded prognosis always should be given with secondary transposition.[3] The potential for full motor recovery after operation is greatly reduced in those patients in whom preoperative symptoms have been present for more than one year or who have intrinsic muscle atrophy before surgery.

References

1. Adelaar RS, Foster WC, McDowell C: The treatment of the cubital tunnel syndrome. J Hand Surg 9A:90, 1984.
2. Apfelbert DB, Larson SJ: Dynamic anatomy of the ulnar nerve at the elbow. Plast Reconstr Surg 51:76, 1973.
3. Broudy AS, Leffert RD, Smith RJ: Technical problems with ulnar nerve transposition at the elbow: findings and results of reoperation. J Hand Surg 3:85, 1978.

4. Burman MS, Sutro CJ: Recurrent luxation of the ulnar nerve by congenital posterior position of the medial epicondyle of the humerus. J Bone Joint Surg 21:958, 1939.

5. Campbell JB, Morantz RA, Post KD: A technique for relief of motor and sensory deficits occurring after anterior ulnar transposition. J Neurosurg 40:405, 1974.

6. Chaplin E, Kasdan ML, Corwin HM: Occupational neurology and the hand: different diagnosis. Hand Clin 2:513, 2986.

7. Childress HM: Recurrent ulnar-nerve dislocation at the elbow. Clin Orthop 108:168, 1975.

8. Craven PR, Green DP: Cubital tunnel syndrome. Treatment by epicondylectomy. J Bone Joint Surg 62A:986, 1980.

9. Del Pizzo W, Jobe FW, Norwood L: Ulnar nerve entrapment syndrome in baseball players. Am J Sports Med 5:182, 1977.

10. Eaton RG, Crowe JF, Parkes JC III: Anterior transposition of the ulnar nerve using a non-compressing fasciodermal sling. J Bone Joint Surg 62A:820, 1980.

11. Eisen A, Danon J: The mild cubital tunnel syndrome: Its natural history and indications for surgical intervention. Neurol 24:608, 1974.

12. Eversmann WW Jr: Entrapment and compression neuropathies. In DP Green (ED): Operative Hand Surgery. New York, Churchill Livingstone, 1982, chap 29, pp 957.

13. Eversmann WW Jr: Compression and entrapment neuropathies of the upper extremity. J Hand Surg 8:759, 1983.

14. Feindel W, Stratford J: Cubital tunnel compression in tardy ulnar palsy. Can Med Assoc J 78:351, 1958.

15. Feindel W, Stratford J: Cubital tunnel palsy in tardy ulnar palsy. Can J Surg 1:287, 1958.

16. Froimson AI, Zahrawi F: Treatment of compression neuropathy of the ulnar nerve at the elbow by epicondylectomy and neurolysis. J Hand Surg 5:391, 1980.

17. Gay JR, Love JG: Diagnosis and treatment of tardy paralysis of the ulnar nerve. J Bone Joint Surg 29A:1087, 1947.

18. Gilliatt RW, Thomas PK: Changes in nerve conduction with ulnar nerve lesions at the elbow. J Neurol Neurosurg Psychiatry 23:312, 1960.

19. Harrison MJG, Nurick S: Results of anterior transposition of the ulnar nerve for ulnar neurotis. Br Med J 1:27, 1970.

20. Hecht O, Lipsher E: Median and ulnar nerve entrapment caused by ectopic calcification. J Hand Surg 5:30, 1980.

21. Holmes JC, Hall JE: Tardy ulnar nerve palsy in children. Clin Orthop 135:128, 1978.

22. Inglis AE, Kinnett G: Ulnar neuropathy at the elbow. Proceedings of American Society for Surgery of the Hand. J Hand Surg 3:290, 1978.

23. Jones RE, Gauntt C: Medial epicondylectomy for ulnar nerve compression syndrome at the elbow. Clin Orthop 139:174, 1979.

24. King T, Morgan F: The treatment of traumatic ulnar neuritis. Aust NZ J Surg 20:33, 1950.

25. Lazaro L III: Ulnar nerve instability: ulnar nerve injury due to elbow flexion. South Med J 70:36, 1977.

26. Learmonth JR: A technique for transplanting the ulnar nerve. Surg Gynecol Obstet 75:792, 1943.

27. Levy DM, Apfelberg DB: Results of anterior transposition for ulnar neuropathy at the elbow. Am J Surg 123:304, 1972.

28. Lulch AL: Ulnar nerve entrapment after anterior transposition at the elbow. NY State J Med 75:75, 1975.

29. Lundborg G, Gelberman RH, Minteer-Convery M, Lee YF, Hargens AR: Median nerve compression in the carpal tunnel—functional response to experimentally induced controlled pressure. J Hand Surg 7:252, 1982.

30. Mackinnon SE, Dellon AL: Experimental study of chronic nerve compression. Hand Clin 2:639, 1986.

31. Macnicol MF: The results of operation for ulnar neuritis. J Bone Joint Surg 61B:159, 1979.

32. Mass DP, Silverberg B: Cubital tunnel syndrome: anterior transposition with epicondylar osteotomy. Orthopaedics 9:711, 1986.

33. McFarland GB: Entrapment syndromes. *In* C McEvarts, RI Burton (Eds): Surgery of the Musculoskeletal System. New York, Churchill Livingstone, 1983, chap 20:2, pp 521-540.

34. McGowan AJ: The results of transposition of the ulnar nerve for traumatic ulnar neuritis. J Bone Joint Surg 32B:293, 1950.

35. Neblett C, Ehni G: Medial epicondylectomy for ulnar palsy. J Neurosurg 32:55, 1970.

36. Omer GE Jr: Pitfalls in the management of peripheral nerve injuries. Bull NY Acad Med 55:829, 1979.

37. Omer GE Jr: The ulnar nerve at the elbow. *In* JW Strickland, JB Steichen (Eds): Difficult Problems in Hand Surgery. St. Louis, C.V. Mosby Co., 1982, chap 44, pp 374.

38. Osborne GV: Compression neuritis of the ulnar nerve at the elbow. Hand 2:10, 1970.

39. Payan J: Electrophysiological localization of ulnar nerve lesions. J Neurol Neurosurg Psychiatry 32:208, 1969.

40. Pechan J, Julis I: The pressure measurement in the ulnar nerve: a contribution to the pathophysiology of the cubital tunnel syndrome. J Biomechanics 8:75, 1975.

41. Platt H: The operative treatment of traumatic neuritis at the elbow. Surg Gynecol Obstet 47:822, 1928.

42. Rolfsen L: Snapping triceps tendon with ulnar neuritis. Acta Orthop Scand 41:74, 1970.

43. Spinner M: Injuries to the Major Branches of Peripheral Nerves in the Forearm, 2nd Ed. Philadelphia, W.B. Saunders Co., 1978.

44. Spinner M: Management of nerve compression lesions of the upper extremity. *In* GE Jr Omer, M Spinner (Eds): Management of Peripheral Nerve Problems. Philadelphia, W.B. Saunders Co., 1980, chap 34, pp 569.

45. Spinner M: Management of nerve compression lesions. Instructional Course Lecture, Academy of American Orthopaedic Surgeons 33:461, 1984.

46. Sunderland S: The intraneural topography of the radial, median, and ulnar nerves. Brain 68:243, 1945.

47. Vanderpool DW, Chambers J, Lamb DW, Whiston TB: Peripheral compression lesions of the ulnar nerve. J Bone Joint Surg 50B:792, 1968.

48. Wadsworth TG: The external compression syndrome of the ulnar nerve at the cubital tunnel. Clin Orthop 124:189, 1977.

49. Wadsworth TG: The Elbow. Edinburgh, Churchill Livingstone, 1982.

50. Wilson DH, Krout R: Surgery of ulnar neuropathy at the elbow: 16 cases treated by decompression without transposition. Technical Note. J Neurosurg 38:780, 1973.

CHAPTER 11

Radial Tunnel Syndrome/Posterior Interosseous Nerve Compression

Clayton A. Peimer, M.D.
Dale R. Wheeler, M.D.

Radial tunnel syndrome is a compression neuropathy involving the posterior interosseous branch of the radial nerve; it may present as a variety of clinical complaints, the most frequent being pain about the proximal lateral forearm. Symptoms are exacerbated by forearm rotation. In severe cases, patients may have weakness or progressive paralysis of the finger, thumb, and wrist extensors.

Case reports of posterior interosseous nerve (PIN) palsy, not associated with trauma, dot the literature. Agnew, in 1963, first described a patient with a bursal tumor which caused both median and PIN paresis and weakness.[2] Since that time, "spontaneous" PIN palsy or compression associated with a variety of tumors (lipoma, fibroma, aneurysm), Monteggia and supracondylar fractures, and rheumatoid arthritis has been reported.[1,3,5,8,12,20,23,34,35,41,41,46-48,50-52,57,58,62,65,70,76] Anatomic variations have also been suggested as etiologic factors.[71]

Whiteley implicated the "upper medial edge" of the supinator as the point of constriction in a 45-year-old male with antecubital pain and progressive extensor weakness.[75] Exploration revealed a neuroma in continuity. Capener and Somerville suggested that persistent tennis elbow pain might be due to compression of the posterior interosseous nerve as it passed between the supinator and its aponeurosis, reporting that some patients' symptoms were relieved by decompression.[13,61] A variety of other causes of "tennis elbow" have been described, serving only to cloud the hypothesis that posterior interosseous neuropathy exists as a separate clinical entity.[7,9,16,24,37,38,56]

In 1963 Kopell and Thompson postulated that PIN compression and pain were due to "a tightening of the fibrous edge of the extensor carpi radialis brevis and the fibrous edge of the supinator slit with creasing of the nerve."[39] Sharrard described four patients who progressed from a painful elbow following minor hyperextension injuries to weakness and paralysis of the posterior interosseous nerve.[60] On exploration, all were noted to have adhesions or fibrous bands entrapping the nerve anterior to the radial head and capsule. In his anatomic study of 25 adult and 10 fetal specimens, Spinner found that in 30% of the adult specimens the medial half of the superficial head of the supinator had a firm tendinous consistency, and suggested that this fibrous arcade of Frohse is probably formed in "response to repeated rotary movement" of the forearm.[63]

The term *radial tunnel syndrome* was first used by Roles and Maudsley who, in 1972, described the course of the radial nerve and its branches in relation to the radial tunnel.[59] Basing their observations on operative and cadaveric dissections, they described similar areas of compression, and reported that surgical release produced good or excellent results in 92% of 38 cases of "resistant tennis elbow."

That PIN compression, or radial tunnel syndrome, is a diagnosis distinct from lateral epicondylitis and radiohumeral synovitis, was established by two papers published in 1979.[43,74] Although not in total agreement on the anatomical structures that most often cause posterior interosseous nerve compression, both studies clearly revealed that lateral elbow or forearm pain may be caused by a compression neuropathy at this zone, which can be relieved by PIN decompression. Both groups of authors also proposed that this diagnosis may be distinguished clinically from other causes of elbow pain in the majority of cases by specific signs and symptoms, although other causes such as lateral epicondylitis may coexist, perhaps as primary etiologies.

Anatomy

The radial nerve pierces the lateral intermuscular septum, entering the anterior compartment of the arm approximately 10 cm above the lateral epicondyle; it then proceeds distally to enter the radial tunnel. The capitellum is posterior to the radial nerve; the brachialis and biceps tendon are medial to it; and brachioradialis (BR) and the extensor carpi radialis longus (ECRL) are anterolateral.[71] The most proximal motor branches are to the BR, then to the ECRL, and occasionally medially to the brachialis. Sensory branches pass to the periosteum of the lateral epicondyle, the radiocapitellar joint, and the orbicular ligament.[37,59] The radial nerve then usually divides into two large (terminal) branches, one superficial sensory and the other deep motor, 4 to 5 cm proximal to the radiocapitellar joint (sometimes at the joint or up to 2 cm distally).[37,71] These two terminal branches pass distally, anterior to the radiocapitellar joint, 1 cm lateral to the biceps tendons in fatty tissue tethered to the joint capsule. These tethering bands, which may be either rather flimsy or substantial, may cause compression. The posterior (motor) branch (the PIN) of the radial nerve then passes beneath the edge of the ECRB, which originates from the lateral epicondyle, and extends medially, blending into the deep fascia of the forearm flexors. The superficial branch usually passes anteriorly, lying on the underside of the brachioradialis.[39] At the radial neck, the PIN is crossed superficially by a fan of radial recurrent vessels. Then this nerve courses laterally and posteriorly, passing beneath the superficial medial edge of the supinator, the arcade of Frohse. Lister et al. have suggested that these vessels are also a potential site of nerve construction.[43]

The nerve then courses between superficial and deep muscle layers as it winds dorsally around the radius to emerge at the lower border of the supinator under the superficial extensors. The motor branch to the ECRB arises from the posterior interosseous branch prior to entering the supinator, or as a branch from the superficial trunk in the same region. The branches to the supinator arise from the PIN proximal to its entrance into the muscle layers. Additional branches may arise as the deep branch passes through the muscle.[33] Coursing through the supinator, the posterior interosseous nerve may come into contact with a bare area of the radius, so that it lies directly on the periosteum deep to the superficial supinator, in the region between the insertion of the deep and superficial components of the supinator, somewhat distal to the lower border of the radial tuberosity.[18]

As the PIN exits from the supinator, the variability of its branches becomes so great that only generalizations can be made.[71] The basic pattern recapitulates phylogeny: the superficial extensors are the more proximally innervated muscles representing the distally migrated brachial-antebrachial extensors, the extensor humero-dorsalis, the extensor digitorum communis (EDC), the extensor humero-ulnaris, the extensor carpi ulnaris (ECU), and the extensor digiti quinti (EDQ). The deeper, more distally innervated muscles, representing the proximally migrated antebrachial manual muscle, and the ulno-carpal extensors, the abductor pollicis longus (APL), extensor pollicis brevis (EPB), extensor pollicis longus (EPL) and extensor indicis proprius (EIP), are all innervated by the more distal division of the posterior interosseous nerve.[69] On emerging from the supinator, the nerve lies between these superficial and deep muscle groups beside the posterior interosseous artery. From this point, two branches, one heading proximal, traverse to the mid- to upper third of the EDC. The ECU is supplied by one or more branches extending horizontally to it, and running just distal to the anconeus. Similarly, branches go to the EDQ. These may all arise from the PIN or from the division to the superficial muscles. The distal division consists of at least two branches, one to the APL, sometimes to the EPB, and a second to the EPL and EIP, and sometimes also to the EPB. The most distally innervated muscle is usually the EIP. The terminal portion of the nerve passes deep to the EPL on the interosseous membrane to provide sensory innervation to the wrist.

Anatomic variations involving the supinator are pertinent to the development of radial tunnel syndrome. The superficial portion of the supinator arises from the lateral epicondyle in a semicircular fashion, arching distally, then regaining attachment to the medial aspect of the epicondyle adjacent to the capitellum.[63] The posterior branch of the radial nerve passes beneath this margin, or arcade of Frohse, anterior to the radiocapitellar joint between superficial and deep components of the supinator and gains access to the posterior forearm. In Spinner's study, previously cited, the medial half of the arcade of Frohse was a firm, fibrous band in 30% of the adult specimens.[63] The proximal edge in fetal specimens was always muscular, as it was in the other 70 percent of adults, all "presumed" to be asymptomatic. Of 90 operative cases of posterior interosseous nerve entrapment, Werner noted that 80 (89 percent) had a "well developed fibrous edge at intersection with the nerve," and that with passive pronation the nerve was compressed in 83.[74] Seventy-eight of those with compressed nerves had fibrous margins and five did not, firmly supporting the assumption that the fibrous margin is a site of compression.

Another anatomic variation related to a major proposed compression site is the fibrous medial edge of the ECRB. Kopell and Thompson describe the origin of the ECRB as a fibrous band stretching from the lateral epicondyle to the deep fascia over the midvolar aspect of the forearm; the posterior interosseous nerve crosses beneath the fibrous edge.[39] They postulated that this fibrous edge may be a site of compression in some patients when the forearm is fully pronated. There is some disagreement about the role that the ECRB actually plays in this compression neuropathy. Spinner noted that in three of his adult specimens full pronation caused compression of the posterior interosseous nerve by the fibrous margin of the ECRB.[63] Lister et al., noted this fascial extension to be a site of compression in 14 of 20 operated cases.[43] Werner, however, noted that, although there was a fascial extension of the brevis over the PIN in 54 of 90 cases, none of these caused dynamic compression with passive pronation and wrist flexion, nor was any a site of static compression.[74] Sunderland also disputes Spinner and Lister's description of the anatomic basis for nerve compression.[71]

There are several other reported anatomic variations. In some documented cases, a branch or all of the posterior interosseous nerve was noted to pass superficial to the entire supinator.[77] Other reports describe nerve impingement by fibrous bands at the distal margin of the supinator in addition to, or instead of, impingement at the proximal margin.[19,67] There may also be muscular variations, for example, a bifid extensor carpi radialis brevis, which may cause entrapment.[53] The clinical examination may also be clouded by a possible distal communication between branches of the anterior and posterior interosseous nerves in the forearm as described by Rauber.[64]

Etiology

The described sites of compression include the leash of recurrent vessels, fibrous bands anterior to the radiocapitellar joint, the fibrous medial edge of the ECRB, and the arcade of Frohse. Anatomic dissections and series of operative cases support the theory that repetitive forearm rotation and microtrauma are the most likely etiologies.[29,60,63] Data from four large surgical series revealed that 82 percent of patients had jobs requiring repetitive rotatory or hyperextension motions, and 83 percent of the procedures were performed on the dominant or most utilized arm.[30,43,59,74] A microtraumatic or occupational etiology is consistent with findings for carpal tunnel disease. Werner found that pressure increased with passive forearm pronation.[74] Active supination (by radial nerve stimulation) produced pressures five times greater than passive pronation. This intermittent dynamic compression by the edge of the supinator could cause PIN irritation and compression.

Other causes for compression may be appreciated preoperatively by clinical examination or radiographs. Soft tissue masses, which may compress or stretch the posterior interosseous nerve, particularly lipomata, are common about the proximal radius and radial neck region. Other reported masses include ganglia or aneurysms.[3,8,20,48] Generally, patients with these tend to present with paralysis and weakness rather than pain. Some may present with pain which then progresses to a pain-free paralysis. In a review of the literature, Wu noted that functional loss preceded awareness of a mass in 8 of 12 cases.[78]

Radial or posterior interosseous nerve injuries may occur acutely as a consequence of elbow fracture dislocations, particularly Monteggia fractures characterized by anterior dislocation of the radial head and supracondylar humerus fracture.[23,42,52,65,70] Such palsies resolve without intervention other than reduction of the fracture dislocation. Chronic radial head dislocations that cause tardy nerve palsy should be easily identified radiographically. Treatment would require radial head resection and/or standard nerve decompression.[1,34,41]

Elbow synovitis in rheumatoids, causing a PIN palsy with loss of finger extension, was first reported by Marmor in 1967.[46] The extensor retinaculum (at the wrist) of this patient was explored, with the expectation of finding tendon rupture, before the correct diagnosis was made. Millender described three additional cases in 1973, one of which was explored, but all of whom were initially misdiagnosed as tendon ruptures.[50] These cases emphasized that it is necessary in rheumatoids to differentiate among compression neuropathy, extensor tendon rupture or subluxation, and metacarpal-phalangeal (MP) joint dysfunction as the cause of loss of MP extension. Synovitis usually produces increasing elbow pain and swelling preceding weakness and paralysis. Extensor rupture is an abrupt event, usually presaged by (visible, but often painless) dorsal wrist tenosynovitis. Chronic metacarpal-phalangeal joint synovitis, ulnar drift, and progressive extensor lag are accompanied by extensor subluxation and MCP dislocation. When active MP extension is lost but extensor tenodesis is still present at the MP joints in passive palmar flexion, EMG studies may useful. Synovitis-induced nerve compression should be managed initially with splinting, anti-inflammatory agents and possibly steroid injections. If these modalities are unsuccessful, synovectomy, radial head resection, and nerve decompression are indicated.

Diagnosis

SIGNS AND SYMPTOMS: The typical patient presents with complaints of dull, aching, lateral forearm and elbow pain which worsens with activity and may occur frequently. Patients admit to weakness of the arm and of grip, but not to sensory loss. There may be intensification of complaints with repetitive movements incorporating forearm pronation and often with wrist flexion. Prior treatments may include physical therapy, splints, anti-inflammatory agents, steroid injections, and surgical procedures for tennis elbow. The duration of symptoms typically averages two or more years. Pain as a primary symptom of a compression neuropathy of a motor nerve may be confusing until one recognizes that motor nerves contain not only large myelinated efferent fibers but also many thin myelinated afferent fibers of muscular and extramuscular origin, many of which are nociceptive. The irritation of such fibers is presumably responsible for the discomfort.[74]

A "pathognomonic sign" proposed by Lister is maximum tenderness over the posterior interosseous nerve at and just distal to the radial head; pain in this region is also caused by resisted supination with the elbow extended, which is believed to represent impingement by the arcade of Frohse.[43] In administering this test, Werner noted intense pain in 51 and slight pain in 33 patients. Intraoperative findings revealed that 80 of 90 patients had a fibrous arcade, and 83 had dynamic compression caused by forearm rotation.[74] Forearm pain produced by resisted extension of the middle finger with the elbow extended represents compression of the nerve by the fibrous medial extension of the ECRB.[39,59] Werner noted that in 39 of 67 patients for whom this test was positive and in 15 of 23 patients for whom it was negative, there was a medial fibrous extension of the ECRB.[74] In none could he demonstrate nerve compression with passive forearm rotation or wrist flexion convincingly. Lister et al. describe passive impingement in 14 of their 20 cases, and believed it to be important.[43] This test may also be more indicative of tears in the origin of the ECRB or of lateral epicondylitis.[13]

Infrequently, patients with radial tunnel syndrome present primarily with actual weakness. Complete dorsal interosseous nerve palsy does not eliminate radially deviated wrist dorsiflexion (the ECRL is innervated proximally), or finger and thumb IP extension (action of the distal intrinsics, and abductor pollicis brevis [APB] and adductor pollicis[AddP], respectively). If the thumb is stabilized by the examiner in radial abduction-extension, the APB and AddP can no longer extend the thumb IP joint. Weakness without paralysis and with preserved motion represents a more subtle but important sign of compression that should be considered.

Moss and Switzer described two other symptoms in patients with radial tunnel syndrome.[53] One was a presentation of radial paresthesias and the "feeling of a mass" in the first web space, or decreased sensibility in the radial sensory nerve distribution; the anatomic cause of such symptoms is not clear, but their patients improved following PIN decompression. They also noted complaints of "popping" about the elbow which, on exploration, revealed the ECRB to be subluxating over the radial head.

Diagnostic Testing

Neurophysiologic testing may not be of great benefit in radial tunnel syndrome. Gassel and Diamantopoulos, who determined the PIN conduction velocity to the EDC as 72 m/sec, presented a case in whom they were able to show polyphasic potentials but normal amplitude and latency on distal recording, despite complete paralysis.[26] They concluded that this "indicates a discrepancy between the nerve's capacity for the conduction of voluntary or reflexly inaugurated impulses and electrically executed impulses." Jebsen describes the technique for measuring distal radial nerve conduction velocity and found it to be 58.4 m/sec., similar to the conduction velocity of the distal median and ulnar nerves.[36]

Werner's series, which produced the only large collection of data, involved the testing of 25 of his 90 cases electromyographically (EMG) and for nerve conduction velocity (NCV).[74] Conduction velocity was determined from a point proximal to the elbow to a point distal to the supinator. EMG recordings were obtained from muscles innervated by branches both proximal and distal to the supinator. In 13 of the 25, the conduction velocity was slowed, and in eight a slight increase in size of motor unit potentials was measured in EDC and EIP. Good results from decompression were obtained in 11 of the 13 with abnormal NCV and in 7 of 8 of those with abnormal EMG findings. However, good results were also obtained in seven of eight patients with normal neurophysiologic data. Testing while the patient actively supinates may expose more alterations in nerve conduction. The EMG/NCV studies may support the diagnosis in perhaps one-third to one-half of cases; but a negative exam, at the current level of sophistication, clearly does not exclude this diagnosis.

Thermography has also been suggested as a possible aid in differentiation of nerve entrapment versus tennis elbow or lateral epicondylitis. One report without specific data states that 82 patients with tennis elbow had a hot spot on thermogram whereas seven with a compression neuropathy did not.[22]

Differential Diagnosis

Radial tunnel syndrome is differentiated from lateral epicondylitis primarily by the location of the pain and by the physical findings and signs; but, it is important to remember that these two lesions can coexist. Werner estimated that 5 percent of patients with tennis elbow had posterior interosseous nerve compression, and Lister reported that three of twenty patients had both.[43,74] Systemic causes of peripheral neuropathy or a more proximal site of partial radial nerve compression could be misinterpreted as a more distal posterior interosseous nerve compression.[44,45] Polyarteritis may present (uncommonly) as a mononeuritis, with sudden onset of pain and paresthesia followed by motor weakness. Paralysis of the radial nerve from lead or other heavy metal intoxication is an atypical presentation, although isolated instances of posterior interosseous nerve paralysis have been reported. Parsonage and Turner in 1957 reported eight cases involvinng the deep branch of the radial nerve, and Burns and Lister in 1984 reported four more, all requiring long periods (up to three years) for recovery. Allergic angioneuropathy, a problem resembling Parsonage-Turner syndrome, presents with the sudden onset of intense pain followed by weakness and paralysis, frequently following medical illnesses or anesthesia.[11,72]

Treatment

Nonsurgical Modalities

Splinting, activity modification, anti-inflammatory medication, and steroid injection are the initial steps in managing the patient with pain from any compression neuropathy, including radial tunnel syndrome. Spontaneous recovery from paralysis of the entire nerve after periods of splinting and anti-inflammatory medication has been reported. Symptoms are generally present 2 to 6 months prior to surgical intervention.[30,43,59,74] If nonoperative treatment is unsuccessful, further care requires a thorough exploration and decompression of the nerve.

Surgery

The brachioradialis (BR) splitting approach (Lister), provides the best and easiest exposure of the four usual sites of nerve compression at the proximal margin of the supinator (Fig. 11-1).[43] The incision is made under tourniquet control 3 to 4 cm lateral to the biceps tendon, over the BR, extending distally in an S for about 6 cm from a level about 5 cm distal to the lateral epicondyle. The muscle fascia is split longitudinally, and then blunt dissection is directed deeply in line with the muscle fibers, constantly aiming toward the radial neck. As Lister has noted, "It is one of those very rare situations in which one sees no landmarks (for about a minute) and should not." Immediately beneath the brachioradialis are the obliquely oriented supinator fibers and the superficial branch of the radial nerve; deep retractors will add to the exposure. The posterior interosseous nerve is seen proximal to the medial edge of the supinator, surrounded by fat and crossed by the radial recurrent vessels. Filmy adhesions usually cover the entire region. Bipolar electrocautery of the crossing vessels is followed by mobilization and lysis of the nerve, with the result that the (fibrous) edge of the supinator and, if needed, the ECRB can be released.[17,43] Following adequate decompression, the tourniquet is released and hemostasis obtained prior to closure, which includes only an approximation of the subcutaneous layer and skin. Wound dressing includes modest compression about the lateral aspect of the arm and the use of a sling for comfort. A gradual resumption of normal daily activities is allowed. Return to heavy work and lifting may take 8 to 12 weeks, or more.

Complete proximal exposure of the nerve can be obtained at surgery by extending the skin incision above the elbow (crossing the antecubital crease transversely) and dissecting *between* the brachioradialis and the

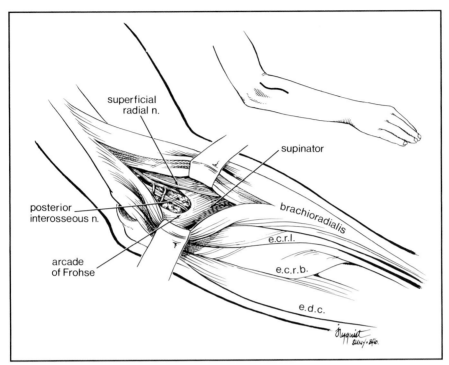

Figure 11-1. The PIN is best approached by splitting the brachioradialis fibers bluntly with a clamp and dissecting toward the radial neck. The PIN is dorsal to the sensory branch and is traced under the (fibrous edge) supinator and ECRB.

brachialis/biceps (Fig. 11-2). Exposure of the nerve more distally can be achieved by dissecting the fascia between the EDC and ECRL, exposing the distal margin of the supinator and the emerging terminal branches of the PIN (Fig. 11-3). In patients having lateral epicondylitis and radial tunnel syndrome, both can be addressed through a single exposure that requires only that the proximal extent of the skin incision be swung posteriorly over the lateral epicondyle to expose the common extensor origin (Figs. 11-1, 11-2). Other primary surgical exposures are described and advocated by other authors.[14,31,64] Any surgery about the elbow may lead to a hypertrophic, widened scar, which is the most frequent postoperative problem.

All authors recommend release of the medial edge of the supinator. Eversman suggests that the entire superficial supinator be sectioned.[22] Practically, release of the medial edge (arcade) is necessary, following which the nerve should be inspected in its course into the supinator. At a minimum, the distal margin should be inspected if no dynamic or static nerve compression can be demonstrated at the arcade. If there is significant nerve flattening or narrowing, an epineurotomy and, possibly, an internal neurolysis should be performed. Narrowing is seen in a relatively low proportion of cases and may be attributed to the fact that a greater number

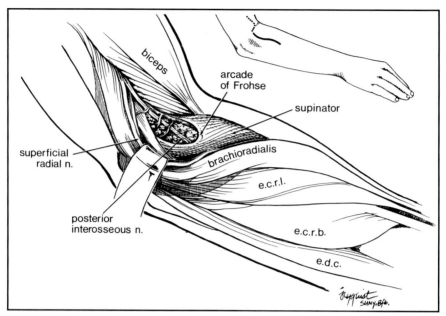

Figure 11-2. The radial nerve proper and proximal PIN are exposed by extension of the skin incision and dissection in the intermuscular plane *between* brachioradialis and brachialis/biceps. The lateral epicondyle can be exposed, if needed, by turning this extended skin incision posteriorly instead of anteriorly and proximally.

of these patients have intermittent compression which, unlike other neuropathies, allows the patient to "decompress" the nerve by rotating the forearm. Evaluation of the compressed nerve under the operating microscope in five cases by Hagert revealed differing extents of compression in separate parts of the nerve, which helps to explain the variety of presentations and symptomatology from pain to weakness to paralysis.[30]

Results of Treatment

The late results of decompression of pain due to radial tunnel syndrome are quite good in our own experience. Relief of pain, except for mild, occasional discomfort, was achieved in 169 of 198 (85 percent) of the combined series of patients (Table 11-1). The best results were obtained if the nerve appeared normal at surgery. Relief of the epicondylar pain frequently occurs within days, although the muscular aching may take several months or a year to resolve fully. Recurrence is discussed only by Werner, who noted problems in 6 of 90 (7 percent) cases.[74] Reoperation and decompression were performed on these patients, with good results in five, although scar surrounded the nerve of each.

Even if patients present with complete paralysis, function may return as much as 18 months following decompression. If patients present with incomplete paralysis, the prognosis may be considerably better.[64] However,

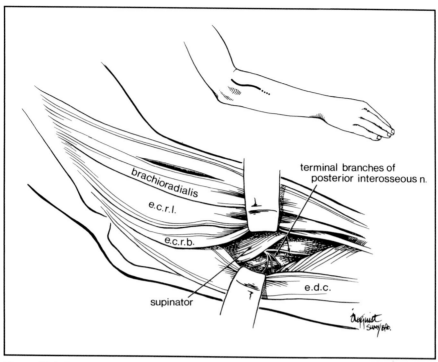

Figure 11-3. The distal portion of the PIN on exit from the supinator is found by extending the skin incision and opening the fascia between EDC and ECRL.

Table 11-1			
	Nerve Tenderness (N = 198)	**+ Resisted Supination (N = 198)**	**+ Resisted Mid. Finger (N X= 160)**	**Epicondylar Pain (N = 198)**
---	---	---	---	---
Lister et al.[43]	19	19	20	3
Roles/ Maudsley[59]	38	38	Not recorded	38
Hagert et al.[30]	50	43	29	20
Werner[74]	90	84	67	61
	197(99%)	192(97%)	116(72%)	122(62%)

if a patient is followed for 8 to 12 weeks after presentation with a complete PIN palsy with no sign of recovery, the nerve should be tested and then decompressed to maximize return of function.

Summary

Radial tunnel syndrome is a distinct clinical entity caused by a compression neuropathy of the posterior interosseous nerve. It presents with signs and symptoms correlating to the nerve and its innervations. Treatment of the neuropathy requires decompression of the nerve, whether by nonoperative means or by surgical decompression. The results of surgery are quite good with respect to relief of pain in 85 percent; the most common complication of this procedure is an unsightly scar.

We wish to acknowledge John A. Nyquist for the medical illustrations for this chapter and Frances S. Sherwin for assistance with the preparation of the manuscript.

References

1. Adams JP, Rizzoli HV: Tardy radial and ulnar nerve palsy. J Neurosurg 16:342, 1959.
2. Agnew DH: Bursal tumor producing loss of power of forearm. Am J Med Sci 46:404, 1863.
3. Barber KW, Bianco AJ, Soule EH, MacCarty CS: Benign extraneural soft-tissue tumors of the extremities causing compression of nerve. J Bone Joint Surg 44A:98, 1962.
4. Barton NJ: Radial nerve lesions. Hand 5:200, 1973.
5. Blakemore ME: Posterior interosseous nerve paralysis caused by a lipoma. J Roy Coll Surg 24:113, 1976.
6. Belsole RJ, Lister GD, Kleinert HE: Polyarteritis: A cause of nerve palsy in the extremity. J Hand Surg 3:320, 1978.
7. Bosworth DM: Surgical treatment of tennis elbow. J Bone Joint Surg 47A:1533, 1965.
8. Bowen TL, Stone KH: Posterior interosseous nerve paralysis caused by a ganglion at the elbow. J Bone Joint Surg 48B:774, 1966.
9. Boyd HB, McLeod AC: Tennis elbow. J Bone Joint Surg 55A:1183, 1973.
10. Bryan FS, Miller LS, Panijayanond P: Spontaneous paralysis of the posterior interosseous nerve. Clin Orthop Rel Res 80:9, 1971.
11. Burns J, Lister GD: Localized constrictive radial neuropathy in the absence of extrinsic compression: Three cases. J Hand Surg 9A:99, 1984.
12. Campbell CS, Wulf RF: Lipoma producing a lesion of the deep branch of the radial nerve. J Neurosurg 11:310, 1954.
13. Capener N: Tennis elbow and posterior interosseous nerve. Br Med J 2:130, 1960.
14. Capener N: The vulnerability of the posterior interosseous nerve of the forearm. J Bone Joint Surg 48B:770, 1966.
15. Cohen BE, Cukier J: Simultaneous posterior and anterior interosseous nerve syndromes. J Hand Surg 7:398, 1982.
16. Coonrad RW, Hooper WR: Tennis elbow: Its course, natural history, conservative and surgical management. J Bone Joint Surg 55A:1177, 1973.
17. Crawford GP: Radial tunnel syndrome. J Hand Surg 9A:451, 1984.
18. Davies F, Laird M: The supinator muscle and the deep radial (posterior interosseous) nerve. Anat Rec 101:243, 1948.

19. Derkash RS, Niebauser JJ: Entrapment of the posterior interosseous nerve by a fibrous band in the dorsal edge of the supinator muscle and erosion of a groove in the proximal radius. J Hand Surg 6:524, 1981.

20. Dharapak C, Nimberg GA: Posterior interosseous nerve compression. Clin Orthop Rel Res 101:225, 1974.

21. Engel J, Favin Y, Horozovsky H, Shilo R: Thermography of the Elbow joint. J Bone Joint Surg 58B:382, 1976.

22. Eversmann WW: Compression and entrapment neuropathies of the upper extremity. J Hand Surg 8:759, 1983.

23. Galbraith KA, McCullough CJ: Acute nerve injury as a complication of closed fractures or dislocations of the elbow. Injury 11:159, 1979.

24. Garden RS: Tennis elbow. J Bone Joint Surg 43B:100, 1961.

25. Gardner E: The innervation of the elbow joint. Anat Rec 102:161, 1948.

26. Gassel MM, Diamantopoulos E: Pattern of conduction times in the distribution of the radial nerve. Neurology 14:222, 1964.

27. Giattini JF: The anatomy of the radial nerve at the elbow and its relationship to tennis elbow. Proceedings American Academy of Orthopaedic Surgeons, J Bone Joint Surg 50A:843, 1968.

28. Goldman S, Honet JC, Sobel R, Goldstein AS: Posterior interosseous nerve palsy in the absence of trauma. Arch Neurol 21:435, 1969.

29. Guillain G, Courtellement: L'action du muscle court supinator dans la paralysie du nerf radial. Presse Med 13:50, 1905.

30. Hagert C-G, Lundborg G, Hansen T: Entrapment of the posterior interosseous nerve. Scand J Plast Reconstr Surg 11:205, 1977.

31. Hall HC, MacKinnon SE, Gilbert RW: An approach to the posterior interosseous nerve. Plast Reconstr Surg 74:435, 1984.

32. Heyse-Moore GH: Resistant tennis elbow. J Hand Surg 9B:64, 1984.

33. Hollinshead WH, Markee JE: The multiple innervation of limb muscles in man. J Bone Joint Surg 28:721, 1946.

34. Holst-Nielsen F, Jensen V: Tardy posterior interosseous nerve palsy as a result of an unreduced radial head dislocation in Monteggia fractures: A report of two cases. J Hand Surg 9A:572, 1984.

35. Hustead AP, Mulder DW, MacCarty CS: Nontraumatic, progressive paralysis of the deep radial (posterior interosseous) nerve. AMA Arch Neurol Psych 79:269, 1958.

36. Jebsen RH: Motor conduction velocity of distal radial nerve. Arch Phys Med Rehab 47:12, 1966.

37. Kaplan EB: Treatment of tennis elbow (epicondylitis) by denervation. J Bone Joint Surg 41A:147, 1959.

38. Kaplan EB: The etiology and treatment of epicondylitis. Bull Hosp Joint Dis 29:77, 1968.

39. Kopell HP, Thompson WAL: Peripheral Entrapment Neuropathies. Baltimore, The William & Wilkins Company, 1963, pp 121.

40. Kruse F Jr: Paralysis of the dorsal interosseous nerve not due to direct trauma. A case showing spontaneous recovery. Neurology 8:307, 1958.

41. Lichter RL, Jacobsen T: Tary palsy of the posterior interosseous nerve with a Monteggia fracture. J Bone Joint Surg 57A:124, 1975.

42. Lipscomb PR, Burleson RJ: Vascular and neural complications in supracondylar fractures of the humerus in children. J Bone Joint Surg 37A:487, 1955.

43. Lister GD, Belsole RB, Kleinert HE: The radial tunnel syndrome. J Hand Surg 4:52, 1979.

44. Lotem M, Fried A, Levy M, Solzi P, Najenson T, Nathan H: Radial palsy following muscular effort: J Bone Joint Surg 53B:500, 1971.
45. Manske PR: Compression of the radial nerve by the triceps muscle. A case report. J Bone Joint Surg 59A:835, 1977.
46. Marmor L, Lawrence JF; Dubois EL: Posterior interosseous nerve palsy due to rheumatoid arthritis. J Bone Joint Surg 49A:381, 1967.
47. Marshall SC, Murray WR: Deep radial nerve palsy associated with rheumatoid arthritis. Clin Orthop Rel Res 103:157, 1974.
48. Mass DP, Tortosa R, Newmeyer WL, Kilgore ES: Compression of posterior interosseous nerve by a ganglion—Case report. J Hand Surg 8:92, 1982.
49. Mayer JH, Mayfield FH: Surgery of the posterior interosseous branch of the radial nerve. Surg Gynecol Obstet 84:979, 1947.
50. Millender LH, Nalebuff EA, Holdsworth DE: Posterior interosseous-nerve syndrome secondary to rheumatoid synovitis. J Bone Joint Surg 55A:753, 1973.
51. Moon N, Marmor L: Parosteal lipoma of the proximal part of the radius. A clinical entity with frequent radial-nerve injury. J Bone Joint Surg 46A:608, 1964.
52. Morris AH: Irreducible Monteggia lesion with radial-nerve entrapment. J Bone Joint Surg 56A:1744, 1974.
53. Moss SH, Switzer HE: Radial tunnel syndrome: A spectrum of clinical presentations. J Hand Surg 8:414, 1983.
54. Mulholland RC: Non-traumatic progressive paralysis of the posterior interosseous nerve. J Bone Joint Surg 48B:781, 1966.
55. Nielsen HO: Posterior interosseous nerve paralysis caused by fibrous band compression at the supinator muscle. A report of four cases. Acta Orthop Scand 47:304, 1976.
56. Nirschl RP, Pettrone FA: Tennis elbow. The surgical treatment of lateral epicondylitis. J Bone Joint Surg 61A:832, 1979.
57. Popelka S, Vainio K: Entrapment of the posterior interosseous branch of the radial nerve in rheumatoid arthritis. Acta Orthop Scand 45:370, 1974.
58. Richmond DA: Lipoma causing a posterior interosseous nerve lesion. J Bone Joint Surg 35B:83, 1953.
59. Roles NC, Maudsley RH: Radial tunnel syndrome. Resistant tennis elbow as a nerve entrapment. J Bone Joint Surg 54B:499, 1972.
60. Sharrard WJW: Posterior interosseous neuritis. J Bone Joint Surg 48B:777, 1966.
61. Somerville EW: J Bone Joint Surg 45B:621, 1963.
62. Spar 1: A neurologic complication following Monteggia fracture. Clin Orthop Rel Res 122:207, 1977.
63. Spinner M: The Arcade of Frohse and its relationship to posterior interosseous nerve paralysis. J Bone Joint Surg 50B:809, 1968.
64. Spinner M: Injuries to the Major Branches of Peripheral Nerves of the Forearm. Philadelphia, W.B. Saunders Company, 1978, pp 80.
65. Spinner M, Freundlich BD, Teicher J: Posterior interosseous nerve palsy as a complication of Monteggia fractures in children. Clin Orthop 58:141, 1968.
66. Spinner M, Spencer PS: Nerve compression lesions of the upper extremity. A clinical and experimental review. Clin Orthop 104:46, 1974.
67. Sponseller PD, Engber WD: Double-entrapment radial tunnel syndrome. J Hand Surg 8:420, 1983.
68. Strachan JCH, Ellis BW: Vulnerability of the posterior interosseous nerve during radial head resection. J Bone Joint Surg 53B:320, 1971.

69. Straus WL Jr: The phylogeny of the human forearm extensors. Human Biology 13:23-50, 203, 1941.
70. Stein F, Grabias SL, Deffer PA: Nerve injuries complicating Monteggia lesions. J Bone Joint Surg 53A:1432, 1971.
71. Sunderland S: Nerves and Nerve Injuries. Edinburgh, Churchill Livingstone, 1978, pp 802.
72. Turner JWA, Parsonage MJ:: Neuralgic amyotrophy (paralytic brachial neuritis). Lancet 2:209, 1957.
73. Van Rossum J, Buruma OJS, Kamphuisen HAC, Onvlee GJ: Tennis elbow—A radial tunnel syndrome? J Bone Joint Surg 60B:197, 1978.
74. Werner C-O: Lateral elbow pain and posterior interosseous nerve entrapment. Acta Orthop Scand Suppl 174:1, 1979.
75. Whiteley WH, Alpers BJ: Posterior interosseous nerve palsy with spontaneous neuroma formation. AMA Arch Neurol 1:118, 1959.
76. White WL, Hanna DC: Troublesome lipomata of the upper extremity. J Bone Joint Surg 44A:1353, 1962.
77. Woltman HW, Learmonth JR: Progressive paralysis of the nervus interosseous dorsalis. Brain 57:25, 1934.
78. Wu K-T, Jordan FR, Eckert C: Lipoma, a cause of paralysis of deep radial (posterior interosseous) nerve: Report of a case and review of the literature. Surgery 75:790, 1974.

CHAPTER 12

Superficial Radial Nerve Compression Syndrome

Robert M. Szabo, M.D.

Compression neuropathy of the sensory branch of radial nerve is uncommonly recognized and, at times, misdiagnosed. Wartenberg described five cases in 1932 and suggested the condition be named "cheiralgia paraesthetica" because of its similarity to the isolated involvement of the lateral cutaneous nerve of the thigh which had been called meralgia paraesthetica.[13] Cheiralgia paraesthetica, however, has since become known as "Wartenberg's Disease." Wartenberg, and later Sprofkin,[12] both wrote that cheiralgia paraesthetica is second only to meralgia paraesthetica in frequency among the modern neuropathies. It is interesting to note that this was the opinion of the day prior to the enlightenment of the medical community in 1959 by George Phalen with his description of carpal tunnel syndrome. While compression of the median nerve at the wrist is far more commonly recognized today, the true incidence of radial sensory nerve entrapment is unknown because many cases are overlooked and the diagnosis probably confused with de Quervain's disease.

Anatomy

The radial nerve branches into the posterior interosseous nerve and the superficial radial nerve at the level of the lateral epicondyle. It then descends along the lateral side of the forearm approaching the radial artery at the lower border of the supinator muscle and runs parallel to the radial artery in the mid-third of the forearm across the pronator teres. It lies beneath the tendon of the brachioradialis and, several centimeters above the wrist, pierces the deep fascia and crosses the dorsal retinaculum, where it usually divides into a radial and ulnar branch. The two main branches then further divide into five dorsal digital nerves, which are distributed to the dorsal radial aspect of the thumb and thenar eminence and the dorsum of the index, long, and ring fingers as far as the proximal interphalangeal joints.

Near the wrist level, the superficial branch of the radial nerve is applied closely to the dorsal lateral aspect of the radius surrounded by tight strands of fascia. It is cushioned by neither muscle nor fat, and its superficial location makes it easily susceptible to any compressive force, particularly one externally applied. The nerve becomes subcutaneous at the posterior border of the brachioradialis tendon. When the forearm is supinated, the superficial branch of the radial nerve lies between the tendons of the brachioradialis and extensor carpi radialis longus without compression from these two tendons. When the forearm is pronated, however, the extensor carpi radialis longus crosses beneath the brachioradialis tendon, and in a scissor-like fashion creates compression on the superficial branch of the radial nerve.[3] Palmar ulnar flexion of the wrist puts the nerve on maximum stretch.

Clinical Signs of Superficial Radial Nerve Entrapment

Patients with entrapment of the radial sensory nerve complain of pain, numbness, tingling, and dysesthesias over the dorsal radial aspect of the hand. The symptoms are often brought on by, and always made worse by, wrist movement. Vasomotor symptoms and night pain are not part of the symptom complex. The pain intensifies in making a tight grip with the thumb and index finger to the point of limiting the use of the hand.[5]

On physical exam, percussion along the course of the nerve produces paresthesias. This can be greatest either in the midforearm where the nerve exits underneath the tendon of the brachioradialis or more distally where the nerve lies directly over the distal radius. Sensibility may be decreased compared to the opposite hand when tested with Semmes-Weinstein monofilaments. Wartenberg demonstrated that movements of pronation and ulnar flexion of the wrist provokes the symptoms.[13] Dellon describes a provocative test for entrapment of the superficial branch of the radial nerve. The patient is instructed to pronate the forearm. If within 30 to 60 seconds the symptoms of paresthesias or dysesthesias are evoked or exacerbated over the dorsal radial aspect of the hand, entrapment is confirmed.[3]

In Dellon's series of 51 patients with superficial radial nerve entrapment, associated problems were frequent, including carpal tunnel syndrome (57 percent), first dorsal extensor tenosynovitis (17 percent), neuroma of the lateral antebrachial cutaneous nerve (2 percent), other peripheral nerve entrapment syndromes (34 percent), and injury to the terminal branch of the posterior interosseous nerve (6 percent).[3] Ninety-six percent of his patients had a positive "Finkelstein" sign.

The single entity most commonly confused with cheiralgia paresthetica is deQuervain's disease. In 1985 deQuervain described stenosing tendovaginitis at the radial styloid process as a condition affecting the tendon sheath of the abductor pollicis longus and extensor pollicis brevis. The symptom complex of this disease consists of pain at the radial styloid process radiating down the thumb and up the forearm, mild swelling over the first dorsal compartment, and pain on movements of the thumb and wrist along with inability to grasp objects firmly.[6] Finkelstein considered that excruciating pain over the radial styloid produced upon quick ulnar deviation of the hand with the patient's thumb grasped in the palm to be pathognomonic of deQuervain's disease. This same motion produces traction on the superficial branch of the radial nerve, thus also causing pain when entrapment is present. These two entities may be differentiated by the presence or absence of swelling over the first dorsal compartment, a nerve percussion test over the course of the superficial radial nerve, and careful sensory testing. A diagnostic nerve block performed with local anesthetic infiltrated dorsal to the musculotendinous junction of the brachioradialis will also help differentiate these two entities. Electrodiagnostic studies may be performed; however, their yield has not been very high for confirming superficial radial nerve entrapment.[3]

Another entity that must be considered in the presence of dorsal radial wrist dysesthesias and paresthesias is an injured lateral antebrachial cutaneous nerve. MacKinnon has pointed out the anatomic relationship between the lateral antebrachial cutaneous nerve and the superficial branch of the radial nerve in 53 cadaver dissections. Partial or complete overlap of these two sensory nerves occurred in 75 percent of the cases.[8] The terminal branches of the lateral antebrachial cutaneous nerve are also susceptible to injury over the distal radius for the same reasons that the superficial branch of the radial nerve is. The lateral antebrachial cutaneous nerve may be blocked with local anesthetic in the proximal forearm just distal to the cubital crease and adjacent to the cephalic vein. Such a diagnostic block will rule out pathology related to the lateral antebrachial cutaneous nerve. The nerve is fairly deep, and one must confirm numbness in its distribution to be sure of an effective block. I have seen a patient who sustained a contusion injury to her dominant hand which resulted in exquisite pain and dysesthesias over the dorsal radial aspect of her wrist, who had a positive nerve percussion test, a positive Finkelstein's test and decreased sensation over the dorsal radial aspect of her wrist. All of these symptoms temporarily disappeared with a diagnostic block of the lateral antebrachial cutaneous nerve in the proximal forearm.

Etiology

As with other nerve compression syndromes, there are many factors of etiologic importance. Most patients will give a history of either a contusion injury to the wrist or forearm or some job-related activity requiring repetition motion such as using a screwdriver, prolonged writing with a pen, or using a typewriter.[3,5] Dellon has postulated that a distal injury entraping the nerve in scar tissue at the wrist prohibits the superficial branch of the radial nerve to slide and adjust its position as the tendons of the extensor carpi radialis brevis and brachioradialis change positions in pronation and supination. In time, the proximal edema and fibrosis result in chronic nerve compression.[3] Any activities that require repetitive forearm pronation and supination will thus aggravate the disease. Histopathology in at least one case has laid credence to this theory.[9]

Another group of patients have Wartenberg's disease due to external compression. The offending agent most commonly is a tight wristwatch band.[1-3,5,7] The distal branches of the lateral antebrachial cutaneous nerve may also be compressed by the same tight wristwatch band. These cases tend to improve with conservative measures by removing the offending agent. A similar group of patients have been described with Wartenberg's disease secondary to the prolonged application of tight handcuffs.[4,10]

Superficial radial nerve entrapment may result secondary to deQuervain's disease.[11] The inflammed diseased tenosynovial structures over the first dorsal compartment may cause scarring and entrapment of the distal branch of the superficial radial nerve presenting a mixed picture of symptoms of both diseases. I have seen unhappy patients with pain and paresthesias in the distribution of the radial nerve after having their first dorsal compartment released for deQuervain's disease by very careful and reputable surgeons. Many times their symptoms have improved with conservative treatment, and I have often wondered if the insult to the nerve came from the inflammatory disease state or from traction on the nerve during surgery. Unless one specifically tests for and recognizes superficial radial neuritis before surgery for deQuervain's disease, one cannot inform the patient about the prolonged recovery expected.

Treatment

Since the entrapment of the superficial branch of the radial nerve produces a pure pain or sensory syndrome, with no possibility of irreversible motor loss resulting in weakness, conservative therapy should be tried before considering surgical intervention. Certainly in the case of external compression such as that caused by a tight wrist band, elimination of the offending agent usually leads to a cure. If the condition does not subside, it is worth trying a local injection of steroid into the area of maximum pain. Steroid injections have been reported to be effective.[2] When pain due to superficial radial nerve involvement appears in conjunction with deQuervain's disease, the symptoms associated with tendon entrapment may disappear immediately after surgery, but the nerve symptoms may persist for two or three months more.[11] Therefore, once a diagnosis of Wartenberg's disease is confirmed, a program of restricted activities, anti-inflammatory medications and splinting should be instituted for at least several months. It is also worth having the patient perform desensitization on the distal portion of the superficial branch of the radial nerve. This treatment, as with neuromas, may decrease the tenderness and paresthesias.

When nonoperative management fails, then surgery is considered. Surgery can be expected to produce good results in about 85 percent of patients.[3] The operation is directed at releasing the entire nerve from the fascia in the forearm starting at a point where it exits between the tendons of the extensor carpi radialis longus and brachioradialis. Under axillary block anesthesia, a longitudinal incision 3 inches in length is made overlying the midradial aspect of the radius starting about 1 inch proximal from the tip of the radial styloid, centered over the point where the nerve starts its subcutaneous course (Figure 12-1A). The incision must be palmar enough in location so as not to overlie the nerve directly, in which case further scarring may result in further problems. The radial nerve is identified between the extensor carpi radialis longus and the brachioradialis and tagged with a rubber dam. The fascia between the brachioradialis and extensor carpi radialis longus is released proximally and distally (Figure 12-1B-D). The radial sensory nerve should then lie loosely in its bed, and the extensor carpi radialis longus and brachioradialis tendons have independent gliding without constricting the nerve. The nerve should then carefully be examined for any areas of constriction. If none are found, it should be left alone. If an area of constriction is identified, an epineurotomy under magnification is performed. Excess handling of the nerve and extensive neurolysis should be avoided, as both are associated with increased scarring postoperatively. The wound is then closed and a bulky compression dressing applied. At 10 days the sutures are removed, and the patient is allowed unrestricted motion and encouraged to use the hand as much as possible.

The preceding extensive fasciotomy is indicated when symptoms clearly point to compression of the major branch of the senory radial nerve in the midforearm. This can be determined by the presence of the positive nerve percussion test in this area. However, if there is clearly a distal area of constriction and the Tinel is more pronounced at the radial styloid area, I feel that this area should be explored through a less extensive approach. A one-inch longitudinal incision is made centered over the point of maximum tenderness and positive nerve percussion sign distally. The incision is made only through skin and the subcutaneous tissues gently

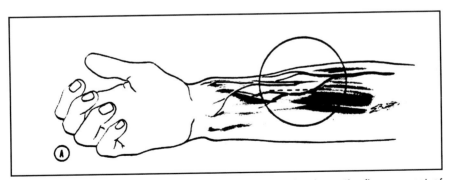

Figure 12-1A. Operative technique. Dotted line for incision is on the flexor aspect of the forearm, centered about the radial sensory nerve (RSN) Tinel sign at point of exit from fascia. Note to avoid injury to overlapping lateral antebrachial cutaneous nerve branch.

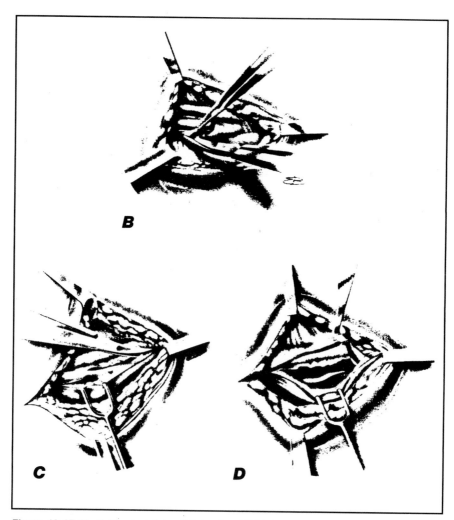

Figure 12-1B-D. *B*, Fascia joining BR tendon–ECRL is divided distally to BR insertion. *C*, This fascia is then released proximally until the RSN is lying loosely in its bed, and the BR and ECRL have independent gliding without constricting this nerve. *D*, The externally neurolysed RSN. Note the area of constriction in the nerve where it traversed from deep to superficial through the fascia (from Dellon, A.L., MacKinnon, S.E.: Radial Sensory Nerve Entrapment in the Forearm. J Hand Surg 11A:201–202, 1986, with permission).

dissected with a blunt scissor and the terminal branches of the radial nerve identified. An area of compression is sought out and released. The branches of the radial nerve are then examined under the microscope and a careful microdissection including epineurotomy is performed. Once again, extensive internal neurolysis and traction on the nerves are avoided. The wound is then closed in a double flapped Z-plasty, suturing skin edges only. A plaster-reinforced bulky hand dressing is applied, and the postoperative course is similar to that already described. There is not usually the same dramatic relief immediately postsurgery as one finds with carpal tunnel releases. Patients might be counseled to anticipate a prolonged course before expecting much relief.

The importance of the relationship between the superficial branch of the radial nerve and the lateral antebrachial cutaneous nerve must always be remembered before advising surgery on the radial nerve. Operative failures may relate to addressing the wrong nerve at the time of surgery. One will not fall into this trap if a careful exam with accompanying diagnostic nerve blocks in the proximal forearm is performed prior to surgery. Resection of the superficial branch of the radial nerve in the proximal forearm is not indicated as the initial treatment of Wartenberg's disease. It may be indicated as a salvage procedure, particularly after failed surgery or when there is an associated neuroma distally.

References

1. Bierman HR: Nerve compression due to a tight watchband. N Engl J Med 261(5):237, 1959.
2. Braidwood AS: Superficial radial neuropathy. J Bone Joint Surg 57B(3):380-383, 1975.
3. Dellon AL, Mackinnon SE: Radial sensory nerve entrapment in the forearm. J Hand Surg 11A(2):199-205, 1986.
4. Dorfman LJ, Jayaram AR: Handcuff neuropathy. JAMA 239(10):957, 1978.
5. Ehrlich W, Dellon AL, Mackinnon SE: Cheiralgia paresthetica (entrapment of the radial sensory nerve). J Hand Surg 11A(2):196-199, 1986.
6. Finkelstein H: Stenosing tendovaginitis at the radial styloid process. J Bone Joint Surg 12A:509-539, 1930.
7. Linscheid RL: Injuries to radial nerve at wrist. Arch Surg 91:942-946, 1965.
8. Mackinnon SE, Dellon AL: The overlap pattern of the lateral antebrachial cutaneous nerve and the superficial branch of the radial nerve. J Hand Surg 10A(4):522-526, 1985.
9. Mackinnon SE, Dellon AL, Hudson AR, Hunter DA: Histopathology of compression of the superficial radial nerve in the forearm. J Hand Surg 11A(2):206-210, 1980.
10. Massey EW, Pleet AB: Handcuffs and cheiralgia paresthetica. Neurology 28:1312-1313, 1978.
11. Rask MR: Superficial radial neuritis and de Quervain's disease. Clin Orthop 131:176-178, 1978.
12. Sprofkin BE: Cheiralgia paresthetica—Wartenberg's Disease. Neurology 4:857-862, 1954.
13. Wartenberg R: Cheiralgia paresthetica. Ztschr Neurol u Psychiat 141:145, 1932.

CHAPTER 13

Lateral Antebrachial Nerve Compression

James A. Nunley, II, M.D., F.A.C.S.
Patricia Howson, M.D., C.M., F.R.C.S.(C)

The musculocutaneous nerve of the upper extremity rarely is involved in compressive neuropathy. Of 14,300 peripheral nerve injuries summarized by Sunderland, 228 involved the musculocutaneous nerve—all being caused by direct trauma, avulsion, or missile forces.[16] Compressive neuropathy to the motor portion of the nerve above the elbow has been reported in only five instances.[3,10] Duke Medical Center lists only 11 cases of sensory compressive neuropathy in some 3000 peripheral nerve injuries seen over a 15-year period;[2] isolated reports confirm its infrequency.[4,7]

The terminal branches of the musculocutaneous nerve, as they come to lie subcutaneous at the level of the cubital fossa, are purely sensory and are variously termed the lateral antebrachial or lateral cutaneous nerve to the forearm. Although compression of the lateral cutaneous nerve of the forearm is not often recognized, the clinical presentation is clear, the treatment specific, and the results reproducible.

Clinical Presentation

Entrapment of the musculocutaneous nerve occurs at the level of the elbow joint where only sensory fibers remain.

History

Characteristically, patients with acute compression give a history of repetitive, specific, forceful exercise of the elbow, with the elbow in a position of extension while the forearm is either pronated or supinated. The time frame of acute compression is usually less than three months duration from the inciting event to clinical presentation. Mechanisms of injury seen have been tennis overhead smashes, backhand stroke or a poorly executed forehand stroke with rolling over from supination to pronation with the elbow extended, a sudden reach behind the back with the arm internally rotated, pronated and extended, or simply sudden actively resisted hyperextension. Complaints are predominately pain on active motion of the elbow, with accompanying burning or numbness in the radial forearm.

In long-standing cases, the history may be rather vague, or even misleading, having been variously diagnosed as cervical radiculitis, resistant tennis elbow, refractory lateral epicondylitis, anterior interosseous nerve compression, or median nerve compression. In chronic cases, the pain is more an aching discomfort of the antecubital fossa region, usually without dysesthesia (Table 13-1).

Table 13.1		
	Acute	**Chronic**
Symptoms	clear event forceful extension elbow	vague repetitive/overuse in extension
Signs	pain — radial forearm ± paresthesias	pain — vague forearm paresthesias prominent
Pathology	impingement by biceps tendon	impingement by biceps tendon

Physical Findings

Although subjectively unaware of it, the patient usually has some limitation of elbow extension which is evident only with the forearm pronated. In supination, where the biceps is somewhat more relaxed, there is full extension. Characteristically, point tenderness is found lateral to the biceps tendon at the elbow crease—the point at which the nerve exits from beneath the muscle and comes to lie superficial. Though the patient may be unaware, objective sensory changes are usually present with hypesthesia along the distal, palmar, radial forearm (Fig. 13-1).

Anatomy and Pathomechanics

Derived from the fifth, sixth and to a lesser extent, seventh cervical roots, the nerve fibers of the musculocutaneous nerve descend in the upper trunk, through the anterior division picking up fibers of C7 to become the lateral cord found lateral to the brachial artery within the sheath at the level of the inferior border of pectoralis minor[5,6] (Fig. 13-2). The musculocutaneous nerve quickly leaves the lateral cord traveling laterally and distally deep to the coracobrachialis muscle while supplying this muscle at the level of the insertion of latissimus dorsi into the humerus. As the nerve continues distally it emerges anterolateral to the coracobrachialis muscle under cover of the biceps. Here the nerve is sandwiched between biceps and brachialis muscle, both of which it supplies with motor fibers. There are no anatomic points of compression down to this level. The musculocutaneous nerve then emerges at the level of the elbow crease *lateral* to the bicipital tendon, but medial to the brachioradialis muscle. It is here that the musculocutaneous nerve containing only sensory fibers is subject to compression. Classic texts describe the terminal portion as emerging several centimeters above the elbow crease at the level of the musculotendinous junction of the biceps. However, anatomic dissections by Olsen have demonstrated that the nerve, emerging more distally, remains under the tendon until it reaches the antecubital crease.[12] The flat, sharp edge of the biceps tendon lies taut with the elbow in extension but becomes even more taut if the biceps tendon is contracting against resisted flexion and pronation. If the arm is passively pronated with the elbow in extension, the tendon is likewise put on stretch. It is at the elbow crease that the unprotected musculocutaneous nerve may be compressed. In fact, violent extension of the elbow has reportedly caused complete severence of the nerve at this level.[16]

From the elbow distally, the sensory portion, termed the lateral antebrachial cutaneous (or lateral cutaneous nerve to the forearm) lies subcutaneously, and is in fact superficial to the antebrachial fascia. Important landmarks used in finding the lateral cutaneous nerve of the forearm are the major forearm veins. In the elbow crease, the nerve lies between the cephalic and median cubital vein about 1.5 cms lateral to the biceps tendon. As it leaves the fossa, the nerve lies parallel and closely allied and in a plane deep to the cephalic vein, which is easily identifiable in most patients. The nerve divides into anterior and posterior divisions at the junction of the middle and distal thirds of the forearm. In 30 percent of cases, it may divide more proximally at the junction of the proximal and middle third of the forearm.[11]

The anterior branch follows the lateral radial border of the forearm supplying the overlying skin and the terminal fibers arborize to innervate part of the radiocarpal joint, the intercarpal joints and the skin overlying the base of the thenar eminence (Fig. 13-1a). There is a significant overlapping of sensory territories of the lateral cutaneous nerve of forearm, the palmar cutaneous branch of the median nerve, and the superficial radial nerve.

The posterior branch of the lateral cutaneous nerve of the forearm curves more posteriorly *along* the cephalic vein and descends on the lateral border of the radius dorsally ending in the area between the dorsoradial wrist and the base of the second and third metacarpals (Fig. 13-1b). It also partially innervates the wrist joint. There is considerable sensory overlap of this branch with the medial and the posterior cutaneous nerves of the forearm, and the sensory contribution of the lateral cutaneous nerve of the forearm may in fact extend medially to the midline of the forearm. The skin sensibility over the dorsal and thenar areas of the hand is variable and may replace much of the territory supplied by the superficial radial nerve (Fig. 13-1).[1,9,14]

Figure 13-1. *a,* Palmar forearm sensory distribution of the anterior and posterior branches of the musculocutaneous nerve. *b,* Dorsal forearm. Sensory distribution of musculocutaneous nerve.

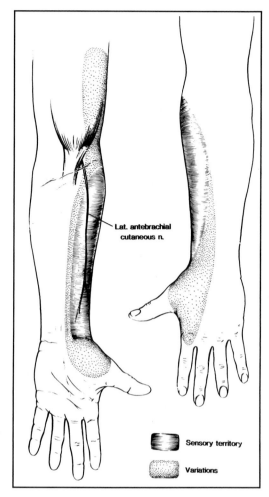

Lat. antebrachial cutaneous n.

Sensory territory

Variations

Occasionally arising from the lateral antebrachial nerve at its emergence from the biceps tendon is a recurrent branch of the musculocutaneous nerve.[16] This cutaneous nerve supplies the skin of the antecubital fossa and the distal one-third of the anterolateral aspect of the arm. This recurrent branch follows the cephalic vein in a retrograde manner. Compression of this branch of the nerve could account for some of the pain that is felt proximal to the elbow in patients with entrapment of the musculocutaneous nerve at the elbow.

Variations of the musculocutaneous nerve are numerous but basically: (1) it may be seen with the median nerve exiting at variable distances proximal to the crease or receiving branches from the median nerve; instances are estimated at 8 to 24 percent; (2) the nerve may leave the coracobrachialis muscle more superiorly and may leave the cover of the biceps tendon more superiorly; (3) it may supply the pronator teres muscle; (4) it may supply the coracobrachialis directly from the lateral cord; (5)

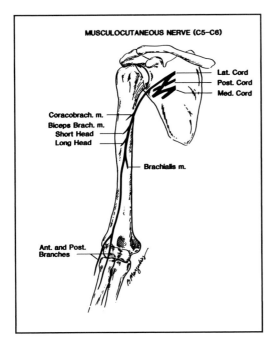

Figure 13-2. The musculocutaneous nerve takes origin from the lateral cord of the brachial plexus. Its course within the arm may be variable as it supplies the coracobrachialis, biceps, and brachialis muscles and terminates as the antebrachial cutaneous nerve.

it may contribute no fibers to the brachialis; instead, all fibers may come from the median nerve; (6) with cutaneous branches it may run with the median and exit distal to the elbow crease. The variations of the nerve above the elbow have been associated with the occasionally seen third head of the biceps.[8,15]

Electrodiagnostic Studies and Differential Diagnosis

Aside from the clinical presentation, confirmation of compression of the nerve at the elbow may be made with sensory conduction velocity studies measured between the elbow crease and the axilla. The reader is referred to Chapter 4 on the general principles of electrodiagnosis in the upper extremity. Trojaborg first determined the sensory conduction velocity for the antebrachial cutaneous nerve using needle electrodes.[17] The far nerve electrode was placed at the elbow crease lateral to the tendon. The near nerve electrode is placed either in the axilla or in the anterior cervical triangle; the position is then adjusted with the amplitude of the sensory potential recording acting as an indicator. The maximum and minimum sensory latencies are determined using 5 to 10 mA current pulse. The average normal value was 63 meters per second (range 51 to 75 meters per second). A decrease in velocity of 2 meters per second per decade of age over 20 is seen, as in most other nerves. Velocities less than this, then, must be considered diagnostic of nerve compression.

Felsenthal has used surface stimulation to measure the sensory nerve conduction velocity of the antebrachial cutaneous nerve.[13] The "distal" cathode stimulator is placed at the elbow crease lateral to the tendon and the "proximal" recording electrode is placed 12 cm distally over the anterior branch of the nerve along a line between the radial artery of the palmar wrist and "distal" electrode at the crease. A ground is placed between the two. The average conduction velocity measured with this method was 65± 3.6 meters per second (range 75 to 57 meters per second).

A later report has demonstrated the decreased amplitude of the action potential to be of more help in diagnosis, particularly if the conduction velocity is normal; the normal mean amplitude is 24 uV (S.D. 7.2 uV).[4] Abnormal values, then, are assessed if there is a 30 percent difference from the contralateral side. There has been little experience with sensory conduction velocities of the lateral antebrachial cutaneous nerve, but it does seem of good potential value.[4]

Differential Diagnosis

Compression of the musculocutaneous nerve at the elbow has frequently been confused with (1) flexor pronator syndrome, (2) radial tunnel syndrome, (3) anterior interosseous nerve compression, (4) lateral epicondylitis, (5) bicipital tendonitis, (6) intra-articular pathology, (7) cervical radiculopathy, and (8) other causes of arm pain such as coronary disease.

Management

Treatment should be directed at conservative measures common to most compressive nerve disorders; splinting or placing the limb in a sling, when combined with oral anti-inflammatories is frequently effective. If the symptoms are not improving by three to six weeks, then a trial injection of corticosteroids and local anesthetic is made, directing the needle locally first over the trigger point and then under the lateral edge of the bicipital tendon.

If by three months symptoms have not resolved, surgical decompression may be warranted. In a small series, 7 of 11 of our patients treated conservatively eventually required surgical decompression.[2]

Surgical Approach

A standard, gentle extensile curving incision is made over the antecubital fossa. The biceps tendon is identified and the nerve is easily found 1.5 cms lateral to the tendon, at the level of the medial condyle (Fig. 13-3). The nerve is traced proximally several centimeters. The entrapment may be easily demonstrated by pronating the arm in extension. Flattening and loss of vascular markings may be seen where the nerve is compressed at the edge of the biceps above and brachialis muscle below. A triangular wedge of biceps tendon (1 × 3 cm) is excised and the decompression checked by pronation/supination motions of the elbow while the arm is in extension

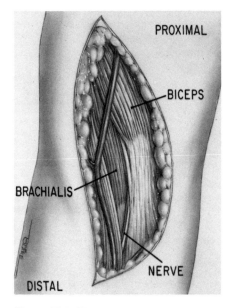

Figure 13-3. The musculocutaneous nerve is emerging at the elbow. The brachialis fascia is below, the brachioradialis muscle laterally and the biceps tendon superiorly and medially.

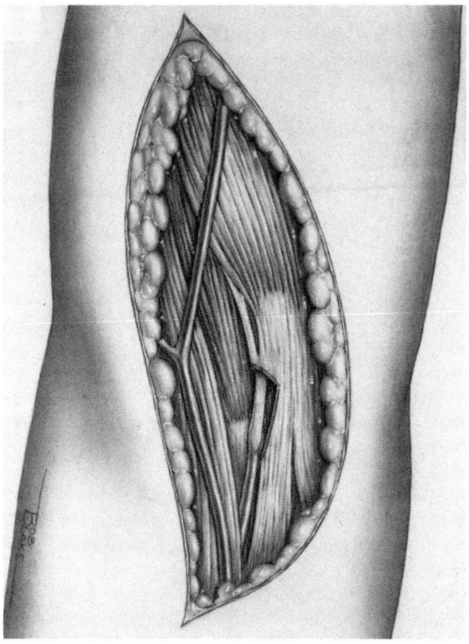

Figure 13-4. Wedge excision of lateral edge of the biceps tendon overlying a compressed lateral antebrachial cutaneous nerve.

(Fig. 13-4). Postoperatively, the elbow is splinted at 90 degrees in neutral rotation for two to three weeks and then full activity is resumed. In all our cases, there has been complete resolution of pain, the flexion contracture resolves and sensation returns.

Summary

    Lateral antebrachial nerve compression is characterized by a history of injury in resisted extension in pronation or supination, pain in the antecubital fossa and lateral forearm and/or dysesthesia of the radial forearm, and local tenderness lateral to the biceps tendon at the elbow crease. Treatment modalities include rest, splinting, oral anti-inflammatories, and local corticosteroid plus anesthetic. If refractory, surgical decompression is then performed by removing a wedge of the lateral edge of the biceps tendon.

References

1. Appleton AB: A case of abnormal distribution of the nerve musculocutaneous, with complete absence of the ramus cutaneous nerve radialis. J Anat Phys 51:89-94, 1911.
2. Bassett RH III, Nunley JA: Compression of the musculocutaneous nerve at the elbow. JBJS 64-A(7):1050-1052, 1982.

3. Braddom RL, Wolfe C: Musculocutaneous nerve injury after heavy exercise. Arch Phys Med Rehabil 59:290-291, 1978.
4. Felsenthal G, Mondell DL, Reischer MA, et.al.: Forearm pain secondary to compression syndrome of the lateral cutaneous nerve of the forearm. Arch Phys Med Rehabil 64:139-141, 1984.
5. Grant, J.C. Boileau: Grant's Atlas of Anatomy. Sixth Edition, Baltimore, Wilkins & Williams Co., 1972.
6. Gray H: Anatomy, Rev. American, from the 15th English Ed. New York, Bounty Books, 1977, pp 770-771.
7. Hale BR: Handbag paresthesia. Lancet 2:470, 1976.
8. Horiguchi M: The recurrent branch of the lateral cutaneous nerve of the forearm. J Anat 132(2):243-247, 1981.
9. Hutton WK: Remarks on the innervation of the dorsum manus, with special reference to certain rare abnormalities. J Anat Physiol 40:326-331, 1906.
10. Kim SM, Goodrich JA: Isolated proximal musculocutaneous nerve palsy: Case report. Arch Phys Med Rehabil 65:735-736, 1984.
11. Mackinnon SE, Dellon AL: The overlap pattern of the lateral antebrachial cutaneous nerve and the superficial branch of the radial nerve. J Hand 5(10A):522-526, 1985.
12. Olson IA: The origin of the lateral cutaneous nerve of the forearm and its anesthesia for modified brachial plexus block. J Anat 105(2):381-382, 1969.
13. Spindler HA, Felsenthal G: Sensory conduction in the musculocutaneous nerve. Arch Phys Med Rehabil 59:20-23, 1978.
14. Stopford JSB: The variation in distribution of the cutaneous nerves of the hand and digits. J Anat 53:14-25, 1918.
15. Serisawa M, Hagure N, Eto M: On the third head to the biceps brachii muscle and its relation to the lateral cutaneous nerve of the forearm. Dokky J Med Sci 5(2):303-312, 1978.
16. Sunderland SS: The musculocutaneous nerve. In Nerves and Nerve Injuries, 1st Ed. Baltimore, Williams and Wilkins Co., 1968, pp 886-893.
17. Trojaborg W: Motor and sensory conduction in the musculocutaneous nerve. J Neurol Neurosurg Psych 39(9):890-899, 1976.

CHAPTER 14

Thoracic Outlet Compression Syndrome

E. Bruce Toby, M.D.,
and L. Andrew Koman, M.D.

The symptom complex of upper extremity pain and paresthesia secondary to vascular or neurologic compression of the subclavian vessels or brachial plexus at the thoracic outlet has been termed "thoracic outlet compression syndrome."[1-12] Symptoms, which vary from inconsequential to incapacitating, have been attributed to venous obstruction,[4,13-15] arterial insufficiency,[4,13,16-21] lymphatic occlusion,[14] and constriction or compression of branches of the brachial plexus.[4,13,19,22-24] Structural anatomic variations, exacerbated by neck or arm position, are identifiable clinically in most patients.[4,12,25]

Despite its being one of the earliest described and most discussed of the compression neuropathies, thoracic outlet compression syndrome remains controversial.[26] In addition to disagreement over its etiology, diagnosis, and treatment, its very existence has been questioned. Estimates of incidence vary significantly, with relatively few surgeons diagnosing and treating large numbers of patients and many surgeons diagnosing and operating upon very few patients. Several investigators have reported excellent results in large series after surgical management; others have expressed concern over the number of complications and the high postoperative recurrence rates. The difficulties and hazards of surgical treatment are suggested by the frequency of liability claims associated with surgical management.[27]

The controversy and confusion are further compounded by the variability of symptom patterns and the lack of objective diagnostic criteria. In reality, the term "thoracic outlet compression syndrome" describes multiple disorders that may be grouped as primarily vascular or primarily neurologic according to the symptoms. Vascular compromise is more readily diagnosed and the results of treatment are more predictable. Unfortunately, the vast majority of symptomatic cases (approximately 90 percent) are neurologic, and it is in this subcategory that the most controversy remains.

The purpose of this chapter is to outline a comprehensive diagnostic and therapeutic approach to this complex subject.

Historical Perspective

The concept of thoracic outlet compression was postulated before the anatomy of that area was well understood, and the persistence of this initial nomenclature in juxtaposition with the true anatomic and physiologic causes of the syndrome contributes to the present confusion. The first description of osseous compression of the thoracic outlet is attributed to Hunald, who in 1743 reported on supernumerary ribs and used their presence to explain cervicobrachial pain and numbness.[1] His findings were echoed by others who placed much emphasis on vascular compression, especially of the subclavian structures.[18,20,28] Early emphasis remained focused on compression by osseous structures, and the etiologic implications of the normal first rib were postulated by Brickner in 1927.[29] Articles placing further emphasis on the importance of the first rib, its anomalies, and their role in neurovascular compression were published by Telford et al. in 1931[21] and 1948.[30]

Extraosseous thoracic outlet compression was first alluded to by Bramwell and Dykes in 1921,[22] and the implications of scalene muscle compression in neurovascular compromise of the thoracic outlet were strongly supported by others.[23,24,31] In 1927, Adson and Coffey reported relief of thoracic outlet compression by division of the scalenus anticus muscle.[31] Wright, in 1945, believed the position of the cervicobrachial anatomic structures to be the cause of symptoms, proposing the mechanism of hyperabduction with the compression of the neurovascular elements by the tendon of the pectoralis minor.[12] In 1956, Peet and colleagues recommended grouping all cervicobrachial pain and numbness syndromes under the common title, "thoracic outlet syndrome,"[3] a title that was modified by Rob and Standeven in 1958 to "thoracic outlet compression syndrome."[32] Excision of osseous structures in the treatment of thoracic outlet compression syndromes has included excision of cervical rib,[13,20] claviculectomy,[8] posterior first rib resection,[33] and transaxillary first rib resection.[5]

Pathophysiology

The neurovascular elements traverse a series of relatively narrow passageways in which traumatic, postural, or inflammatory changes can easily result in compression sufficient to produce symptoms. Areas of compression as the brachial plexus and the neurovascular structures course distally are: (1) the intrascalene space, (2) the costoclavicular space, and (3) the subpectoral area. These areas are potential sites of compression due to their unique anatomic configuration and the dynamic and functional demands of the neck and upper extremity. The presence of congenital anomalies and abnormal clavicular development[34] further complicates matters and may decrease tolerance levels so that symptoms may be precipitated by otherwise inconsequential events or occurrences.

Compression may occur at specific sites, secondary to anatomic structures, or after specific activities (Table 14-1). Compression may be on the basis of bone or nonosseous structures and may be exacerbated by the presence of inflammation, the quality of ligamentous and muscular support mechanisms, and the position of the arm, scapula, and neck.

Intrascalene Space

The intrascalene triangle is bounded anteriorly by the anterior scalene muscle, posteriorly by the middle scalene muscle, and inferiorly by the first rib. The subclavian artery and brachial plexus traverse this triangle, while the subclavian vein generally passes anterior to the anterior scalene muscle and is not affected by compression syndromes (Fig. 14-1). The pathologic processes occurring within the intrascalene area are secondary to mechanical angulation of the structures within the fixed area of the triangle or by space-occupying structures. Significant decreases in the size of the base of the intrascalene triangle have been documented in symptomatic patients.[19] Autopsy studies of normal intrascalene triangles showed the area of the base to average 1.1 cm^2,[17] while intraoperative measurements of symptomatic patients showed a decrease in triangle size of 7.7 to 7.8 mm^2 in men and a decrease of 6.5 to 6.8 mm^2 in women.[19] Since this relatively small degree of narrowing is sufficient to precipitate symptoms, the role played by any space-occupying structure may be significant. Variability in the rapidity

---

Table 14-1. Thoracic Outlet Compression Syndrome
Causes of Compression

A. Osseous
   Cervical rib
   First thoracic rib anomalies
   Large transverse process C7
   Bifid clavicle or clavicular anomaly
   Fractured clavicle
B. Non-Osseous
   Fascial remnants of cervical rib
   Fibrous anlage
   Hypertrophic muscle
   Aberrant vasculature
   Inflammation
   Tumor/neoplasm
C. Mechanical
   Hyperabduction (pectoralis minor)
   Dislocation humeral head

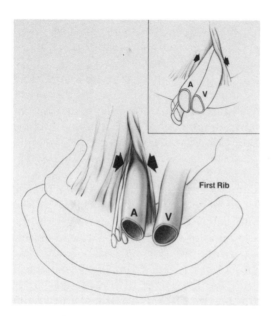

Figure 14-1. Intrascalene triangle bounded by anterior scalene muscle and posterior scalene muscles (arrows) and inferiorly by first ribs. Normally the subclavian vein is outside the triangular space, but if inside anterior scalene (inset) becomes a space-occupying mass.

with which symptoms develop is then explainable by low tolerances for inflammation or further narrowing.

The structures most commonly implicated in compression within the intrascalene triangle are: (1) cervical ribs, (2) cervical rib anlagen or fibrous bands, (3) enlarged cervical transverse processes, (4) abnormalities of the first rib that alter the insertion or position of the scalene muscles, (5) arterial anomalies, (6) venous anomalies traversing the intrascalene space, (7) changes in the size, shape, or position of the scalene muscles. Cervical ribs, which are present in approximately 1 percent of the population, are believed to be symptomatic in less than 10 percent of patients having them.[2] In fact, osseous abnormalities, including cervical ribs, long transverse processes, clavicular abnormalities, bifid first rib, and congenital synostosis of the first and second ribs, account for less than 20 percent of the patients with thoracic outlet compression syndrome seen in surgical series.[2]

Nonosseous structures have been documented to compress externally the intrascalene space and to occur as space-occupying lesions or mechanical obstructions within the intrascalene triangle. Abnormalities of the boundaries of the intrascalene space may themselves account for significant compression.[35] The most common of these problems involve the subclavian artery and the medial cord of the brachial plexus. Anatomic reasons for this are obvious: the subclavian vein generally is not involved because it rarely crosses the intrascalene triangle. The position of the medial cord of the brachial plexus, which lies in an inferior position within the intrascalene triangle, makes it most vulnerable to compression or angulation at the thoracic outlet. For this reason, C8 and T1 (ulnar nerve) symptoms predominate in intrascalene thoracic outlet compression syndromes.

Syndromes related to the intrascalene area include *Naffziger's syndrome*—scalene compression of the thoracic outlet—and *Paget-Schroetter syndrome*—progressive increase in the girth of the upper arm associated with subclavian vein thrombosis.

Costoclavicular Syndrome

Symptoms attributed to compression between the clavicle and first rib have been termed "costoclavicular" in origin. Anatomically, the space between the clavicle anteriorly and the first rib posteriorly has variable dimensions (Fig. 14-2), which depend on the position of the shoulder, the shape of the clavicle and first rib, and the neuromuscular control of the shoulder. Abduction of the upper extremity, backward retraction of the shoulder, and elevation of the first rib with deep inspiration all narrow the space, as does a hypertrophic subclavius muscle. Weakness of the suspensory muscles of the shoulder, which allows the clavicle to rest on the first rib, may further narrow the space.

Hyperabduction Syndrome

In the hyperabduction syndrome, the thoracic outlet entrapment occurs beneath the pectoralis minor, between the clavicle and the first rib, or in both locations. Symptoms are associated with abduction and external rotation of the shoulder and generally occur after or during repetitive activity. At the level of compression below the clavicle, venous engorgement may occur and neurologic symptoms may involve the entire brachial plexus (Fig. 14-3).

Clinical Presentation

The vascular, neurologic, or neurovascular symptom complex associated with thoracic outlet syndrome may be vague, ill defined, and inconsistent. Vascular lesions caused by mechanical compression of the subclavian artery or vein may result in irritation and spasm of the artery with subsequent symptoms of arterial insufficiency of the upper extremity. In addition, vascular compromise may result in an ischemic neuritis of the brachial plexus itself. Involvement of the vein may result in venous engorgement with diffuse compression of neural elements. When the artery is not primarily involved, compression of the lower trunk of the brachial plexus with subsequent degrees of neural compromise produces symptoms. Pain and abnormalities of sympathetic control secondary to the lesion may be complicating factors, with secondary reflex vasomotor and thermoregulatory changes in the upper extremity being present.[36]

Incidence

The incidence of thoracic outlet compression syndromes is difficult to ascertain, since mild and transient clinical manifestations may occur in 0.1 to 0.2 percent of the population; the incidence of symptoms sufficient to require a physician's consultation is less than 0.1 percent of the

Figure 14-2. The area of compression in the costoclavicular syndrome are indicated. Inset shows compressive effects of cervical ribs.

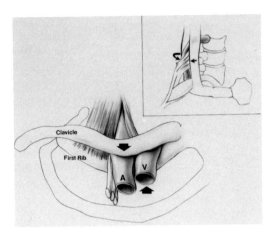

Figure 14-3. Mechanism of hyperabduction syndrome is depicted with compression beneath the pectoralis minor (arrows) and tethering at the costoclavicular area more proximally.

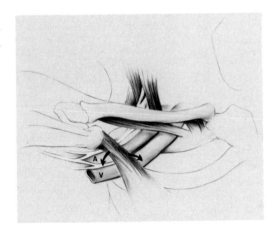

population. This syndrome may present at any age, and has been reported in teenage athletes;[10] the peak incidence of presentation is between 30 and 50 years of age (mean 36 years);[9] and 80 percent of reported cases present before age 50 years.[9,37,38] Men are less frequently symptomatic than women; male:female=1:1.5-3.[9,35,37,38] Either arm may be affected, and in 7 to 10 percent of patients both extremities are symptomatic.[35,37] A history of trauma to the head, neck, or shoulder may be present (2 to 28 percent).[37,38] Thirty to 40 percent of patients have jobs requiring repetitive activity with their arms above the head.[37]

Symptoms

Symptoms associated with thoracic outlet syndrome are those of vascular insufficiency, neurologic compromise, or both. Because the site and degree of compression vary in magnitude, often with postural and positional changes, symptoms tend to be vague and nonspecific. Pain, numbness, tingling, and paresthesias are the most common complaints. Symptoms of vasomotor instability may be present; a history of motor weakness is rarely elicited. Other entities within the differential diagnosis are outlined in Table 14-2.

Table 14-2. Differential Diagnoses

Cervical spondylosis
Apical cell lung carcinomas or lymphomas
Peripheral neuropathy
  —carpal tunnel
  —tardy ulnar palsy
Brachial plexitis/inflammatory
Malignant tumors of the neck or mediastinum
Traction injury of the brachial plexus
Raynaud's disease
Arterial insufficiency
  —atherosclerosis
  —embolic occlusion
Angina
Inflammation (arm)
  —tendinitis
  —fibrositis
  —arthritis
Hysteria

Pain: Pain is the most common finding and usually consists of a dull ache on the ulnar side of the hand. It is generally described as aching or throbbing and may involve the shoulder, arm, or hand; less frequently it may involve the neck, the chest, and even the side of the head. Symptoms may be exacerbated by arm position, particularly when the arms are held overhead. Lying on the involved side may relieve symptoms by increasing the intrascalene area and widening the costoclavicular space.

Pain may be secondary to direct compression of the brachial plexus or intermittent ischemia on the basis of compression at rest or intermittent claudication during exercise. Severe pain on awakening from sleep is often due to sleeping posture, and details of arm position should be elicited in the history.

Numbness, Tingling, Paresthesia: Symptoms of nerve irritation are common and the intensity and pattern of symptoms will depend, in part, on the mechanism. Numbness, tingling, and paresthesias secondary to direct compression are predominantly ulnar (medial cord: C8, T1), while the same neural symptoms secondary to arterial compromise may involve the entire extremity.[35,39]

Isolated median nerve symptoms are rarely due to thoracic outlet compression, and if present as the only symptom should prompt further evaluation for another cause.[25] Symptoms related purely to the radial nerve are seldom elicited.[25]

Vasomotor Disturbances: Cold intolerance, cold sensations, and periodic changes in skin color may occur. Symptoms typical of Raynaud's phenomenon may be present.

Motor Symptoms: Motor weakness is uncommon but when present will generally be manifested as intrinsic weakness. With complete occlusion of the artery, global weakness may be elicited.

Signs

Unfortunately, thoracic outlet syndrome is difficult to diagnose with certainty. The most common objective physical signs, including pulse obliteration, extremity changes with hyperabduction, and weakness, are relatively nonspecific and are found in fewer than 50 percent of patients with this syndrome.[6,12,16,21,39] The most common signs are those seen in conjunction with nerve irritation and arterial abnormalities (Table 14-3).

Table 14-3. Clinical Findings (In Descending Order of Frequency)

Symptoms	Signs
Pain	Pulse obliteration
Paresthesias	Hyperabduction
Hypesthesia	Weakness
Vasomotor weakness	Vasomotor changes
Vascular (claudication)	Hypesthesia
	Mass/bruit
	Raynaud's phenomenon
	Edema
	Gangrene

Nerve Irritation: Evidence of vasomotor instability in conjunction with dryness on the ulnar side of the hand and motor weakness may be elicited. Irritation of the sympathetic nerves may lead to vasomotor changes similar to Raynaud's phenomenon.[36] Objective motor weakness is uncommon, but occasionally may be observed. Motor weakness following abduction maneuvers associated with pulse obliteration may occur, but pulse obliteration is also present in a high percentage of normal subjects.[6,16] Similarly, vasomotor changes with associated hypesthesia are nonspecific and may be seen with a variety of abnormalities.[36]

Arterial: Pulse obliteration with diagnostic maneuvers has long been considered pathognomonic of thoracic outlet syndrome,[31] but, as mentioned, is found in many normal subjects as well. Similarly, supraclavicular bruits may be found in a high percentage of normal subjects as well as patients with thoracic outlet compression syndromes. Occasionally, gangrene and ischemic changes in the digits may be present secondary to occlusion or emboli from a damaged subclavian artery. Edema and venous engorgement are rare.

Diagnostic Maneuvers

The most commonly employed diagnostic maneuvers (Table 14-4) are discussed.

Table 14-4. Diagnostic Maneuvers

Adson test
Shoulder depression test
Hyperabduction arm/shoulder test
Three-minute arm elevation
Supraclavicular palpation

Adson Maneuver

Although the Adson maneuver is considered the classic test for thoracic outlet compression syndrome, its objective diagnostic value is questionable.[5-7,12,21,39] The test is performed in the following manner: the patient sits with hands on knees, inhales deeply, extends the head, and turns the chin toward the affected side. This should result in diminution or obliteration of the radial pulse; simultaneously, a bruit may be present on auscultation of the supraclavicular space. The Adson maneuver is designed to demonstrate the etiologic role of the scalenus anticus muscle in the compression of the subclavian artery, since that muscle is tensed during deep inspiration and extension of the neck.

Shoulder Depression

Compression at the level of the first rib and clavicle may be elicited by depressing the shoulder both backward and downward (military position), and is evidenced by diminution or obliteration of the radial pulse.

Hyperabduction of the Shoulder

With the patient in the sitting position and facing forward, the shoulder is hyperabducted and externally rotated while any changes in symptoms and any radial pulse obliteration are noted. Hyperabduction may be used in conjunction with the Adson maneuver and the shoulder depression test, but, again, it must be remembered that pulse obliteration is observed in many normal patients.

Three-Minute Arm Elevation

Elevating the arms above the head for three minutes with resulting gradual onset of numbness and tingling may be diagnostically helpful.[5-7]

Supraclavicular Brachial Plexus Palpation

Percussion and thumb pressure in the supraclavicular portion of the brachial plexus may cause symptoms and discomfort in patients with thoracic outlet compression syndrome.[5-7]

Laboratory Studies

Routine laboratory evaluations should include standard tests for complete blood cell count and blood chemistry values. Chest x-rays may be useful and may demonstrate a cervical rib, anomalous first rib, or abnormalities of the clavicle. Apical lordotic views of the chest also should be considered to rule out neoplasms. A complete series of cervical spine x-rays should be obtained if neck position influences symptoms, if range of cervical motion is limited, or if symptoms are predominantly radicular.

Special Testing

Because of difficulties in definitively diagnosing thoracic outlet compression syndrome from the history and physical examination, multiple specialized diagnostic tests have been evaluated (Table 14-5).

Table 14-5. Diagnostic Tests

Doppler/ultrasound
Peripheral nerve conduction velocity/electromyography
Arteriography
Somatosensory evoked potentials
Myelography

Doppler Ultrasonography

Doppler ultrasonography provides objective and reproducible evidence of arterial or venous compromise across the thoracic outlet.[40] Utilization of the 5 to 7.5 mHz bidirectional Doppler allows quantitative observation of waveform changes and precise arterial and venous information. Doppler studies may be performed in a noninvasive manner without morbidity or discomfort. Measurements are obtained with the patient's extremity at rest, during deep inspiration, during an Adson maneuver, with shoulder depression, and with hyperabduction of the extremity. Although it provides more precise quantitative information than the various diagnostic maneuvers that have been described, Doppler ultrasonography of the upper extremity has limitations similar to the limitations encountered with those maneuvers: Many normal subjects exhibit changes in arterial and venous flow during provocative maneuvers; vascular information is of limited value in patients who have primarily neurologic symptoms; and Doppler ultrasonography provides no objective evidence of neurologic impairment.

Real-time ultrasonography using 7.5 and 10 mHz recorders has the potential for direct visualization of the neurovascular structures. These techniques allow direct visualization of the brachial artery and surrounding structures during movement of the extremity.[41]

Peripheral Nerve Conduction Velocity/Electromyography

Using measurement of peripheral nerve conduction velocity (PNCV) and electromyography to assess primarily neurologic symptoms has significant potential diagnostic value. Unfortunately, the normal conduction velocities of the brachial plexus and the ulnar nerve vary widely, and measurement of motor conduction velocities across the thoracic outlet is technically demanding. The diagnostic accuracy of PNCV testing is limited by access to the thoracic outlet and the difficulty in evaluating large nerves by conduction velocities of single motor units (e.g., several fibers with normal conduction may prevent observation of compression of the adjacent neural tissue).

The presence of an abnormal motor PNCV is useful corroborative evidence. The addition of sensory PNCV makes this test more accurate.[42] A major role for PNCV testing and electromyography in thoracic outlet compression is the ruling out of other compression neuropathies and evidence of more proximal denervation.[43,44] Carpal tunnel syndrome, when present, generally means that the patient does not have a true thoracic outlet compression syndrome.[39]

Somatosensory Evoked Potentials

By employing the sophisticated equipment necessary to measure conduction velocities across the thoracic outlet to Erb's point or the cerebral cortex, diagnostic accuracy of evaluating neural function is significantly improved. Techniques capable of measuring somatosensory evoked potentials are currently available in most large hospitals, and are of value in assessing thoracic outlet compression syndrome.[45-49] Using these techniques, the distal peripheral nerve relevant to the patient's syndrome is stimulated transcutaneously with a low-stimulus intensity adjusted to produce a minimal twitch of the appropriate muscle. The response is recorded proximally at Erb's point, at a cervical vertebra, and at a midfrontal reference electrode. The low stimulus is averaged and an evoked latency amplitude can be calculated. It is necessary to compare the symptomatic extremity with the asymptomatic extremity in the patient with a unilateral disorder and during provocative maneuvers.

Utilizing this technique, objective evidence can be obtained in approximately 70 percent of patients with a clinical thoracic outlet compression syndrome of neurologic origin.[46] In the presence of muscle wasting or weakness, a reduction in the amplitude of the appropriate sensory evoked potential will be obtained in conjunction with prolongation of the F-wave latency.[49] Somatosensory evoked potential testing, while more sensitive than PNCV testing, has shortcomings similar to those of PNCV testing. Testing of normally conducting fibers in a nerve that has significant compression and slowing of the majority of the fibers may give a "normal" response. "Normal" somatosensory evoked potentials may be recorded in patients with clinical thoracic outlet compression syndrome if the extremity is not stressed.

Provocative tests increase diagnostic accuracy and provide objective identification of peripheral nerve compression in patients with vague symptoms.[43,45,46,49] Although current doctrine dictates that thoracic outlet compression syndrome is primarily a clinical diagnosis, the absence of abnormal somatosensory evoked potentials after provocative testing should prompt a careful re-evaluation of the patient before surgical intervention.

Arteriography

Arteriography is a valuable objective test in patients with suspected vascular compromise due to thoracic outlet compression. Arteriography may reveal compression of the artery with post-stenotic dilatation (Fig. 14-2 **inset**) or minor degrees of stenosis secondary to external compression. Post-stenotic arterial dilatation can be quantitated in the presence of thrombus, and intimal disruption can be ascertained. Venography should be restricted to patients with evidence of venous occlusion or compromise (e.g., formation of venous collaterals around the shoulder, edema, or both signs).[14,15] Arteriography has a low likelihood of providing useful information in patients with primarily neurologic symptoms or findings, and, being an invasive procedure with potential serious side effects, should not be used in those patients. It is essential that diagnostic maneuvers be performed during arteriography in order to substantiate compression.[42] The necessity for multiple tests, each requiring an additional injection of contrast material, prolongs the study and may make it extremely uncomfortable.

Myelography

Although myelography has been listed as a diagnostic test used in the evaluation of thoracic outlet syndrome, it does not, by itself, permit diagnosis of thoracic outlet compression; rather, it excludes cervical disc or tumor as a cause of the symptoms. It is our feeling that myelography is not indicated unless there is objective evidence suggesting that the symptoms have a cervical origin.

Differential Diagnosis

The differential diagnosis of thoracic outlet compression syndrome is outlined in Table 14-2. The syndrome is, by definition, a clinical diagnosis, and exclusion of those listed entities is an important part of the evaluation.

Nonoperative Treatment

Conservative treatment after the initial diagnosis of thoracic outlet compression syndrome is recommended almost universally.[16,37,50-52] Inflammation should be decreased with nonsteroidal anti-inflammatory drugs; changes in postural positions (especially in the patient who tends to drop the shoulder) should be decreased by appropriate scapular elevation exercises and isometric shoulder girdle exercises;[3,26] avoidance of activities requiring elevation of the arms over the head should be tried;[26] and moderate pain medication should be given as indicated.

Conservative management should usually be tried for six weeks to six months, and operative intervention is indicated only if symptoms persist despite all that can be done nonoperatively. Patients with vascular symptoms, especially those with evidence of digital ischemia, may require more immediate operative treatment, and they should be treated as patients with arterial insufficiency rather than thoracic outlet compression. Fifty to 90 percent of patients with primarily neurologic symptoms can be managed successfully with a physical therapy program.[3,16,25]

Operative Treatment

Vascular Symptoms

As stated previously, patients with vascular symptoms and evidence of arterial or venous insufficiency may require early surgical intervention. In this case, the surgical procedures should be directed toward the vascular problem, with removal of the compressive structures and repair, endarterectomy, or grafting of the structures as indicated by arteriography or at exploration.

Neurologic Symptoms

For patients with primarily neurologic symptoms, surgical exploration should be considered only after (1) a course of conservative management comprising shoulder girdle strengthening exercises in conjunction with activities to decrease muscle tension and eliminate faulty posture has been tried, and (2) if symptoms persist, other potential causes of the symptoms have been excluded and objective measurements are consistent with thoracic outlet compression. The potential of serious neurologic sequelae mandates delegating surgical intervention to the position of last resort. Operative alternatives include excision of the first rib or removal of the offending osseous or nonosseous structure.

First Rib Resection

The first rib may be resected by the transaxillary approach,[53] the anterior approach,[5-7] or the posterior approach.[33,54] The most common approach to decompression of the thoracic outlet is a transaxillary resection of the first rib. A cervical rib can be resected through the same approach. First rib resection is theoretically effective for either intrascalene compression or costoclavicular compression. In the former, resection of the first rib effectively decompresses the thoracic outlet by removing the floor of the intrascalene space; in the latter, the primary compressive agent is removed. Patients with significant postural abnormalities may have problems after first rib resection if depression of the shoulder allows the clavicle to abut the second rib. Patients with these postural changes should be treated by decompression of structures above the clavicle in conjunction with postoperative physical therapy to decrease shoulder depression.

Transaxillary First Rib Resection: The patient is positioned in a lateral decubitus position with the affected extremity kept superior. The arm and hand should be prepared free or positioned in an arm-holding device so that the shoulder may be moved through a full range of motion intraoperatively. Through a transverse incision made just below the axillary hairline, access is gained to the plane between the pectoralis major and latissimus dorsi (Fig. 14-4). The dissection is then deepened to the rib cage and continued superiorly until the first rib is encountered. Neurovascular structures are identified as they pass over the first rib and are protected. The anterior scalene muscle can then be visualized and divided at its attachment to the first rib. The first rib is then dissected extraperiosteally to prevent regeneration, divided anteriorly and posteriorly, and removed. At this point the arm can be taken through a full range of motion and potential compression by fibrous bands or a cervical rib anlage, and so forth, can be investigated, and any compression elements that are present can be resected.[2,5-7,55,56]

Potential complications of the transaxillary approach include injury to the long thoracic nerve, injury to the brachial plexus, pneumothorax, and postoperative pain syndrome.[2,5-7,16,55,56] Complication rates have been relatively low in large series, but there is evidence to suggest that they are much higher in smaller series.[16]

Anterior Approach (Supraclavicular): The anterior approach provides the most extensive exposure, ensures the best operative field for vascular control and reconstruction, and provides the best access to a cervical rib, the cervical sympathetic chain, and vascular structures. The major drawback to this approach is the unsightly scar.

Posterior Approach: The posterior approach, while providing easy retraction of neurologic structures, requires a large muscle-splitting incision, provides poor access to vascular structures, and leaves a large posterior scar without providing better long-term results. For these reasons, the posterior incision has largely been abandoned.

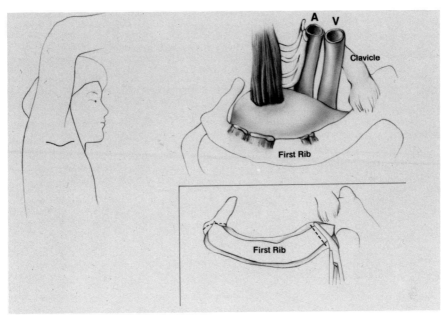

Figure 14-4. Transaxillary first rib dissection. Incision outlined on *left* and with view of first rib (*right*). Inset outlines level of anterior and posterior ribs transection.

Scalenectomy

Supraclavicular exposure of the scalene muscles with excision of compressive elements and resection of the anterior scalene muscle as needed is a safe and straightforward method for the treatment of intrascalene compression. The approach is not commonly used, because of the popularity of transaxillary first rib resection, but it has a definite role in the operative management of thoracic outlet compression syndrome. The exposure is straightforward and without the risks of bony excision.[55]

Choice of Operative Approach

The operative approach chosen should be dictated by the pathophysiology of the symptoms, the experience of the surgeon, and the expectations of the patient. Vascular problems require extensive exposure and necessitate an anterior approach. Osseous intrascalene compression (by cervical ribs) is best approached by a supraclavicular incision. First rib resection remains the most popular technique, and the transaxillary approach for first rib resection is the most frequently used. Unfortunately, first rib resection has not been uniformly successful in relieving neurologic symptoms,[16] a finding that prompts consideration of the simpler anterior scalene resection as a reasonable alternative.[55]

Conclusions

The diagnosis and management of thoracic outlet compression syndrome remains controversial and, with the exception of tests for vascular compromise, there are not diagnostic tests or provocative maneuvers that have high specificity. Measurement of somatosensory evoked potentials provides the best assessment of neurologic involvement but is still in the evolutionary stage. Diagnosis, therefore, remains primarily clinical and one of exclusion. There is uniform agreement that patients with primarily neurologic symptoms should have prolonged *nonoperative* treatment and that surgical intervention should be reserved for patients with ischemic vascular symptoms and as a last resort in patients with neurologic symptoms.

References

1. Hunald cited by Tyson RR, Kaplan GF: Modern concepts of diagnosis and treatment of the thoracic outlet syndrome. Orthop Clin North Am 6:507, 1975.
2. Kelly TR: Thoracic outlet syndrome. Current concepts of treatment. Ann Surg 190:657, 1979.
3. Peet RM, Henriksen JD, Anderson TP, et al.: Thoracic outlet syndrome. Evaluation of a therapeutic exercise program. Mayo Clin Proc 31:281, 1956.
4. Rob C, May AG: Neurovascular compression syndromes. Adv Surg 9:211, 1975.
5. Roos DB: Transaxillary approach for first rib resection to relieve thoracic outlet syndrome. Ann Surg 163:354, 1966.
6. Roos DB, Owens JC: Thoracic outlet syndrome. Arch Surg 93:71, 1966.
7. Roos DB, Congenital anomalies associated with thoracic outlet syndrome. Anatomy, symptoms, diagnosis, and treatment. Am J Surg 132:771, 1976.
8. Rosati LM, Lord JW: Neurovascular compression syndromes of the shoulder girdle. (Modern Surgical Monographs) New York: Grune and Stratton, 1961.
9. Stanton PE Jr, McClusky DA Jr, Richardson HD, et al.: Thoracic outlet syndrome: A comprehensive evaluation. South Med J 71:1070, 1978.
10. Strukel RJ, Garrick JG: Thoracic outlet compression in athletes. A report of four cases. Am J Sports Med 6:35, 1978.
11. Winsor T, Brow R: Costoclavicular syndrome. Its diagnosis and treatment. J Am Med Assoc 196:697, 1966.
12. Wright IS: The neurovascular syndrome produced by hyperabduction of the arms. The immediate changes produced in 150 normal controls, and the effects on some persons of prolonged hyperabduction of the arms, as in sleeping, and in certain occupations. Am Heart J 29:1, 1945.
13. Coote H: Pressure on the axillary vessels and nerve by an exostosis from a cervical rib; interference with the circulation of the arm; removal of the rib and exostosis; recovery. Med Times & Gaz 2:108, 1861.
14. Glass BA: The relationship of axillary venous thrombosis to the thoracic outlet compression syndrome. Ann Thorac Surg 19:613, 1975.
15. Etheredge S, Wilbur B, Stoney RJ: Thoracic outlet syndrome. Am J Surg 138:175, 1979.
16. Dale WA: Thoracic outlet compression syndrome. Critique in 1982. Arch Surg 117:1437, 1982.

17. Daseler EH, Anson BJ: Surgical anatomy of the subclavian artery and its branches. Surg Gynecol Obstet 108:149, 1959.

18. Halsted WS: An experimental study of circumscribed dilation of an artery immediately distal to a partially occluding band, and its bearing on the dilation of the subclavian artery observed in certain cases of cervical rib. J Exp Med 24:271, 1916.

19. Kirgis HD, Reed AF: Significant anatomic relations in the syndrome of the scalene muscles. Ann Surg 127:1182, 1948.

20. Murphy JB: A case of cervical rib with symptoms resembling subclavian aneurism. Ann Surg 41:399, 1905.

21. Telford ED, Stopford JSB: The vascular complications of cervical rib. Br J Surg 18:557, 1931.

22. Bramwell E, Dykes HB: Rib pressure and the brachial plexus. Edinburgh Med J 27:65, 1921.

23. Naffziger HC, Grant WT: Neuritis of the brachial plexus, mechanical in origin: The scalenus anticus syndrome. Surg Gynecol Obstet 67:722, 1938.

24. Ochsner A, Gage M, DeBakey M: Scalenus anticus (Naffziger) syndrome. Am J Surg 28:669, 1935.

25. Stallworth JM, Horne JB: Diagnosis and management of thoracic outlet syndrome. Arch Surg 119:1149, 1984.

26. Crawford FA Jr: Thoracic outlet syndrome. Surg Clin North Am 60:947, 1980.

27. Brookfield WI: Medical malpractice closed claim study, executive summary, 1975-1978. National Association of Insurance Commissioners, 1978.

28. Keen WW: The symptomatology, diagnosis, and surgical treatment of cervical ribs. Am J Med Sci 133:173, 1907.

29. Brickner WM: Brachial plexus pressure by the normal first rib. Ann Surg 85:858, 1927.

30. Telford ED, Mottershead S: Pressure at the cervicobrachial junction: An operative and anatomical study. J Bone Joint Surg 30B:249, 1948.

31. Adson AW, Coffey JR: Cervical rib. A method of anterior approach for relief of symptoms by division of the scalenus anticus. Ann Surg 85:839, 1927.

32. Rob CG, Standeven A: Arterial occlusion complicating thoracic outlet compression syndrome. Br Med J 2:709, 1958.

33. Clagett OT: Presidential address: Research and prosearch. J Thorac Cardiovasc Surg 44:153, 1962.

34. Fawcett (first initials not given): The development and ossification of the human clavicle. J Anat Physiol 47:225, 1913.

35. Thomas GI, Jones TW, Stavney LS, et al.: The middle scalene muscle and its contribution to the thoracic outlet syndrome. Am J Surg 145:589, 1983.

36. Koman LA, Nunley JA, Goldner JL, et al.: Isolated cold stress testing in the assessment of symptoms in the upper extremity: Preliminary communication. J Hand Surg 9A:305, 1984.

37. Hempel GK, Rusher AH Jr, Wheeler CG, et al.: Supraclavicular resection of the first rib for thoracic outlet syndrome. Am J Surg 141:213, 1981.

38. Sällstrom J, Gjöres JE: Surgical treatment of the thoracic outlet syndrome. Acta Chir Scand 149:555, 1983.

39. Carroll RE, Hurst LC: The relationship of thoracic outlet syndrome and carpal tunnel syndrome. Clin Orthop 164:149, 1982.

40. Pisko-Dubienski ZA, Hollingsworth J: Clinical application of Doppler ultrasonography in the thoracic outlet syndrome. Can J Surg 21:145, 1978.

41. Koman LA, Bond MG, Carter RE, et al.: Evaluation of the upper extremity vasculature with high-resolution ultrasound. J Hand Surg 10A:249, 1985.
42. Sadler TR Jr, Rainer WG, Twombley G: Thoracic outlet compression. Application of positional arteriographic and nerve conduction studies. Am J Surg 130:704, 1975.
43. Caldwell JW, Crane CR, Krusen EM: Nerve conduction studies: An aid in the diagnosis of thoracic outlet syndrome. South Med J 64:210, 1971.
44. Urschel HC Jr, Razzuk MA, Wood RE, et al.: Objective diagnosis (ulnar nerve conduction velocity) and current therapy of the thoracic outlet syndrome. Ann Thorac Surg 12:608, 1971.
45. Chodoroff G, Lee DW, Honet JC: Dynamic approach in the diagnosis of thoracic outlet syndrome using somatosensory evoked responses. Arch Phys Med Rehabil 66:3, 1985.
46. Glover JL, Worth RM, Bendick PJ, et al.: Evoked responses in the diagnosis of thoracic outlet syndrome. Surgery 89:86, 1981.
47. Jones SJ: Short latency potentials recorded for the neck and scalp following median nerve stimulation in man. Electroencephalogr Clin Neurophysiol 43:853, 1977.
48. Siivola J, Sulg I, Pokela R: Somatosensory evoked responses as a diagnostic aid in thoracic outlet syndrome. A preoperative study. Acta Chir Scand 148:647, 1982.
49. Yiannikas C, Walsh JC: Somatosensory evoked responses in the diagnosis of thoracic outlet syndrome. J Neurol Neurosurg Psychiatry 46:234, 1983.
50. Hare WSC, Rogers WJ: The scalenus medius band and the seventh cervical transverse process. Diagn Imaging 50:263, 1981.
51. Thompson JB, Hernandez IA: The thoracic outlet syndrome: A second look. Am J Surg 138:251, 1979.
52. Eversmann WW Jr: Compression and entrapment neuropathies of the upper extremity. J Hand Surg 8:759, 1983.
53. Thomas GI, Jones TW, Stavney LS, et al.: Thoracic outlet syndrome. Am Surg 44:483, 1978.
54. Martinez NS: Posterior first rib resection for total thoracic outlet syndrome decompression. Contemp Surg 15:13, 1979.
55. Sanders RJ, Monsour JW, Baer SB: Transaxillary first rib resection for the thoracic outlet syndrome. Arch Surg 97:1014, 1968.
56. Urschel HC Jr in discussion of McGough EC, Pierce MB, Byrne JP: Management of thoracic outlet syndrome. J Thorac Cardiovasc Surg 77:169, 1979.

CHAPTER 15

Compression Syndromes About the Shoulder Including Brachial Plexus

Algiamantas Narakas, M.D.

Among the innumerable causes of neck, shoulder, and arm pain, compressive neuropathies of the cervicobrachial plexus and its terminal rami play a limited role. They are difficult to isolate from the legion of other causes of shoulder pain that may be associated with nerve compression. Being uncommon, they are often not diagnosed and not treated, or come into the hands of the specialist very late. Compressed nerves get damaged in long-standing cases, so that results of surgical decompression performed too late are often poor. All nervous structures involved in these neuropathies are of ardous surgical access as compared to a median nerve in the carpal tunnel. This explains why medical literature is not rich on this subject and why the surgeon is reluctant to perform an exploration without being sure of diagnosis and results.

The aim of this chapter is to describe nerve compression syndromes about the shoulder, excluding the thoracic outlet compression syndrome already treated in Chapter 14.

Nerve fibers are exquisitely sensitive to compression when, for example, nerve roots are not protected by the intermeshing connective tissue of the epineurium. After short periods of compression and without being interrupted anatomically, they may not regenerate at all or only partially. They are very close to the cell body and should benefit early from the regeneration processes the neuron produces. Trunks and individual terminal rami of the cervicobrachial plexus tolerate compression well, as, for example, the axillary nerve does in the narrow quadrilateral space. This can be explained by the fact that at that level the axillary nerve contains up to 90 percent connective tissue investing its fascicles and taking up external mechanical forces.[2] Thus the severity of neuropathy will vary with the amount of protective tissues around the fascicles. Repetitive or chronic compression and/or a friction will induce intrafascicular edema followed in time by fibrosis. Collagen deposited between nerve fibers is not directly accessible to surgery. Therefore, recovery after decompression may require time, provided the patient is young and healthy enough to renew his tissues and eliminate sclerosis. Structures we consider in this chapter are very well vascularized and some of them, such as the dorsoscapular, the axillary, and the accessory nerve are close enough to muscles they innervate to recover quickly. Prognosis after their early decompression should therefore be good. Plexus trunks and cords containing the fibers of the radial, median, and ulnar nerves and those nerves themselves at their departure from the plexus will also recover quite quickly at the site of compression. Nevertheless, regenerating fibers will need months to reach their targets. An axon sprout growing 1 mm per 24 hours requires a daily production of neoaxoplasm equivalent to half of the volume of the neuron which synthesizes it. Patient and doctor may lose confidence in the end result as months go by. Three to four years are necessary after brachial plexus decompression to recover hand intrinsic muscle function if regeneration does not encounter

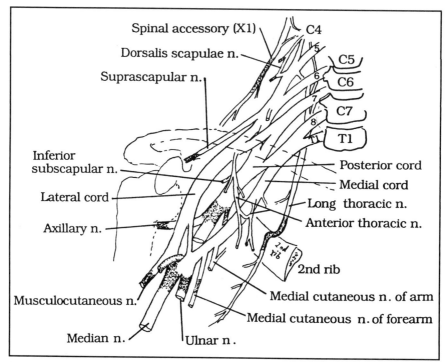

Figure 15-1. General anterior view of the brachial plexus and its branches. Sites of compression pathology are shaded.

obstacles on its way. This is long enough to create a poor reputation for surgical intervention in this type of case (Figure 15-1).

General Etiology And Diagnosis

There are many causes for compression of the nervous structures we are considering. Some are specific to the nerves involved and will be treated in the corresponding paragraphs. Others are general and have to be mentioned in this section. Tumors developing in the vicinity of the brachial plexus, of its terminal branches, or in them will produce progressive symptoms and loss of function. Some will be identified by routine x-rays, others by computerized tomography or magnetic resonance imaging. Patient's history and examination will circumscribe diagnostic possibilities such as presence of café-au-lait spots and familial incidence of Von Recklinghausen's disease. Nerve compression in these cases is only the manifestation of a systemic pathology. Plexiform nerve tumors are more difficult to identify, while pathologic lymph nodes or ganglia (axilla and medial cord; in the neighborhood of joints) have a specific distribution as well as narrow passages where nerves may be compressed, such as the scapular notch and the quadrilateral space.

Very uncommon are compressions by fibrous bands, scar, accessory muscles, and tendons producing symptoms, usually after trauma. In these conditions differential diagnosis becomes difficult and the physician has a tendency to assume that the trouble is related to an atypical thoracic outlet compression syndrome. He will ask for electrophysiologic studies and arteriography. The former will be negative initially in dynamic intermittent compression and vascular problems are seen in only 2 percent of this syndrome.

Nerve compression neuropathy about the shoulder is a diagnosis by exclusion (see Table 15-1). Arthritic changes in the cervical spine, herniated discs, tumors of the spinal cord, muscular dystrophies, and all forms of inflamed musculotendinous insertion, ruptures of the rotator cuff and related pathology, Parsonage-Turner[15]-like syndromes and viral or other diseases have to be ruled out before nerve entrapment or friction neuropathy is considered.

The scapulothoracic, scapulohumeral and glenohumeral joint functions are difficult to understand and to explain consistently. Fifteen muscles provide them with an unequalled range of motion that mobilizes about one-fourth of the myelinated fibers originating in the cervicobrachial plexus. Neurologic or mechanical disturbance of only a part of this system will result in an impairment of function that is real, though masked in the initial stages by compensatory mechanisms.

Cervical Radiculopathy

Shoulder impairment and pain can be caused by C4, C5, C6, and to a lesser extent C7 radiculopathy. A Parsonage-Turner[15] syndrome will be

Continued on page 233

Table 15-1. Differential Diagnosis in Compressive Neuropathies about the Shoulder

Site of Lesion	Causes	Affected Structure	Remarks
Spinal cord & space surrounding it, dural cul-de-sac and medial portion of foraminal canal	Tumors, metastases, syringomyelia, discus hernia, arthrosis, viral & other diseases (Parsonage-Turner), root avulsions	Spinal cord, origin of roots, roots, cervical spine, brachial plexus	Signs of involvement of long presynaptic motor, dissociated hetero-lateral sensory pathways EMG-disturbances (deep muscles of the neck affected). CT-scan and MRI and myelography ascertains clinical diagnosis.
Transverse process and foraminal gutter	Interpeduncular fibrous and muscular bands, arthritis, tumors (metastases) fractures of cervical spine, stab wounds, lacerations, traction injuries.	C5, C6 (C7) spinal nerves, serratus anterior	Structures depending on the posterior ramus of concerned spinal nerves are not affected. Rhomboids and serratus anterior can be paralyzed. Investigations as above will help diagnosis
Interscalenic space	Fibrosis of scaleni, tumors, metastases stab wounds and lacerations. Traction injuries, post-radiation fibrosis and neuropathy	Upper primary trunk, sometimes medial trunk	TOCS suspected. Adson test and similar may be positive. Carpal tunnel syndrome or/and epicondylalgia may be present.
Scaleni	Fibrosis after trauma or X-ray therapy. Stab wounds	n. dorsalis scapulae and long thoracic nerve	Isolated paralysis of corresponding muscles

Table 15-1. Differential Diagnosis in Compressive Neuropathies about the Shoulder (Continued)

Site of Lesion	Causes	Affected Structure	Remarks
Costo-clavicular space	Sequelae of fractured clavicle or 1st rib. Paralysis of trapezius, drooping shoulder, traction injuries	Distal part of primary trunks and origin of cords	Positive clinical tests involving several plexual structures. Possibly positive arteriogram. TOCS to be considered
Scapular notch	Irritation by excessive shoulder movements. Scapular fractures. Ossification of notch. Traction injuries	Supra-clavicular nerve	Pain in shoulder exacerbated by cross-body-adduction test or isolated paresis/paralysis of spinati. No signs of rotator cuff rupture. Positive anaesthetic infiltration test.
Quadrilateral space	Direct trauma; hematoma, scar, fibrous bands; traction or contusion injury, iatrogenic lesions, (rarely shoulder dislocation)	Axillary and teres minor nerves; rarely nerve to triceps	Pain on latero-anterior aspect of shoulder. Abduction-external rotation test positive. Doppler and arteriography positive. Sometimes muscular wasting. EMG positive only then.
Shoulder	Degenerative processes, trauma	Acromio-clavicular joint, gleno-humeral joint, rotator cuff, biceps tendon, tumor of humeral head	Often limitation of passive movements. Positive X-rays, arthrography, arthroscopy, negative EMG

Table 15-1. Differential Diagnosis in Compressive Neuropathies about the Shoulder (Continued)

Site of Lesion	Causes	Affected Structure	Remarks
Infraclavicular fossa	Traction injuries. Post-radiation fibrosis (pect-minor). Metastases. Gun shot wounds	Infraclavicular plexus, mostly lateral and post. Cords medial cord mostly affected by radiation or metastases	TOCS like syndrome, several nerves affected, mostly positive EMG; Ct-scan shows fibrosis and/or metastases. Phlebography may be positive in fibrosis.
Infraclavicular fossa	Traction injuries, iatrogenic	Isolated axillary, nerve or posterior cord lesions. Sometimes association of supra scapular, axillary, and musculo-cutaneous nerve palsy	History, clinical examination, EMG will establish diagnosis
Axilla	Direct trauma (contusion, laceration) post-radiation fibrosis, metastases, fibrous bands, or anomalous muscle	Any nerves or vessels passing in the axilla: mostly musculo-cutaneous median,ulnar, thoraco-dorsal	History, clinical examination, EMG, sometimes CT-scan and/or MRI will establish diagnosis
Triangular space between humerus triceps and latassimus dorsi tendon	Muscular imbalance? over-activity, compression, direct trauma	Isolated rami to long and medial triceps or whole radial nerve	Only 3 cases observed by author (1 operated); not yet well established syndrome

Abbreviations: TOCS: thoracic outlet compression syndrome

recognized because of the sudden onset of excruciating pain, which subsides when paralysis sets in. It is too extended to suggest a typical compression syndrome. Patients with apparently post traumatic neck and shoulder pain fill the consultation rooms of neurologic clinics.

About 40 percent show arthritic changes of the cervical spine on X-rays but only 3 percent of them will present a root compression by a herniated intersomatic disc or a bony spur. Less than a few in a thousand may have an associated peripheral nerve compression syndrome. Routine neurologic examination followed by CT scan, EMG, and myelography in selected cases will circumscribe diagnosis and treatment. Suspicion of the presence of the syndromes we are interested in will arise only when other diagnoses have been ruled out.

Spinal Accessory Nerve Compression

This nerve ought not to be considered in this chapter, but as palsy of the trapezius causing drooping of the shoulder may contribute to creation of a thoracic outlet syndrome or irritation of the supra-scapular nerve and may cause compression of the long thoracic nerve, a few lines have to be devoted to it. Compression of this nerve in its peripheral segment was seen in the past when tuberculosis affected cervical lymphatic ganglions. It is observed today only in tumorous conditions and postirradiation sclerosis. It is important to note if the sternocleidomastoid muscle is involved or not, that is, if the lesion is peripheral or near the base of the skull. In distal lesions only the upper trapezius is usually involved. Because loops from the cervical plexus participate to the formation of the XIth nerve and sensory rami run close to it, pain on top of the shoulder and in the scapular region is a common symptom.

Iatrogenic lesions to that nerve in cervical lymph node biopsy are too well known to be mentioned here. In some instances the nerve is not severed during biopsy but slightly contused and does not recover because it gets caught in scar. Neurolysis and padding the liberated nerve with healthy tissue from the neighborhood will solve the problem. If neurolysis or repair by grafting is carried out before six months have elapsed since injury, prognosis is excellent. Quality of results diminishes when delay is over a year.

We have seen severe compression of the XIth nerve under a total fibrotic sternocleidomastoid muscle caused by radiotherapy for Hodgkin's disease or cancer of the pharynx and tonsils. Prognosis in these cases is poor, as the nerve itself may be damaged by radiation. It should be covered by vascularized omentum if neurolysis is performed.

Dorsal Scapular Nerve Compression

The dorsal scapular nerve (n. dorsalis scapulae) is a posterior motor branch originating usually from C5, but quite often receiving a ramus of C4, and very rarely of C3. It perforates the medial scalene, follows its medial border to innervate the levator scapulae a few centimeters above its insertion to the superior angulum of the scapula, then descends along its medial margin to innervate the rhomboid muscles. The latter receive usually additional direct motor rami from C3 and C4, explaining recovery of these muscles in traumatic root avulsions of C5. Levator scapulae and rhomboidei pull the scapula medially in diverging directions; they are together antagonists of the serratus anterior. Isolated lesions of the dorsoscapular nerve are very rare. They occur after stab wounds or iatrogenic injuries. Even if the nerve is purely motor, they cause a dull ache in the lower posterior aspect of the neck radiating toward the medial margin of the scapula, under it, and in two cases seen by the author, to the posterior aspect of the shoulder. This could be explained by participation of the posterior cervical sensory rami traveling together with the dorsoscapular nerve. This nerve participates often in Parsonage-Turner[15] syndromes and traumatic brachial plexopathies (Figure 15-2).

Compression neuropathies of the dorsoscapular nerve have not been described in medical literature. We have diagnosed only a few cases. In one patient elective compression with pathologic EMG of levator scapulae and rhomboidei was caused by a lipoma 4 by 6 cm in size situated between the medial and posterior scaleni, pushing the levator scapulae outwards. Pain in the scapular and posterior shoulder area was the chief complaint

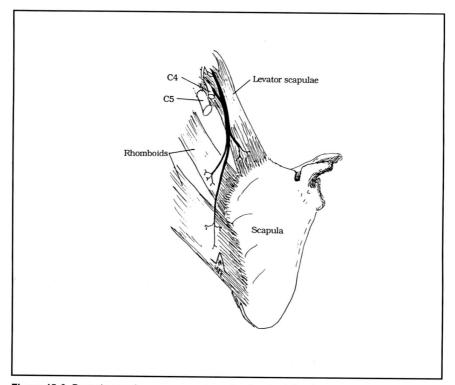

Figure 15-2. Dorsal scapular nerve seen from the front originating on the posterior aspect of C4 and C5 and innervating levator scapulae and rhomboids.

of the patient. C5 seemed symptomatically involved but presented no pathological signs. In three patients with supraclavicular postradiation plexitis the nerve was found at operation compressed when crossing a fibrotic medial scalene and was probably internally damaged.

Long Thoracic (Bell's) Nerve Pathology

This nerve originates on the posterior aspect of the anterior spinal nerves C5, C6, and C7. In some instances C4 contributes to it directly or indirectly through the C4-C5 juncture even when the brachial plexus is not prefixed. In a few cases of postfixation, C8 may provide a ramus to Bell's nerve. It crosses the medial scalene and runs downwards behind and laterally to the plexual trunks to reach each digitation of serratus anterior. Its course adopts a sharp S-shape when crossing the second rib. The serratus anterior attracts the scapula to the thoracic wall and is able to move its tip laterally and anteriorly. It participates in abduction of the arm and forward elevation (flexion), which are impaired and painful when it is paralyzed.

The long thoracic nerve is well known for traumatic and iatrogenic injuries;[9] its involvement in Parsonage-Turner[15] syndromes, in infections and viral illnesses, and in reactions to serum and various immunizing injections.

Compression or entrapment syndromes of the long thoracic nerve have not been described, though the nerve may be imbedded in scar in traction injuries of the brachial plexus or in sclerosis caused by irradiation. In trapezius palsy it may suffer progressively either because of friction or compression when it passes the second rib because of the drooping shoulder. Conversely, acute compression of friction neuropathies of this nerve causing paresis or palsy have been described in patients subjected to depression of the shoulder while carrying loads (dock workers, rucksack paralysis, and so on) or carrying out repeated violent movements in the scapulo-thoracic joint, such as performed by handball, basketball and tennis players. It was also observed in patients after cutting trees with an ax, in miners, in railway workers and smiths using heavy picks or hammers.

Partial or complete palsy is usually accompanied by pain in the whole scapular and shoulder area. It may radiate to the axilla and below. Diagnosis is rendered easy by the winging of the scapula (scapula alata) when the arm is elevated in front of the body or when the patient leans against the wall with outstretched arms. Push-ups will exaggerate the deformity and may not be possible to perform. In the thin normal patient, it is easy to palpate the digitations of the muscle on contraction.

When the cause of friction or repeated compression is stopped, recovery will commence. In complete palsies, two or three years will be required for complete healing. The pain may be long lasting and difficult to treat. In acute compression or friction neuropathies, there is no indication for surgery. It is well known that secondary correction by musculotendinous transfers using pectoralis minor[4] or the lower portion of pectoralis major[9,13,20] is not always satisfactory. Nevertheless, a conservative attitude prevails even in traumatic and iatrogenic injury.

The reluctance to proceed to surgical repair of this nerve not only relates to the late referral of cases but also to the difficult approach to the course of Bell's nerve, requiring a supraclavicular and an axillary route.

Suprascapular Nerve Compression

This nerve arises from the lateral aspect of the upper trunk C5-C6, getting most of its fibers from the cranial fascicles of C5. In prefixed plexuses it may get a distinct ramus from C4 in addition to some fibers coming from the C4-C5 anastomosis. Leaving the upper trunk, it runs loosely under the trapezius forming a concave arch behind the clavicle and reaches the scapular notch. The omohyoid muscle lies in front of it, and the arteria transversa scapulae and its satellite veins run above it. An arteriole and venules accompany it within the same sheath. Actually the nerve fascicles occupy only about one-third of its apparent diameter (Figure 15-3).

The nerve passes in the scapular notch under the superior transverse ligament of the scapula while the vessels pass over it. Sometimes it is accompanied by a small arterial branch. In the supraspinatus fossa it gives off a medially running branch that innervates the supraspinatus and some rami to the subacromial bursa and the upper and posterior aspect of the glenohumeral joint. Actually it innervates with its sensory and sympathetic fibers two-thirds of this joint. Some rami ascend from the subacromial bursa to the deep aspect of the acromioclavicular joint. The main trunk of the nerve turns around the base of the acromion, passes under the inferior transverse scapular ligament where it is relatively free, and innervates the infraspinatus by a main horizontally running ramus, almost parallel to the spina scapulae, and a small oblique ramus parallel to the lateral margin of the scapula. Both motor rami are on the deep aspect of spinati. The nerve does not provide sensory rami to the skin.

The supraspinatus initiates abduction in the shoulder for the first 20 or 30 degrees. When the arm is along the thorax, the deltoid has a very small moment for abduction, the vectors of its contraction being almost vertical. It elevates the humeral head instead of rotating it. The infraspinatus is primarily an external rotator of the humerus together with the teres minor. A complete rotator cuff rupture or suprascapular nerve palsy renders the slight abduction of an elevation of the humerus impossible and significantly diminishes external rotation. The patient may swing his arm outwards by trick movements reaching a sufficient degree of abduction to allow the deltoid to take over. At about 140 degrees abduction, the pectoralis major supplements the movement as its tendon moves above the center of rotation of the humeral head and becomes an abductor. The patient has difficulty in reaching full abduction and elevation when no powerful external rotators are present because the tuberculum majus has a tendency to impinge in the subacromial passage. The suprascapular nerve turns inward by approximately 90 degrees at the scapular notch being against the medial border of it, which is always sharp. The notch itself is either widely open, narrow, or completely closed by an ossified superior ligamentum transversum scapulae. The notch may even be divided in two compartments.

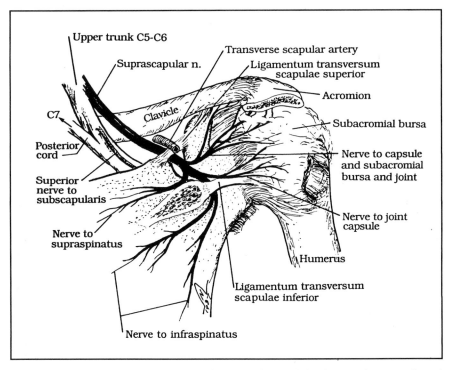

Figure 15-3. Suprascapular nerve seen from the front originating on the anterolateral aspect of the upper trunk, passing under the superior transverse ligament of scapula innervating the supraspinatus, the subacromial bursa, the acromioclavicular and glenohumeral joints, then passing under the inferior transverse scapular ligament and innervating the infraspinatus.

Normally the notch moves along the nerve in scapular movements and contraction of the spinati like a ring around a string. The nerve is brought under tension when the shoulder is depressed or the scapula travels to the front—that is, in active cross-body adduction, in extreme scapulothoracic movements, and when rhomboids and trapezius are paralyzed, with the serratus anterior remaining active.

It is possible, though not proven, that in frozen shoulders the suprascapular nerve is either an initial causative agent or a secondary victim. In traction lesions of the brachial plexus, the fascicles of the nerve are interrupted in the upper trunk but the nerve can be also ruptured at the notch, behind it, and even avulsed from muscle. Thomas[19] focused attention on the suprascapular nerve neuralgia in infraspinatus palsy. Kopell and Thompson[10] described the etiology and pathology of this syndrome and performed the first surgical releases. Mansat[12] (working under Ficat) described additional cases and proposed a new surgical approach to the nerve. Since then, this syndrome has become well known by rheumatologists and orthopaedic and peripheral nerve surgeons. Pain and disturbance of function motivate the patient to seek medical help. The type of pain, acute in extreme movements in the shoulder or dull, permanent, and excruciating when trying to sleep on the affected shoulder (this produces a forward projection of the scapula and adduction putting the nerve under tension) is not characteristic enough to suspect suprascapular nerve entrapment. The pain may radiate along the inner margin of the scapula and under it, but usually patients localize it in the posterior, the subacromial part of the glenohumeral joint, sometimes in the acromioclavicular joint, and often in the posterolateral aspect of the arm, radiating down to the elbow. This could mislead the physician to suspect a C5, C6, and C7 radiculopathy.

Diagnosis is based on the cross-body adduction test, which can be enhanced by simultaneous external rotation of the humerus. In that situation the supra and infraspinatus muscles are put under tension and, thus, pull on their motor branches, which accentuates the impingement of the suprascapular nerve on the medial border of the scapular notch. Direct pressure with the finger above the notch, while the shoulder is elevated will elicit the spontaneous pain. In long-standing cases, atrophy of the spinati will be seen, particularly of the infraspinatus which is less masked by the trapezius; the power of abduction at 30 to 45 degrees as well as of external rotation will be diminished. In two-thirds of the cases the syndrome will be associated with degenerative changes at the shoulder joint (Neer's types I, II, and III) and pathology of the long head of biceps. Diagnosis will be confirmed by injection of local anesthetics or corticoids[17] and by electromyography, which will show increased conduction time between Erb's point and muscles, a latency above 3.7 msec, diminished amplitude or polyphasic motor units, and fibrillations in late cases.

Treatment consists in avoidance of movements that cause pain and that were by their repetition initially responsible for the neuropathy. Corticoid injections in the region of the scapular notch can be attempted. Surgical treatment is indicated when severe symptoms persist in spite of conservative measures or when muscular atrophy is present.

The author prefers the trans-trapezial postero-superior exposure of Mansat to all other approaches. The purely posterior approach of Post[17] is reserved for isolated atrophy of the infraspinatus. The incision bisects the angle formed by the clavicle and spina scapulae. The trapezius is split along its fibers. The supraspinatus is exposed and retracted dorsally. Injury to the transverse scapular vessels is avoided, and when difficulties in orientation arise, the omohyoid muscle is used as a landmark. Meticulous hemostasis with a bipolar microcoagulation is mandatory, as even minimal bleeding will mask the essential structures. The suprascapular nerve is identified in front of the scapular notch. It may be swollen to three to four times its normal size. The well vascularized superior transverse ligament of the scapula is microcoagulated, then incised. The nerve is taken out of the notch, which is widened considerably by a rongeur. When required, the nerve is followed around and inferiorly to the base of the acromion, which demands a much wider incision deflected posteriorly along the spina, reflecting when necessary the dorsal part of the deltoid downwards or upwards.

However simple it seems, exposure of the scapular notch and of the more distal course of the suprascapular nerve is not easy at all. Any surgeon attempting it ought to undertake several cadaveric dissections beforehand. Pitfalls are lesions to the transverse scapular vessels and laceration of muscle fibers, causing a scar which remains painful for months. Closure is easy in the superior approach, as only muscular fibers have been separated along their axis. Careful reinsertion of the trapezius on the spina scapulae is carried out when a posterior approach has been added. Postoperative immobilization should not exceed one week.

Surgery is carried out in about one patient out of five referred for this syndrome and is successful in two-thirds of cases. Failures were due to improper selection or incomplete diagnosis. Patients had unrecognized pathology besides a suprascapular nerve syndrome or an associated pathology that was not or could not be treated. Some were referred very late and so atrophy of spinati existed for more than a year. These patients may improve with time, their symptoms gradually disappearing in two to three years. The supraspinatus recovers often, the infraspinatus seldom.

Quadrilateral Tunnel Syndrome
Causing Axillary Nerve Compression

Axillary nerve fibers originate in roots C5 (for anterior and lateral deltoid according to Foerster,[8]) and C6 (for the posterior deltoid), very seldom from C7. Containing approximately 6700 myelinated[2] and around 30,000 unmyelinated fibers, the nerve fascicles leave the posterior aspect of the upper trunk through the upper division of the posterior cord close to the origin of the suprascapular nerve, level with the clavicle in the majority of cases. The nerve fascicles run in the posterolateral portion of the cord near those of the radial nerve. The origin proper of the axillary nerve is very variable. It may leave the posterior cord already at the lower margin of the clavicle, alone or together with the inferior ramus to the subscapular muscle and the thoracodorsal nerve, or more distally, 2 cm below the coracoid process where it emerges under the axillary artery and is often covered by the anterior circumflex vessels, those for the biceps and the coracobrachialis neurovascular pedicle. It enters the quadrilateral tunnel (foramen of Velpeau) together with the posterior circumflex artery and a venous plexus. Invested by subscapularis muscle fascia and tethered by it, it turns around the posterior aspect of the humeral neck covered by the vessels. In the tunnel the nerve starts to split into terminal rami presenting approximately eight different distribution patterns. The ramus to teres minor is often already individualized at that level, taking a cranial course. There is a ramus for the joint capsule innervating its anterior and inferior portion. An inferior ramus descends along the posterior margin of the deltoid to innervate the skin on the lateral part of the shoulder. The rami to the deltoid distribute themselves to the deep aspect of the muscle. Some give off secondary twigs piercing the muscle to innervate the skin over the deltoid. The length of the nerve from its origin to the deltoid varies from 11 to 15 cm and from the quadrilateral tunnel's entrance to the muscle from 40 to 60 millimeters.[5] (Figure 15-4)

The roof of the tunnel is formed in front by the subscapularis fascia, in its midportion by the inferior glenohumeral ligament and the joint capsule, dorsally by the teres minor muscle and tendon. There is no floor to the tunnel in front and in the middle, but a plexus of venous rami and lobules of fat, sometimes a lymph node or two. Dorsally the floor is made by the teres major tendon. The lateral or humeral wall of the tunnel is formed in front by the sometimes sharp fascia of the coracobrachialis muscle, then the periosteum of the humeral neck and very often by accessory insertions of the triceps on the humerus close to the capsule. The medial or scapular wall is formed in front by the inferior glenoid rim and in the back by the long head of the triceps passing dorsally to the teres major. The axillary nerve is tethered in the tunnel by muscular fascia, joint capsule, and periosteum. It is anchored dorsally by its terminal rami. During surgery a normal quadrilateral tunnel admits an index finger along the vasculonervous pedicle in a relaxed patient with his arm along the thorax. In abduction the tunnel is narrowed by the scissorlike effect of triceps and teres major, while the nerve is put under tension by its distal anchorage point, thus getting away from the origin of the nerve at the posterior cord.

When the limb is lifted above the head with elbow flexed (as when falling forward) the subscapularis, teres major, and triceps tendons are put under tension, narrowing considerably the tunnel while the humeral head

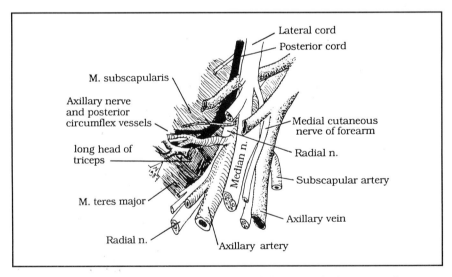

Figure 15-4. Anterior view of the axillary nerve. It originates on the lateroposterior aspect of the posterior cord and enters the quadrilateral tunnel with the nerve to teres minor and circumflex vessels.

protrudes below the glenoid rim, impinging on the nerve. In abduction and external rotation the subscapularis and teres major tendons are put on further tension, closing the tunnel if it is already narrow. In internal rotation and dorsal projection of the humerus (as when falling backwards), the axillary nerve is wound around the humerus and, thus, put under tension while the distance between the tunnel and the origin of the nerve is increased, and teres minor tension is moderately augmented. These dynamic modifications explain traction lesions and ruptures of the axillary nerve and the rationale of tests to prove narrowness of the quadrilateral tunnel.

Idiopathic axillary nerve compression in the tunnel is a rare entity and goes usually unrecognized for long periods. In all of our cases, referral was delayed by over a year. By contrast, post traumatic compression is seen more often, symptoms and signs are more dramatic, and the specialists sees the patients within months of trauma. In the latter case, a hematoma confined to the tunnel is often evoked to explain the pathology. The majority of patients are young, male, and athletic, but older patients with chronic pain in the anterior and lateral aspect of shoulder and multiple alterations of the joint function may present this syndrome also.

The syndrome has been described by Koppel and Thompson,[10] Batemen and Cahill,[3] among others. The patient's history is always confused as, for instance, in one of our patients who complained of not being able to change light bulbs overhead nor to sleep on the affected shoulder. Pain and paresthesias begin progressively, located in the autonomous axillary nerve area but often descending to the elbow and even to the hand on the dorsoulnar border, which adds to the confusion. Extreme movements in the shoulder, particularly abduction and external rotation as when serving at tennis or throwing a ball, exacerbate symptoms. The shoulder feels weak. On examination there is a typical tenderness at the posterior outlet of the tunnel, rarely some weakness of deltoid, teres minor, and even triceps, while other radial-nerve-innervated muscles are normal. In post traumatic cases seen within weeks of injury, discoloration by diffused hematoma can be seen on the scapular and humeral sides of the arm pit. In late cases, some muscular atrophy may be present.

Electromyographic investigations are initially normal, and when no explanation to the patient's complaints is found, particularly after a minor accident at work, a neurosis is suspected, given the unusual distribution of symptoms. Arteriography of the artery with the arm in abduction and external rotation shows an interruption of the dye in the posterior circum-flex artery at the tunnel with possible distal filling through anastomoses with the circumflex scapular or deep humeral arteries.

This is an invasive procedure only recommended to document surgical decompression in disabling cases resistant to conservative therapy. Occlusion of the artery by movements can be easily demonstrated by appropriate investigation with a Doppler. On the other hand, in post traumatic and iatrogenic lesions the clinical diagnosis is evident enough to avoid arteriograms.

When avoidance of aggravating movements, anti-inflammatory drugs, corticoid injections, and so on, have failed; when no other reason for disabling symptoms and signs has been found; and when diagnosis is certain; surgical decompression is carried out.

The patient lies on his healthy side in order to allow approach from the front (see later discussion) and the back. The dorsal outlet of the tunnel is exposed by an incision along the posterior border of the deltoid. The muscle is lifted together with teres minor, relaxing both by bringing the arm slightly backwards and sideways in indifferent rotation. The quadrilateral tunnel is identified (the posteriolateral sensory ramus may serve as a guide), taking care not to confuse it with the triangular space on the medial side of the long head of the triceps crossed by the scapular circumflex artery or the more distal triangular space on the lower border of the teres major and latissimus crossed by the main trunk of the radial nerve, its numerous rami, and the deep humeral artery. When necessary, the affected upper rami to the triceps are identified. Care is taken not to injure the delicate veins around the nerve and its rami. The natural and pathologic adherences and septae are separated by scissors or the index finger which is pushed gently into, then through the tunnel, palpating the arterial pulse. The arm is mobilized to extreme ranges of motion to ascertain decompression. If a compressing structure remains, it is incised for a few millimeters. The compressing structures are, in order: scarred inferior glenohumeral ligament, teres minor, triceps, teres major, and subscapularis fascia. Desinsertion of teres minor does not always solve the problem of persisting compression after liberation of the tunnel. In one case, we had to displace the fibrotic subglenoidal insertion of the triceps, and various situations can be encountered requiring eventually an anterior approach also. In one case there was an accessory tendon of subscapularis crossing the axillary nerve, impossible to sever under the control of the eye. A transposed subscapularis tendon from an improperly performed Magnuson-Stack[11] operation for recurrent dislocation of the shoulder, a latisimus dorsi tendon after reconstruction of the breast, and teres minor and/or teres major tendons after various operations on the shoulder, were identified as causes of axillary nerve compression with palsy. Extended fibrosis of the muscular walls of the tunnel was seen after axillary irradiation. In obstetrical palsy showing poor recovery of the deltoid in addition to elongation of deltoid fibers in the upper trunk, an analogous quadrangular space syndrome was seen several times caused by a short and fibrotic teres minor and teres major (Figure 15-5).

After surgery, the arm is put at rest for a week, then mobilization encouraged. Return to manual work requires three to six weeks, and patients ought to refrain from violent activities requiring full abduction of the arm with powerful downward movement for three months.

Results of surgical decompression are excellent provided the nerve has not been severely contused, crushed, or stretched. There seems to be no time limit for duration of symptoms in cases without palsy beyond which healing is not obtained. However, experience with over a hundred cases

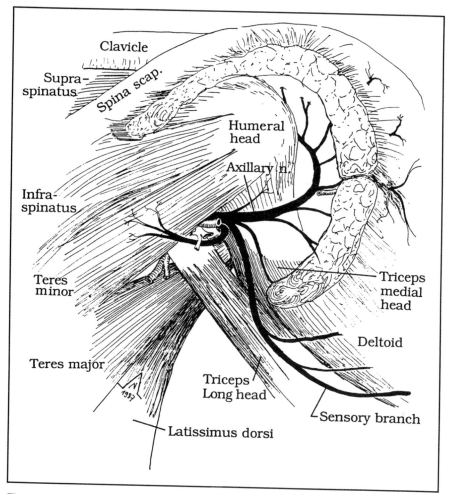

Figure 15-5. Posterior view of the axillary nerve innervating the glenohumeral joint (posteroinferior portion) the skin over the inferior portion of the deltoid, the muscle itself and partially the skin overlying it.

of traumatic injuries to the axillary nerve operated on by the author[5] indicates clearly that when surgery is performed after a delay of six months no excellent result, and after a year no good result is obtained, whether the nerve is grafted or only neurolysis is performed. These facts demonstrate dramatically that static, severe compression resulting in paralysis is not tolerated either by nerve or by muscle as compared to dynamic intermittent compression.

Compression of Musculocutaneous, Thoracodorsal, Median, Ulnar and Radial Nerves

The distal plexus and its many terminal branches are indeed very rarely compressed, excepting cases involving important modifications of the anatomy caused by surgery or trauma. Ligatures or sutures have been seen by the author on the distal lateral and posterior cords, on the axillary nerve after operations for anterior dislocation of the shoulder, some of which implied vascular lesions as after axillary artery catheterizations, and so on. An arterial thrombosis near a nerve in the axilla caused by trauma, surgical instrument or ligature, missile, and so on, produces an acute palsy with a lot of pain in the nerve or nerves touching the artery. This is a phenonmenon very similar to ulnar artery thrombosis in the Guyon's canal producing a distal ulnar nerve palsy. We have treated cases showing compression palsies in the axillary region of the ulnar, the median, the radial and the thoracodorsal nerves.

Vascular pathology includes aneurysms and anomalous distribution of the axillary artery well studied by Miller.[14] An arterial ramus may cross the lateral origin of the median nerve, go through it, cross the distal portion of the lateral cord above the origin of the musculocutaneous nerve or a juncture between the latter and the median, the deep brachial artery may have a proximal origin crossing the medial cord, and so on. These anomalies can be perfectly quiescent or produce symptoms in particular positions of the arm, usually in abduction, and are of a difficult diagnosis requiring detailed arteriography and surgical exploration because in these situations a thoracic outlet compression syndrome will be the most likely diagnosis.

There are numerous muscular anomalies crossing the axilla and having the potential to compress the neurovascular infraclavicular bundle. Their embryologic origin and their attachments are too complex to be exposed here. More or less they produce a transverse arc going from the pectoralis major to the latissimus or from the latter to the coracobrachialis or humerus. They can be assimilated to the axillary arch of Langer containing muscular fibers.

These structures produce atypical nerve irritation or venous compression syndromes. In the cases operated by the author, the level of nerve irritation could be established by clinical examination but the cause remained unknown until the exposure had been performed.

Musculocutaneous nerve compression could theoretically be caused by a very tight fascia of the coracobrachilais under which the nerve passes. Though this is with certainty a rupture spot of the nerve in traumatic lesions, a compression was seen at that level only in one patient in whom the detached coracoid was screwed under strong tension of the coracobrachialis and short head of biceps to the clavicle to treat an acromioclavicular dislocation. It was also observed in postradiation sclerosis.

Proximal radial nerve compression by the latissimus dorsi tendon was seen in a case of breast reconstruction with that muscle. The question is still open whether this nerve is not compressed in the triangular opening between the above tendon, humerus and triceps in some obscure cases of radial nerve "neuritis" we see in middle-aged people.

Notalgia Paraesthetica

This is a rare compression syndrome of the posterior rami of the upper dorsal roots at the level where they cross the multifidus spinae muscle.[16] It produces an interscapular burning pain and paraesthesias similar in nature to the pain felt in meralgia paraesthetica. Sensory disturbances can be elicited in the paravertebral skin. The author has seen only two cases: one in a cello player (associated with a supra-scapular nerve friction neuropathy) and the other in a patient working in front of him 8 hours a day with horizontally abducted arms. In the latter case there was also an associated mild, bilateral thoracic outlet syndrome. Three corticoid paravertebral infiltrations associated with proper exercises healed both patients.

Conclusion

Nerve compression syndromes about the shoulder are infrequent clinical entities but great in their variety, as numerous nerves traverse that region. Diagnosis in these cases is always difficult as they are often associated with other neuropathies in the upper limb and the wide pathology of neck, shoulder, and arm pain. However, once identified, their treatment is relatively easy and rewarding, provided severe compression has not persisted for too long.

References

1. Bateman JE: The shoulder and neck. 2nd ed: Philadelphia, W.B. Saunders, 1978, pp 608.
2. Bonnel F, Rabischong PL: Anatomy and systematisation of the brachial plexus in the adult. Anat Clin 2:289, 1981.
3. Cahall BR: Quadrilateral space syndrome. *In* Omer GE, Spinner M (ed): Peripheral nerve problems. Philadelphia, W.B. Saunders Company, 1980, pp 602.
4. Chaves P: Pectoralis minor transplant for paralysis of the serratus anterior. J Bone Joint Surg (Br) 33B:228, 1951.
5. Coene LN, Narakas AO: Surgical management of axillary nerve lesions, isolated or combined with other infraclavicular nerve lesions. Peripheral Nerve Repair and Regeneration 3:47, 1986.
6. Coene LH: Axillary nerve lesions and associated injuries. Thesis directed by C.W. Bruyn and A.O. Narakas. University of Leyden, 1985, pp 27.
7. Ficat P, Mansat C, Roudil J: Neurolyse du nerf sus-scapulaire Rev Med Toulouse, 3:229, 1967.
8. Foerster O: Anatomie und physiologie des plexus brachialia, *In* Bumke O, Foerster O (ed): Handbuch der Neurologie Teil II, Berlin, Julius Springer, 1929, pp 942.
9. Gozna ER, Harris WR: Traumatic winging of the scapula. J Bone Joint Surg 61A:1230, 1979.
10. Kopell HP, Thompson WAL: Peripheral entrapment neuropathies. Baltimore, William and Wilkins, 1963.
11. Magnuson PB, Stack JK: Recurrent dislocation of the shoulder. JAMA 123:889, 1943.

12. Mansat M, Mansat CH, Guiraud B: Pathologie de l'épaule et syndromes canalaires. *In* Souquet R. (ed): Syndromes canalaires du membre supérieur. Expansion Scientifique, Paris, 1983, pp 31.

13. Marmor L, Bechtol CO: Paralysis of the serratus anterior due to electric shock relieved by transplantation of the pectoralis major muscle: A case report. J Bone Joint Surg 45A:156, 1963.

14. Miller R: Observation upon the arrangement of the axillary artery and brachial plexus. Am J Anat 64:143, 1939.

15. Parsonage MJ, Turner JWA: Neuralgic amyotrophy: The shoulder girdle syndrome. Lancet 1:973, 1948.

16. Pleet AB, Massey EW: Notalgia paresthetica. Neurology 28:1310-1313, 1978.

17. Post M: The shoulder: surgical and non-surgical management. Philadelphia, Lea and Febiger, 1978.

18. Rose DL, Kelly CR: Shoulder pain. Suprascapular nerve block in shoulder pain. J Kansas Med Soc 70:135, 1969.

19. Thomas A: Paralysie du sous-épineux. Presse méd. 64:1283, 1936.

20. Tubby AH: A case illustrating the operative treatment of paralysis of the serratus magnus by muscle grafting. Br Med J ii:159, 1904.

CHAPTER 16

Spinal Nerve Root Compression

Bjorn Rydevik, M.D., Ph.D.
Steven R. Garfin, M.D.

Introduction

Spinal nerve roots are often involved in disease processes such as disc herniation and spinal stenosis. In these situations the nerve roots may be mechanically deformed by surrounding structures, occasionally resulting in neurologic deficit and/or pain. The mechanical compression may lead to a series of changes involving nerve tissues, including edema formation, demyelination, and fibrosis which by various mechanisms can cause functional changes. Interestingly, even with known instances of spinal root compromise, pain and/or neurologic deficit may subside without relieving the compression.

In this chapter, the pathophysiology associated with spinal nerve root compression is reviewed and related to clinical symptoms, diagnosis and treatment of degenerative spinal disorders.

Anatomical and Physiological Aspects

Neural Tissue

Spinal nerve roots form the anatomical connection between the central nervous system and the peripheral nervous system (Fig. 1). Structurally, unlike peripheral nerves, nerve roots within the spinal column are not homogenous: a nerve root in the cauda equina (Fig. 2) is completely different from its extention that exits through the intervertebral foramen. At this level, within the neuroforamen each nerve root is surrounded by dura and composed of a sensory and a motor root, and a dorsal root ganglion. Consequently nerve root compression may involve anatomically distinct components of nerve tissue when comparing, for example, the histopathol-

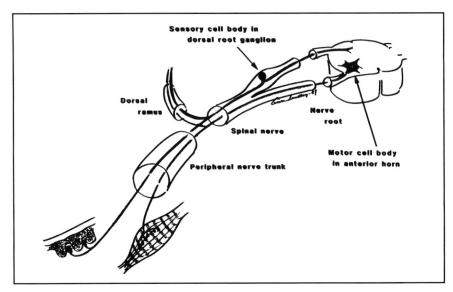

Figure 16-1. Schematic drawing of the anatomical arrangement of nerve roots, spinal nerve and peripheral nerve. (From Rydevik et al., Spine 9:7-15, 1984, reproduced by permission).

Figure 16-2. Cross-section of a fresh human cadaver lumbar spine specimen. The nerve roots in the cauda equina are located in the central spinal canal. (From Rydevik et al., Spine 9:7-15, 1984, reproduced by permission).

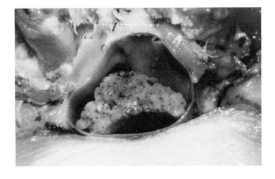

ogy of the compression that occurs with central spinal stenosis and that caused by disc herniation (see also below).

Unlike peripheral nerves, nerve roots of the cauda equina are devoid of perineurium and have a very loose, thin "epineurial" covering, corresponding to the pia mater of the spinal cord. Additionally, the nerve roots are surrounded by cerebrospinal fluid, arachnoid membrane, and dura. These structures act, together with the bony elements, to mechanically protect the nerve roots. Moreover, the cerebrospinal fluid seems to have a nutritional role for the nerve roots at this level (see below). Within the neuroforamen the sensory and motor root for each level are adjacent to each other, with the sensory root dorsal to the motor root. Here they are surrounded by the root sheath and other connective tissue components. The dura of the root sheaths is continuous with the epineurium of the peripheral nerves.[55,56] Traced laterally, the nerve roots gradually assume the micro-anatomical characteristics of peripheral nerves. The dorsal root ganglion tends to be the dividing point.

Blood Supply

The blood supply of the nerve roots is derived both from arteries which enter the spinal nerves lateral to the foramen and from central arteries coursing caudally from the spinal cord.[41,42] There is a region of relative hypovascularity in the nerve roots in the cauda equina where these two vascular supply systems approach each other.[42] Analyses of the number of microvessels per cross-sectional area in these areas of lumbar nerve roots, compared to human peripheral nerves, demonstrate a decreased arterial supply.[42] An additional nutritional support system is necessary in this area. Studies suggest that the nerve roots in this "watershed area" derive a significant portion of their nutrition through the surrounding cerebrospinal fluid.[18,45,48] Thus, the intrathecal parts of the nerve roots have dual nutritional pathways: 1) through the intraneural microvessels and 2) through diffusion from the cerebrospinal fluid.

The blood supply of the dorsal root ganglia differs from other parts of the nerve roots in that the ganglia have a very rich microvascular networks. Furthermore, the blood vessels at this location are more permeable than the intraneural blood vessels at other levels.[2,39] The extensive vascular supply and the higher vascular permeability of the microvessels in the dorsal root ganglia may reflect the increased metabolic demand at this level, where the sensory nerve cell bodies are located (Fig. 1). These cell bodies are the site of the synthesis of several essential substances, for example the proteins needed for the maintenance of structural and functional integrity of the sensory neuron.

Axonal transport

Proteins and organelles which are synthesized in the nerve cell bodies in the dorsal root ganglia (sensory neurons), or in the anterior horn of the spinal cord (motor neurons), are transported antegrade through the axons by axonal transport systems. Interference with the axonal transport as a result of nerve root compression may deplete the distal parts of the axons of proteins and other essential subcellular components.[46] This phenomenon might be the basis for the so-called double- crush-syndrome.[8,9,57] In this syndrome there is a double nerve compression which occurs proximally along a spinal nerve, and distally across the peripheral nerve containing fibers from the compressed spinal nerve. Presumably the proximal constriction of the neurons leads to accumulation of proteins which are normally axonally transported (and therefore deficient distally). Without these transported chemical components the distal parts of the axons may be more susceptible to compression.

Motion of spinal nerve roots

The nerve roots are not static structures in the spine; they move relative to the surrounding tissues with every spinal movement. This phenomenon requires a gliding capacity of the nerve roots in, among other areas, intervertebral foramina. Chronic irritation of the nerve roots, in association with disc herniation or foraminal stenosis, could result in inflammation, edema formation and fibrosis in and around the nerve roots, further impairing the gliding capacity of the nerve roots relative to the surrounding tissues. Such fibrotic adhesions between the nerve roots and the surrounding tissues might cause repeated "micro-stretching" injuries of the nerve roots during normal spinal movements, leading to further tissue irritation (Fig. 3). The normal movements of nerve roots in the lumbar spine has been assessed in cadaver experiments by Goddard and Reid.[13] These authors found that with, for example, straight leg raising, the nerve roots at the level of the intervertebral foramen move approximately 2-5 mm. Therefore, straight leg raising (with extended knee and flexed hip) can, in cases of disc herniation with adhesions and nerve root edema, lead to pathologic nerve root tension and cause pain (straight leg raising test).

Biomechanics of Nerve Root Compression

Nerve root compression syndromes are complex issues from anatomical and physiological points of view. Additionally, there are also biomechanical factors involved in nerve root deformation in association with disc herniation and spinal stenosis.[46,49,53] In cases of disc herniation, the nerve

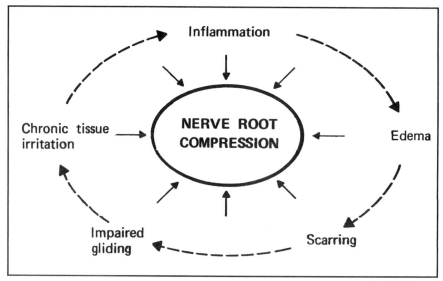

Figure 16-3. Schematic representation of the tissue reactions induced in nerve roots by compression, resulting in a vicious circle.

root is subjected to unilateral compression. Because individual nerve roots are normally adherent to the surrounding tissues above and below the intervertebral disc it transverses[52] compression might give rise to intraneural tension.[47,53] The contact pressure between a simulated disc herniation and the compressed nerve root has been measured as high as 400 mmHg in human cadavers.[53] This pressure could be reduced, if the disc height was experimentally decreased. These findings might explain some of the sciatic pain relief seen following chemonucleolysis and possibly also the "spontaneous" relief of sciatic pain over time as disc degeneration progresses, and disc height decreases.

In cases of central spinal stenosis, the mechanics of nerve root compression are entirely different. In these situations pressure is applied to the nerve roots in the cauda equina at a gradual, slow rate and in a circumferential manner. These factors, together with the fact that the nerve tissue and roots centrally within the cauda equina differ from the spinal nerve roots located more laterally at the location where disc herniation often occurs, may explain why the symptomatology of spinal stenosis is completely different from that of disc herniation.

Effects of Compression on Nerve Roots

There is relatively little information in the literature regarding the reaction of spinal nerve roots to compression, especially when compared to the large number of investigations available on experimental peripheral nerve compression (see Sunderland 1968; Rydevik et al., 1984; and Chapter 2 in this book for references). Schonstrom et al.[49] measured pressure among the nerve roots in the cauda equina related to experimental constriction of the canal in cadaver lumbar spines. Though pressures increased as available room for the neural elements decreased, no correlation with neurophysiologic activity was developed.

Previous data in the literature on experimental nerve root compression are mainly based on studies by Gelfan and Tarlov[12] and Sharpless.[50] These authors made observations which might indicate that nerve roots are more susceptible to compression than peripheral nerves, findings which could be based on the differences in microanatomy between intrathecal nerve roots and peripheral nerves. Recently, a model has been developed for graded nerve root compression in the pig lumbo-sacral spine.[35] This model allows a broad-spectrum approach to the complex issues of nerve root compression, including analyses of intraneural blood flow, solute transport to the nerve roots, impulse conduction and structural properties.[36-38,40] Initial observations indicate that the nutritional supply to the nerve roots in the cauda equina, in terms of reduced solute transport to the roots and impaired intraneural blood flow, can be acutely affected at pressure levels of 20-30 mmHg or greater.[35,36] Longstanding compression of nerve roots at these pressure levels, might, therefore, lead to a reduction of the nutritional supply to the nerve fibers and accumulation of waste-products within the nerve root tissue. These factors could cause various kinds and degrees of functional changes, including pain.

Pain Mechanisms in Nerve Root Compression

Acute compression of a normal peripheral nerve does not cause pain, but rather numbness, paresthesiae, motor weakness and related signs and symptoms. This can be seen in common situations such as when the peroneal nerve is compressed when an individual sits with crossed legs and also from studies involving acute experimental compression of the median nerve in the carpal tunnel.[26] Mechanical compression of *normal* spinal nerve roots also seems to induce similar sensory and motor dysfunctional symptoms without associated pain.[27,51] These observations, regarding the reaction of human spinal nerve roots to compression, were obtained by placing small inflatable catheters[27] or threads[51] close to, or around, nerve roots following laminectomies. Postoperatively, mechanical deformation of *normal* nerve roots caused mainly numbness and pareasthesiae. However, if the nerve root had been compressed by a herniated disc before this test was performed, i.e. the root was irritated, even minimal mechanical deformation resulted in reproduction of the sciatic pain. Recently Brown and co-workers[7] have reported that compressed nerve roots in patients undergoing laminectomy and disc excision under epidural anaesthesia were very sensitive to mechanical manipulation. It was found that even though all tissues in the lumbar spine were well-anesthetized, even careful retraction of an inflamed nerve root caused radiating leg pain. These observations on human subjects are supported by experimental investigations on the neurophysiological response of normal versus inflamed nerves and nerve roots.[19] Thus, it seems, inflammation of the nerve root tissue is a significant factor, which has to be present before mechanical nerve root deformation gives rise to pain.

What is the cause for the inflammation in and/or around nerve roots and can it be treated if it is established? Knowledge of this topic is limited. From the previous discussion, however, it is obvious that mechanical factors, such as compression and/or traction of the nerve roots, can induce the sequence of tissue reactions in the nerve roots which leads to "intraneural inflammation." The exact nature of this inflammation is not known, but it is likely to be characterized by edema, inflammatory cell reaction, and local demyelination.

It has been suggested that chemical, as well as mechanical, factors might be involved in the production of nerve root inflammation. Marshall and others have proposed that breakdown products from a degenerating nucleus pulposus might leak out and induce a "chemical radiculitis" along the root.[28,29] Intraoperative measurements of pH in the nucleus pulposus at the level of disc herniation have demonstrated low pH values, particularly in patients who had extensive adhesion formations around the nearby nerve root.[32,33] These findings might indicate a chemical interaction between the degenerating intervertebral disc and the nerve root which courses over it. This "radiculitis" may be initiated by direct irritating effects of proteoglycans from the disc[28] and/or by an autoimmune reaction from exposure to disc tissues.[5,15] There are, however, no conclusive experimental or clinical studies available which demonstrate that these mechanisms actually exist. On the other hand, current knowledge does not exclude the possibility that "chemical radiculitis" may be of significance in the pathophysiology of nerve root pain.[44,46] If these mechanisms are important in pain development, a better understanding of them, their mode of occurrence, as well as prevention may allow the development of new treatment modalities, for example pharmacologic substances which would interfere with the chemical nerve root irritation. Further research in these areas is essential.

The tissue reactions which occur in a nerve root in association with mechanical compression, for example by disc herniation, have a complex background where mechanical and possibly also chemical factors are involved and interact. The functional changes induced may be of two different modalities: 1) *loss of nerve function*, seen as sensory deficits and muscle weakness, and/or 2) *hyperexcitability* of the nerve tissue (Fig. 4). The latter phenomenon means that the nerve root is easily excited by further

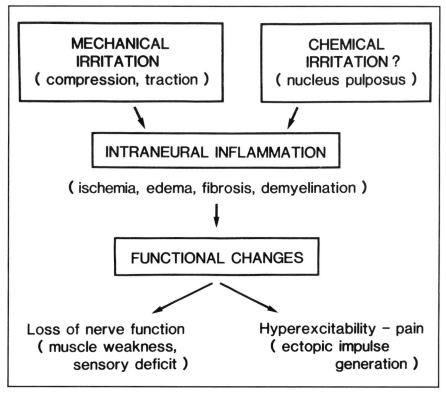

Figure 16-4. Schematic representation of the pathophysiology of functional changes induced by nerve root compression. See text for details.

mechanical stimulus, and becomes a site of ectopic impulse generation,[43] which may be related to pain.[19] The two kinds of functional changes (loss of nerve function and hyperexcitability) can be present at the same time, with the involved nerve roots demonstrating impaired electrophysiologic parameters (block of nerve fiber transmission and/or decreased conduction velocity) at the site of injury, though still being hypersensitive to further mechanical stimulus along the injured segment (Fig. 4). Clinically, the loss of nerve function can be assessed by observing EMG abnormalities and impaired sensory nerve conduction. However, these neurophysiological phenomena may not correlate with the degree of nerve root pain experienced by the patient. It must be remembered that neurophysiologic evaluations merely give information as to whether a nerve root is "affected" or not, and only allow some degree of quantification of this involvement. Experimentally, there is no information available regarding the possible correlation between loss of nerve conduction and hyperexcitability in association with nerve root injury, as for example by disc herniation.

Dorsal root ganglion

Dorso-lateral disc herniations in the lumbar spine often impinge upon the dorsal root ganglion (DRG) of the nerve root.[25] These observations are interesting when related to experimental studies, showing that compression of *normal DRG* may produce a neurophysiological response which corresponds to the neural activity induced when an *irritated nerve or nerve root* is compressed.[19] Thus, there are reasons to believe that compression of a normal DRG, as distinct from compression of a *normal* spinal nerve more proximally, may induce radiating pain. Recent investigations by Weinstein and co-workers[61,62] have indicated a possible role of neuropeptides such as substance-P and vaso-active intestinal peptides (VIP) in the DRG, in the production of low back pain.

Diagnosis and Treatment

It is beyond the scope of this chapter to give a detailed description of various diagnostic procedures and treatment modalities for spinal nerve root compression. Some practical aspects are summarized here and related to the background data on pathophysiology.

The diagnosis of central spinal stenosis or disc herniation with nerve root compression is made by a combination of clinical and radiological examinations and sometimes also neurophysiological investigations.

Disc herniation

The most common anatomic location of disc herniation in the lower lumbar spine is through the dorso-lateral aspect of the intervertebral disc.[49] This can be explained biomechanically by stress-concentrations at this location during loading of the discs.[31,33] Additionally, anatomically the posterior longitudinal ligament is thinner here than directly posteriorly over the disc, which also may favor a dorsolateral extrusion. Occasionally the midline portion of the anulus fibrosus ruptures causing a central, sometimes "massive", disc prolapse with acute compression of the cauda equina (cauda equina syndrome). This lesion, involving the majority of the nerve roots in the cauda equina, including the sacral nerve roots to the urogenital and rectal organs, should be considered an emergency, and very different from the dorso-lateral disc prolapse in terms of treatment and prognosis. The clinical symptoms of cauda equina syndrome include bilateral sciatica and/or leg paralysis, bladder paralysis, loss of rectal tone, and "saddle" anaesthesia, typically located in the perineum around the external genitals and buttocks. The diagnosis and treatment must be undertaken as soon as possible. Computerized tomography (CT), magnetic resonance imaging (MRI) or myelography of the lumbar spine are, together with a detailed neurologic (and urologic) examination, important diagnostic tests. There does not seem to be any generally accepted time limit beyond which irreversible neurological deficit occurs in these situations.[24] One should try to minimize the time interval to treatment, i.e. surgical decompression. The central disc prolapse with cauda equina compression is, however, a rare condition.

The more typical dorso-lateral disc herniation usually involves mainly one nerve root. However, depending on location, multiple roots may be compressed. A disc herniation at L4-L5 may, for example, compress the L5 nerve root and, to some degree, also the S1 nerve root if the disc fragment extends centrally. Rarely, a very laterally positioned disc fragment may compress the exiting nerve root from the level above, e.g. for a lateral L5-S1 disc herniation the L5 nerve root may be entrapped laterally. The clinical examination should include careful neurologic examination of the lower extremities, i.e. sensory and motor evaluation according to nerve root distribution, together with tension tests directed at the sciatic nerve (or femoral nerve if appropriate). This examination, of course, should always be preceded by a detailed history of the pain location and factors which precipitated the symptoms. Any spinal examination for pain should also, if indicated, include tests for possible non-organic pain components.[58] Pain drawings by the patients may also be valuable tools to rule out non-organic components in the pain syndrome.

In many institutions the prime radiologic investigation for detecting disc herniations is a CT scan. Currently, however, the MRI of the lumbar spine is increasing in popularity and usefulness. The non-invasive nature of the CT and MRI is, of course, an advantage. Occasionally, however, CT should be combined with a contrast injection into the subarachnoid space ("CT-myelo") or intravenously, especially when it is used to evaluate recurrent symptoms in patients who previously have undergone laminectomy and disc excision.[14] In the future, the MRI may prove to be of greater value in this regard. At this time, however, myelography remains a reliable diagnostic study.[3] Also, it must be emphasized that the findings on the radiologic evaluation must be consistent with the clinical picture in terms of level and side of the disc herniation. Studies in asymptomatic individuals have shown that approximately one-third of humans have radiographic (myelogram and CT) evidence of nerve compression without any signs or symptoms of it.[17,63] Increasingly, the above listed studies are supplanting plain lumbo-sacral radiographs by many physicians. We feel that the more easily obtained and interpreted routine studies (plain lumbo-sacral spine radiographs) should always be performed prior to more sophisticated ones.

If, after obtaining the history, physical exam and appropriate radiographic and metabolic studies there are still doubts about the exact diagnosis, further information may be gained from electrodiagnostic tests (see Kimura, 1983; Haldeman, 1984 for references).[16,22] For the diagnosis of nerve root involvement in disc herniations, the prime electrophysiologic investigation is a needle EMG of the lower extremity muscles, according to the specific spinal level of innervation (usually L4, L5, and S1). Additionally, para-vertebral muscles should be studied to determine if the posterior rami of the spinal nerves show evidence of dysfunction. The EMG may demonstrate evidence of a polyneuropathy and explain the leg pain or weakness on a basis other than spinal nerve root mechanical compression. We feel, however, unlike peripheral nerve entrapment/compression syndromes, elec-trophysiologic studies are not essential, unless the history, neurologic examination and radiographic studies do not completely correlate and explain the patients complaints. Additionally, along with electrophysio-logic studies, blood hematologic and chemical evaluations should be performed to look for a metabolic cause for the "radicular" signs and symptoms.

Treatment modalities should almost always start with bedrest for a few days, analgesia, and perhaps non-steroidal antiinflammatory drugs.[3,33,34] If these standard, relatively safe treatments fail, physical therapy, epidural steroids, transcutaneous electro-neuro stimulators (TENS), etc. may be considered.[10] If after 4-6 weeks on conservative therapy, pain persists, and the clinical and radiographic studies demonstrate root compression at the appropriate *level and side*, laminectomy and discectomy should be recom-mended.[54,59] Studies have shown that root decompression performed up to 3-6 months following disc herniation, in properly selected individuals, has a nearly 95% chance of relieving the leg pain. Surgery performed 1 year after symptoms develop, or in inappropriate patients (e.g. signs, symptoms and radiographic findings are not consistent, patients on workers compen-sation or who have litigation pending, etc.) is not nearly as successful. From these studies it is important to note: 1) except for a cauda equina syndrome, herniated discs should rarely, if ever, be considered an emergency, and surgery should be delayed at least 3-4 weeks to determine if symptoms will resolve; 2) leg pain is better treated by laminectomy than back pain; 3) unlike peripheral nerves, muscle weakness and symptoms from spinal nerve root compression have a high likelihood of resolution without surgery.

Chemonucleolysis, using chymopapain, and to some extent collagenase, has had varying popularity over the last few years.[6,11,30] There has been controversy as to the detailed mechanism of action of these enzymes, as well as the clinical results and complications. However, in properly selected patients studies have shown an approximately 60%-70% chance of relieving leg pain following chemonucleolysis. This suggests a true usefulness of this modality, but exact indications and long term follow-up are still lacking.

If surgery is performed it should be done with adequate hemostasis, magnification, and illumination. 3.5 power loupes and a head-lamp give improved visualization and should be used whenever possible. Microsurgical approaches using an operating microscope and "micro-" instruments may also be of value in selected cases. However, before deciding on any surgical intervention, the natural history of the disorder should be considered.

Spinal stenosis

For spinal stenosis there is less detailed information available regarding the natural history, as well as the results of various treatment modalities.[20,21]

The clinical picture of central spinal stenosis is typically present in the older patient and is usually characterized by pain radiating into the legs during walking. Unfortunately, this pain may be non-specific, difficult for the patient to fully characterize, and is frequently associated with a normal, or symmetric lower extremity neurologic examination. Tension signs are almost always absent.

Spinal stenosis can be caused by any disorder which narrows the spinal canal. Here, however, our focus is on narrowing of the spinal canal by the degenerative process. The most common cause for spinal stenosis is related to degenerative discs and the associated changes in the facet joints and surrounding/adjacent tissues.[1,23,60] The compression, therefore, may involve several nerve roots, often at multiple levels. Back pain is frequent because of the degenerative disc related changes (degenerative discs, osteophytes, facet arthritis, segmental instability, nerve irritation, etc.). However, pain radiating into one or both of the legs is usually what brings the patient to a physician. The pain usually is aggravated by exercise, or activities causing back extension (e.g. sitting in a car). The clinical syndrome may resemble vascular claudication. The mechanical nature of the pain, pain associated with spine position (lumbar flexion may decrease the symptoms of spinal stenosis), neurologic alterations, and/or peripheral vascular examinations, combined with appropriate findings on plain radiographs, CT, MRI and/or myelograms usually help differentiate these syndromes.

The diagnosis is made by a combination of clinical examination, myelogram, CT and/or MRI. As with pain related to herniated discs, rest, anti-inflammatories, epidural steroids, TENS units, corsets, physical therapy, etc. can be considered. Also advice to try to counteract back muscle extension (hyperlordosis) and improve abdominal muscle tone may help to reduce symptoms, since extention of the spine tends to decrease the volume of the spinal canal, and increase leg pain complaints.

The definitive treatment is, however, a multi-level laminectomy. In properly selected patients (i.e. history, physical exam and radiographic studies which are consistent, the patient is medically stable and well-motivated, and the leg pain exceeds back pain) there is an 85-90% chance of relieving the patient's leg pain with an appropriately performed, wide laminectomy. In this population, unlike those with herniated discs, the symptoms may improve over months, rather than hours or days.

Acknowledgements

The support by the Swedish Medical Research Council (7095), the Swedish Medical Society and the Folksam Research Foundation, Stockholm, Sweden and the Veterans Administration is gratefully acknowledged.

References

1. Arnoldi CC, et al.: Lumbar spinal stenosis and nerve root entrapment syndromes—definition and classification. Clin Orthop Rel Res 115:4-16, 1976.
2. Arvidson B: Distribution of intravenously injected protein tracers in peripheral ganglia of adult mice. Exp Neurol 63:388-410, 1979.
3. Bell G, Rothman R: The conservative treatment of sciatica. Spine 9:54-59, 1984.
4. Bell GR, Rothman RH, Booth RE, Cuckler JM, Garfin SR, Herkowitz H, Simeone FA, Dolinskas C and Han SS: A study of computer assisted tomography: II. Comparison of Metrizamide Myelography and Computed Tomography in the Diagnosis of Herniated Lumbar Disc and Spinal Stenosis. Spine 9:552-556, 1984.
5. Bobechko WP, Hirsch L: Auto-immune response to nucleus pulposus in the rabbit. J Bone Joint Surg 47B:574-580, 1965.
6. Brown MD: Intradiscal therapy—chymopapain or collagenase. Yearbook Medical Publishers Inc., Chicago, IL, 1983.
7. Brown MD, Gepstein R, Pallares V: Somatosensory evoked potentials during epidural anaesthesia. Paper presented at the 32nd Annual Meeting of the Orthopaedic Research Society, New Orleans, LA. Feb., 1986 (ORS Trans, p 62, 1986).
8. Dahlin LB, Rydevik B, McLean WG, Sjostrand J: Changes in fast axonal transport during experimental nerve compression at low pressures. Exp Neurol 84:29-36, 1984.
9. Dahlin LB: Nerve compression and axonal transport. Experimental studies on anterograde and retrograde axonal transport and nerve cell body changes in peripheral nerves subjected to graded compression. Doctoral thesis, University of Gothenburg, Sweden, 1986.
10. Deyo RM: Conservative Therapy for Low Back Pain. JAMA 250:1057-1062, 1983.
11. Editorial: Chymopapain and the intervertebral disc. The Lancet 843-845, Oct. 11, 1986.
12. Gelfan S, Tarlov JM: Physiology of spinal cord, nerve root, and peripheral nerve compression. Am J Physiol 185:217-229, 1956.
13. Goddard MD, Reid JD: Movements induced by straight leg raising in the lumbosacral roots, nerves and plexus, and in the intrapelvic section of the sciatic nerve. J Neurol Neurosurg Psych 28:12-18, 1965.
14. Genant HK: Spine Update—perspectives in radiology, orthopaedic surgery and neurosurgery. Radiol Res Educ Found, San Francisco, 1984.
15. Gertzbein SD, Tile M, Gross A, Falk R: Auto-immunity in degenerative disc disease of the lumbar spine. Ortho Clin North Am 6:67-73, 1975.
16. Haldeman S: The electrodiagnostic evaluation of nerve root function. Spine 9:42-47, 1984.

17. Hitselberger WE and Witten RM: Abnormal myelograms in asymptomatic patients. J Neurosurg 28:204-206, 1968.
18. Holm S, Rydevik B: Nutrition of spinal nerve roots—quantification of the contribution from intraneural microvessels and cerebrospinal fluid (to be published).
19. Howe JF, Loeser JD, Calvin WH: Mechanosensitivity of dorsal root ganglia and chronically injured axons: A physiological basis for the radicular pain of nerve root compression. Pain 3:25-41, 1977.
20. Johnsson K-E, Willner S, Pettersson H: Analysis of operated cases with lumbar spinal stenosis. Acta Orthop Scand 52:427-433, 1981.
21. Johnsson K-E, Willner S, Johnsson K: Postoperative instability after decompression for lumbar spinal stenosis. Spine 11:107-110, 1986.
22. Kimura J: Electrodiagnosis of diseases of nerve and muscle. F.A. Davis Co., Philadelphia, 1983.
23. Kirkaldy-Willis WH, Paine KWE, Cauchoix J, McIvor GWD: Lumbar spinal stenosis. Clin Orthop Rel Res 99:30-39, 1974.
24. Kostuik JP, Harrington I, Alexander D, Rand W and Evans D: Cauda equina syndrome and lumbar disc herniation. J Bone Joint Surg 68A:386-391, 1986.
25. Lindblom K, Rexed B: Spinal nerve injury in dorso-lateral protrusions of lumbar discs. J Neurosurg 5:413-432, 1948.
26. Lundborg G, Gelberman RH, Minteer-Convery M, Lee YF, Hargens A: Median nerve compression in the carpal tunnel: the functional response to experimentally induced controlled pressure. J Hand Surg 7:252-259, 1982.
27. MacNab I: The mechanism of spondylogenic pain. *In*: Cervical Pain. Ed.: Hirsch C, Zotterman Y. New York, Pergamon Press, 1972, pp 89-95.
28. Marshall LL, Trethewie ER: Chemical irritation of nerve roots in disc prolapse. The Lancet 2:320, 1973.
29. Marshall LL, Trethewie ER, Curtain CC: Chemical radiculitis—a clinical physiological and immunological study. Clin Orthop Rel Res 129:61-67, 1977.
30. McCulloch JA, MacNab I: Sciatica and chymopapain. Williams and Wilkins, Baltimore/London, 1983.
31. Nachemson A: The load on the lumbar spine in different positions of the body. Clin Orthop Rel Res 45:107-122, 1966.
32. Nachemson A: Intradiscal measurements of pH in patients with lumbar rhizopathies. Acta Orthop Scand 40:23-42, 1969.
33. Nachemson A: The lumbar spine—an orthopaedic challenge. Spine 1:59-71, 1976.
34. Nachemson A: Advances in low back pain. Clin Orthop Rel Res 200:266-278, 1985.
35. Olmarker K, Holm S, Hansson T, Rydevik B: Experimental graded compression of the pig cauda equina: effects on nerve root nutrition. Paper presented at the International Society for the Study of the Lumbar Spine, Annual Meeting, Dallas, Texas, May 1986.
36. Olmarker K, Rydevik B, Holm S, Bagge V, Hargens AR, Garfin SR, Glover M, Moore M, Swenson M: Graded compression of the porcine cauda equina causing modified nerve root nutrition, blood flow and impulse propagation. Paper presented at the 33rd Annual Meeting of the Orthopaedic Research Society, San Francisco, January, 1987 (Trans. ORS p 427, 1987).
37. Olmarker K, Holm S, Hansson T, Rydevik B: Effects of acute, graded compression on the nutritional supply of spinal nerve roots. An experimental study of the pig cauda equina. (Submitted) 1988.

38. Olmarker K, Bagge U, Holm S, Rydevik B: Effects of Experimental Graded Compression of Blood flow in Spinal Nerve Roots 1988. (Submitted) 1988.

39. Olsson Y: Vascular permeability in the peripheral nervous system. *In*: Peripheral neuropathy. Eds.: Dyck PJ, Thomas PK, Lambert EH, Bunge RP; WB Saunders Co., Philadelphia, 1984, Vol. I, pp 579-598.

40. Pedowitz RA, Rydevik B, Hargens AR, Swenson MR, Garfin SR: Motor and sensory nerve root conduction deficit induced by acute, graded compression of the pig cauda equina. Paper presented at 33rd Annual Meeting of the ORS, Atlanta GA Jan, 1988. (Trans. ORS 134, 1988).

41. Parke WW, Gammell K, Rothman RH: Arterial vascularization of the cauda equina. J Bone Joint Surg 63A:53-62, 1981.

42. Parke WW, Watanabe R: The intrinsic vasculature of the lumbosacral spinal nerve roots. Spine 10:508-515, 1985.

43. Rasminsky M: Ectopic generation of impulses in pathological nerve fibers. *In*: Nerve repair and regeneration—its clinical and experimental basis. Ed.: Jewett DL, McCarroll HR; CV Mosby, St. Louis, Missouri, 1980, pp 178-185.

44. Rydevik B, Brown MD, Ehira T, Nordborg C, Lundborg G: Effects of graded compression and nucleus pulposus on nerve tissue—an experimental study in rabbits. Acta Orthop Scand 54:670-671, 1983.

45. Rydevik B, Holm S, Brown MD, Lundborg G: Nutrition of spinal nerve roots. Paper presented at the 30th Annual Meeting of the Orthopaedic Research Society, February, 1984 (Trans ORS, p 276). (1984)

46. Rydevik B, Brown MD, Lundborg G: Pathoanatomy and pathophysiology of nerve root compression. Spine 9:7-15, 1984.

47. Rydevik B, Lundborg G, Skalak R: Biomechanics of nerves. *In*: Basic biomechanics of the musculoskeletal system, 2nd edition. *Eds*: Frankel VH, Nordin M, Lea and Febiger, Philadelphia, 1988.

48. Rydevik B, Holm S, Lundborg G, Brown MD: Diffusion from the cerebrospinal fluid as a nutritional mechanism for spinal nerve roots. (Submitted) 1988.

49. Schonstrom N, Bollender NF, Spengler DM, Hansson T: Pressure changes within the cauda equina following constriction of the dural sac. An in vitro experimental study. Spine 9:604-607, 1984.

50. Sharpless SK: Susceptibility of spinal nerve roots to compression block. *In*: The research status of spinal manipulative therapy. NIH Workshop, February 2-4, 1975. *Ed*: Goldstein M. NINCDS Monograph No. 15, pp 155-161.

51. Smyth MJ, Wright V: Sciatica and the intervertebral disc. An experimental study. J Bone Joint Surg 40A:1401-1418, 1958.

52. Spencer DL, Irwin GS, Miller JAA: Anatomy and significance of fixation of the lumbosacral nerve roots in sciatica. Spine 8:672-679, 1983.

53. Spencer DL, Miller JAA, Bertolini JE: The effects of intervertebral disc space narrowing on the contact force between the nerve root and a simulated disc protrusion. Spine 9:422-426, 1984.

54. Spengler DM, Freeman C, Westbrook R, Miller J: Low back pain following lumbar spine procedures. Failure of initial selection? Spine 5:356-362, 1980.

55. Sunderland S: Nerves and nerve injuries. Churchill and Livingstone, 2nd Ed., Edinburg, London, New York, 1978.

56. Thomas PK and Olsson Y: Microscopic anatomy and function of the connective tissue components of peripheral nerve. *In*: Peripheral neuropathy. Eds.: Dyck PJ, Thomas PK, Lambert EH, Bunge RP; WB Saunders Co., Philadelphia, 1984, pp 97-120.

57. Upton RM, McComas AJ: The double-crush in nerve entrapment syndromes. Lancet 2:359-362, 1973.

58. Waddell G, McCulloch JA, Kummel E, Wenner RM: Non-organic physical signs in low back pain. Spine 5:117-124, 1980.

59. Weber H: Lumbar disc herniation. A controlled prospective study with ten years of observation. Spine 2:131-139, 1983.

60. Wedge JH, Kirhaldy-Willis WH, Kinnard P: Lumbar spinal stenosis. *In*: Disorders of the Lumbar Spine. Eds: Helfet AJ and Gruebel DM. JB Lippincott Co., Philadelphia/Toronto, 1978.

61. Weinstein JN: Mechanisms of spinal pain—the dorsal root ganglion and its role as a mediator of low back pain. Spine 11:999-1001, 1986.

62. Weinstein JN, Pope M, Schmidt R, Serroussi R: Effects of low frequency vibration on the dorsal root ganglion. Neuroorthopaedics, 4:24-30, 1987.

63. Wiesel SW, Tsourmas N, Feffer HL, Citrin CM and Patronas N: A study of computer-assisted tomography: 1. The incidence of positive CAT scans in an asymptomatic group of patients. Spine 9:549-551, 1984.

CHAPTER 17

Compression of the Lumbosacral Plexus and the Sciatic Nerve

Franklin C. Wagner, Jr., M.D.

Anatomy

The susceptibility of the sciatic nerve to injury is commonly determined by its location at various levels within the pelvis and the lower extremity. A brief review of the anatomy of the sciatic nerve therefore would be worthwhile.[26]

Within the pelvis the components of what are to become the sciatic nerve are a part of the sacral plexus. This plexus is comprised of the lumbosacral trunk, the ventral rami of the first, second, and third sacral nerves, and part of the ventral ramus of the fourth sacral nerve. The lumbosacral trunk is composed of a part of the ventral ramus of the fourth lumbar nerve and the entire ventral ramus of the fifth lumbar nerve. It arises at the medial margin of the psoas major muscle and descends over the brim of the pelvis anterior to the sacroiliac joint where it joins the first sacral nerve. The ventral rami of the second and third sacral nerves converge at the greater sciatic foramen to form with the lumbosacral trunk and the first sacral nerve a large band which is united to a smaller lower band composed of contributions from the second, third, and fourth sacral nerves. While the lower, smaller band is prolonged as the pudendal nerve, the upper, larger band continues as the sciatic nerve.

The sciatic nerve usually divides in the thigh into the tibial and common peroneal nerves. Before this occurs these two nerves can be separated to their roots of origin. When this is done it is found that the tibial nerve is formed from the union of the ventral divisions of the lumbosacral trunk and the first three sacral nerves and the common peroneal nerve by the dorsal divisions of the lumbosacral trunk and first two sacral nerves.

While the sciatic nerve commonly divides in the thigh, this may take place anywhere along its course from the pelvis. When this occurs at the level of the sacral plexus the common peroneal nerve usually pierces the piriformis muscle in the greater sciatic foramen.

Lying on the posterior wall of the pelvic cavity the sacral plexus is located in front of the piriformis muscle and behind the internal iliac vessels, the ureter, and the sigmoid colon on the left side, and the terminal coils of the ileum on the right side. The lumbosacral trunk and the first sacral nerve, or the first and second sacral nerves, are transversed by the superior gluteal vessels, and the ventral rami of the first and second, or second and third sacral nerves by the inferior gluteal vessels.

As a continuation of the upper band of the sacral plexus the sacral nerve leaves the pelvis through the greater sciatic foramen beneath the piriformis muscle and descends between the greater trochanter of the femur and the tuberosity of the ischium. It continues down the back of the thigh until approximately the lower third of the thigh where it divides into its two large branches, the tibial and the common peroneal nerves. During its course in the thigh, the sciatic nerve initially lies deep to the gluteus maximus muscle and rests upon the posterior surface of the ischium. It then passes on to the quadratus femoris muscle, which separates the nerve from the obturator externus and the hip joint. More distally the nerve lies upon the adductor magnus and is crossed by the long head of the biceps femoris. As Williams and Warwick have pointed out, the course of the sciatic nerve in the thigh can be represented by drawing a line from the midpoint between the ischial tuberosity and the apex of the greater trochanter to the top of the popliteal fossa.[26]

As with the sciatic nerve, its larger terminal branch, the tibial (medial popliteal) nerve, can be represented in the lower thigh and in the leg by a line drawn in the midline from the apex of the popliteal fossa to the level of the neck of the fibula and then continued to a point halfway between the medial malleolus and the tendo calcaneus. The tibial nerve in its course is covered by the medial margins of the two heads of the gastrocnemius in the lower part of the popliteal fossa. Distally in the upper part of the leg, the nerve is covered by the soleus and the gastrocnemius muscles, but in the lower third of the leg it becomes more superficial and is covered only by the fascia and skin. It bifurcates under the flexor retinaculum at a point between the heel and the medial malleolus into the medial and lateral plantar nerves.

The smaller of the two terminal branches of the sciatic nerve, the common peroneal (lateral popliteal), arises from the dorsal branches of the ventral rami of the fourth and fifth lumbar and the first and second sacral nerves. From the lateral side of the popliteal fossa, it descends to the head of the fibula between the tendon of the biceps femoris laterally and the lateral head of the gastrocnemius medially. It then winds around the lateral surface of the neck of the fibula deep to the peroneus longus and divides into the superficial and deep peroneal nerves.

The sciatic nerve in the thigh supplies motor branches to the semitendinosus, semimembranosus, the long and short heads of the biceps, and part of the adductor magnus muscles. All of the muscles below the knee are innervated by the terminal branches of the sciatic. The superficial and deep peroneal derived from the common peroneal supply the peroneus longus and brevis and the tibialis anterior, extensor digitorum longus, extensor hallucis longus, peroneus tertius, and extensor digitorum brevis muscles, respectively. The tibial nerve provides motor branches to the gastrocnemius, popliteus, plantaris, soleus, tibialis posterior, flexor digitorum longus, and flexor hallucis longus muscles. The medial and lateral plantar nerves into which the tibial nerve divides supply the small muscles of the feet.

Injuries to the Lumbosacral Plexus and the Sciatic Nerve

The largest experience with injuries to the sciatic nerve and its branches, the tibial and common peroneal nerves, has come from wartime. The series that describe this experience indicate that the sciatic and common peroneal nerves may be injured with approximately the same frequency, while the tibial nerve is less commonly damaged.[22] While differences in the relative position of the tibial and common peroneal nerves in the sciatic trunk, in the muscles that the two branches supply, and in their respective blood supply have been offered as explanations for the greater susceptibility of the common peroneal nerve to injury than the tibial nerve, the reason for this difference remains uncertain. Sunderland, while acknowledging that the factors just mentioned may be important in individual cases, has suggested that the more tightly packed funiculi and the degree to which the nerve may be fixed by its muscular branches more generally explains the greater vulnerability of the common peroneal nerve to injury.[22]

A more realistic picture of the causes in civilian practice of injuries to the sciatic nerve and its branches may be derived from the experience of Seddon.[19] This investigator lists missile injuries; dislocations of the hip, with or without fracture; injection injuries; fractures of the acetabulum and the femur; and injuries of the knee causing traction lesions as common causes of nerve injury. Less frequently, injuries may result from incised wounds, lacerations, surgical operations, compression, and ganglia and tumors.

The review that follows will be limited to a description of the syndromes that may result from compression of the lumbosacral plexus and of the sciatic nerve.

Fractures

It has been estimated that between 1.2 and 3.5 percent of all pelvic fractures and dislocations are complicated by nerve injuries.[18] When the posterior pelvic ring made up of the sacroiliac joint and the posterior and posterolateral walls of the pelvis is involved, the incidence of nerve injuries increases because of the proximity of the lumbosacral trunk.[5] The damage that occurs to the trunk is usually secondary to compression or traction.

Determining that there has been a nerve injury may be difficult due to the presence of injuries to the bone, soft tissue, and viscera. When a neurologic deficit is found to be present, it is most likely to be on the side of the major fracture. The extent and the mixed pattern of the deficit usually implicates a pelvis injury rather than a single intervertebral disc lesion. Furthermore, the degree of recovery suggests peripheral damage rather than a root avulsion.[18]

Electrodiagnostic testing is of value in documenting the extent of nerve damage and in establishing a prognosis. Early myelography may be helpful in confirming the level of nerve damage and in determining the advisability of surgical exploration. The presence of large irregular diverticula near the lumbosacral level when this is done is likely to be the result of a lumbosacral avulsion at or beyond the intervertebral foramen rather than at the spinal cord.[18]

After leaving the pelvis the sciatic nerve in its position on the posterior surface of the ischium between the ischial tuberosity and the greater trochanter can be injured in posterior dislocations of the hip. In those patients with advanced osteoarthritis of the hip, with a marked deformity or hypoplasia of the pelvis, or in whom the buttock is compressed on the operating table and the hip placed in marked flexion, the nerve is susceptible to injury when a closed ischiofemoral arthrodesis by nail and graft is undertaken.[1] It is also possible for a posterior fragment of acetabulum to either stretch or lacerate the peroneal portion of the nerve.[6]

More distally the nerve lies well protected on the adductor magnus under the biceps femoris, therefore making injuries here unusual.[6] Fractures of the femur, though, may result in the sciatic nerve, which is located close to the bone in the thigh, being stretched or injured by the fractured ends of the bone.[16,21] An open reduction of the fracture may be necessary if the nerve is entrapped between the bone ends. Although most nerve injuries associated with a closed fracture of the femur are mild and therefore will recover spontaneously, the complete severance of the nerve has been described.[21]

Pregnancy

During pregnancy the lumbosacral trunk may be compressed within the pelvis by the fetal head or by the buttock of the fetus during a breech delivery.[25] A straight pelvis, a flat wide posterior pelvis, a prominent sacroiliac joint, posterior displacement of the transverse diameter of the inlet, prominent ischial spines and wide sacrosciatic notches are anatomic features that may contribute to such an occurrence.[23]

The protrusion of an intervertebral disc has been offered as an alternative explanation for the neuritis involving the lower extremities associated with pregnancy.[17] This was done after it was observed that only one oblique diameter of the pelvic inlet is occupied by the greatest diameter of the fetal head, that the lumbosacral trunk is protected by the iliac vessels, that there may be no pelvic disproportion, that forceps may not have been used, that labor may have been short, that symptoms may develop some days after labor, and that those symptoms may occur in the distribution of the femoral nerve. Where a herniated intervertebral disc is determined to be the cause, surgery is indicated in those women whose motor disturbances are severe and persistent or in those whose pain does not respond to bed rest.

Entrapment by the Piriformis Muscle

The sciatic nerve in the majority of cases leaves the pelvis below the piriformis muscle.[26] In approximately 10 percent of cases, though, the nerve may pass through the muscle or its common peroneal division may either run through or over the muscle. When either nerve passes through the muscle it may potentially be compressed. In the situation where the common peroneal nerve runs over the muscle it may be entrapped between the muscle and the bone of the greater sciatic notch.[9,10,14]

Vascular

Symptoms of claudication occurring in the distribution of the sciatic nerve may be due to atheromatous narrowing of major vessels in the pelvis such as the iliac arteries.[11] When endarterectomy and vascular reconstruction is carried out, the relief of such symptoms can be anticipated.

Foot drop may follow occlusion of the femoral or popliteal arteries due to thrombosis or embolism. Why the common peroneal nerve should be more susceptible to ischemia developing in this way is uncertain.[4]

Bleeding into the muscles approximating the sciatic nerve and its branches with hematoma formation into the nerve sheaths with resulting nerve impairment has been reported as a complication of hemophilia and of anticoagulant therapy.[3,12,20]

Systemic

Systemic diseases can result in the production of symptoms secondary to the entrapment of the peripheral nerves in the lower extremities. Rheumatoid arthritis may be complicated by the development of a popliteal (Baker's) cyst.[15] This may occur when an effusion develops in those instances where the gastrocnemius-semimembranous bursa communicates with the knee joint. A Baker's cyst may then entrap the lower sciatic nerve. Either the common peroneal or the tibial nerves may be involved separately or together.

Diagnosis

As with injuries to other peripheral nerves, impairment of sciatic nerve function is determined by the level and the extent of the injury and by the degree to which other nerves can compensate for the sensory and motor functions normally performed by the sciatic nerve.[24]

When the sciatic nerve is completely interrupted, paralysis of flexion of the knee, which is carried out by the hamstrings, and of all the muscles below the knee results. Since the branches to the hamstrings, with the exception of those that innervate the short head of the biceps, usually originate near the ischial tuberosity, the lesion of the sciatic nerve must be high in order for knee flexion to be lost. For this reason, injuries to the sciatic nerve in the upper thigh may leave the hamstrings functioning.

A lesion of the common peroneal nerve, which paralyzes the anterior tibial and the peroneal muscles, produces a foot drop. While the patient can stand and walk, the toes of the affected foot are dragged.

Below the branches to the gastrocnemius and soleus, lesions of the tibial nerve do not seriously affect the function of the leg, but, nonetheless, may have grave consequences. Due to rendering the heel insensitive, this region is predisposed to trophic changes and pressure sores, and secondary to the paralysis of the intrinsic muscles, stability of the foot may be altered.

The sensory distribution of the sciatic nerve lies entirely below the knee. The sensory modality most widely affected by the complete division of the nerve is light touch. With the exception of a zone about four centimeters wide along its inner aspect and extending approximately five centimeters distal from the medial malleolus, the whole foot is anesthetic to light touch. The area of anesthesia for light touch on the leg involves the lateral aspect and extends laterally from the midline anteriorly to the midline posteriorly and rostrally to a point about five centimeters below the upper end of the fibula. The loss of superficial pain is less extensive than that of light touch. Position and vibratory sense are lost in the foot with the exception of the proximal two-thirds of its inner aspect.

The reflexes in the lower extremity are affected as well by the division of the sciatic nerve. Both the ankle jerk and the plantar reflex are lost, but the knee jerk is unaffected.

Electromyography

The judicious use of electromyography (EMG) and nerve conduction studies helps distinguish between central and peripheral causes of sciatic nerve impairment, and among peripheral causes of decreased sciatic nerve function.[2]

The piriformis syndrome in which the sciatic nerve becomes entrapped as it leaves the pelvis through the greater sciatic notch and crosses the sharp lower edge of the piriformis muscle is an example of a high sciatic neuropathy. In this instance, the electromyogram will demonstrate normal activity in the gluteus medium, gluteus minimus, and tensor fasciae latae muscles, while abnormalities are likely to be apparent in muscles below this level, such as in the gluteus maximus. In distinction to lumbar disc disease, in which abnormalities of the paravertebral lumbosacral muscles are seen due to innervation of these muscles by the posterior rami of the affected nerve root, in the piriformis syndrome an EMG of these same muscles will be normal.[14]

Distinguishing between a lesion of the sciatic nerve in which the fibers that will ultimately become the common peroneal nerve are selectively involved and a peroneal neuropathy may be clinically impossible. Electromyography of the short head of the biceps femoris muscle may be helpful, for abnormalities in this muscle will indicate a proximal lesion and thereby implicate the sciatic nerve.[2]

Since a popliteal (Baker's) cyst may compress both the tibial and the common peroneal nerves or only one of these branches of the sciatic nerve, electromyography will assist determining the extent of involvement.[14,15] Among the muscles likely to display abnormalities when the tibial nerve is involved are the gastrocnemius, soleus, tibialis posterior, flexor digitorum longus, flexor hallucis longus, and the intrinsic muscles of the foot. Whereas, with compression of the common peroneal, abnormalities in the tibialis anterior, extensor hallucis longus, extensor digitorum longus, and extensor digitorum brevis muscles are likely to be detected.

Treatment

Experience indicates that the most efficacious treatment for injuries of the sciatic nerve and its branches is determined by the pathology of the injury.[8] Understanding what the pathology of a particular nerve is likely to be has been aided by the classifications developed by Seddon and Sunderland.[19,22]

Mild nerve injuries in which axonal flow is interrupted and paranodal or segmental demyelination occurs produce a prolongation in nerve conduction and clinical disability. In such injuries, though, the regeneration of myelin by the extension of adjacent Schwann cells or by the interposition of new Schwann cells results in a restoration of nerve fiber function. Whenever present in mild nerve injuries, the relief of whatever may be compressing the nerve is likely to be of benefit.

More severe nerve injuries result in an interruption of axons, but preservation of basement membranes. While Wallerian degeneration follows in those axon cylinders that have been interrupted, the intact basement membranes permit the regenerating axon sprouts to be guided by the enclosed chain of Schwann cells. Surgery on the damaged nerve in this instance is not indicated, since the prognosis cannot be improved.

The severest injuries produce an interruption of both axon cylinders and basement membranes. The absence of a guidance system in the form of intact basement membranes makes effective regeneration difficult. The removal of obstructing scar tissue and the realignment of nerve fascicles may be of value.

When surgery is undertaken directly on a damaged sciatic nerve or its branches, the recording of nerve action potentials intraoperatively can provide useful information.[13] This is especially true of lesions in continuity where as soon as two months after injury regeneration may not have reached distal motor end-plates and cannot be demonstrated by any other means.

The recording of intraoperative action potentials can be accomplished by bipolar stimulation and recording from electrodes applied directly to the nerve on each side of the lesion. Computer averaging is not required. By comparing the amplitude of the distal evoked response to the proximal response, the quality of regeneration can be estimated. Where the distal action potential is absent, nerve resection and suture is appropriate.

Surgery on proximal sciatic nerve lesions (especially complete lesions) is usually unsuccessful. Associated injuries to soft tissue, bone, and blood vessels may delay axonal regeneration, and by the time the ordinary 12 to 24 months required for axons to reach the muscles of the leg have elapsed, irreparable degenerative changes may have already taken place in those muscles. In contrast, a partial injury to the sciatic nerve is frequently complete to either the common peroneal or tibial division, and partial or nonexistent to the other division. In such an instance neurolysis of the partially involved division and resection and suture of the completely involved division rather than a suture repair of the entire sciatic nerve are indicated.[7]

Injuries of the tibial nerve, even when proximal, do comparatively well, provided early exploration is carried out and the correct decision regarding neurolysis or suture repair is made. Injuries of the peroneal nerve do not do as well, but their prognosis may be enhanced when the nerve has been sharply transected, when a blunt injury to the nerve is located distally, or when the patient is young.[8]

When the sciatic nerve becomes entrapped by the piriformis muscle, conservative measures will usually provide relief. Rarely is surgical exposure of the sciatic notch for neurolysis required.[9,14]

Drainage of a popliteal (Baker's) cyst or injections of corticosteroids effectively reverse the symptoms resulting from the compression of the lower sciatic nerve or its branches.[15] Occasionally, a synovectomy may be necessary in refractory or recurrent cases.

References

1. Adams JC: Vulnerability of the sciatic nerve in closed ischio-femoral arthrodesis by nail and graft. J Bone Joint Surg 46B:748, 1964.
2. Aminoff MJ: Electromyography and nerve conduction studies. *In:* A Crockard, R Hayward, JT Hoff (Eds): Neurosurgery: The Scientific Basis of Clinical Practice. Oxford, Blackwell Scientific Publications, 1985, pp 530.
3. Arbuse DI, Locascio NR: Neurological manifestations in hemophilia. Med Rec NY 146:377, 1937.
4. Ferguson FR, Liversedge LA: Ischaemic lateral popliteal nerve palsy. Br Med J 2:333, 1954.
5. Huittinen V-M: Lumbosacral nerve injury in fracture of the pelvis. A post-mortem radiographic and patho-anatomical study. Acta Chir Scand, (Suppl) 429, 1972.
6. Johnson EW: Nerve injuries in fractures to the lower extremity. Minn Med 52:627, 1969.
7. Kline DG: Operative management of major nerve lesions of the lower extremity. Surg Clin North Am 52:1247, 1972.
8. Kline DG, Hudson AR: Surgical repair of acute peripheral nerve injuries: Timing and technique. *In:* TP Morley (Ed): Current Controversies in Neurosurgery. Philadelphia, W.B. Saunders Co., 1976, pp 184.
9. Kopell HP, Thompson WAL: Peripheral entrapment neuropathies of the lower extremity. N Engl J Med 262:56, 1960.
10. Kopell HP, Thompson WAL: Peripheral entrapment neuropathies. Baltimore, Williams and Wilkins, 1963.

11. Lamerton AJ, Bannister R, Withrington R, Seifert MH, Eastcott HHG: "Claudication" of the sciatic nerve. Br Med J 286:1785, 1983.
12. Leonard MA: Sciatic nerve paralysis following anticoagulant therapy. J Bone Joint Surg 54B:152, 1972.
13. Miller CF, Kline DG: Peripheral-nerve injury. *In:* CB Wilson, JT Hoff (Eds): Current Surgical Management of Neurologic Disease. New York, Churchill Livingstone, 1980, pp 249.
14. Nakano KK: The entrapment neuropathies. Muscle Nerve 1:264, 1978.
15. Nakano KK: Entrapment neuropathy from Baker's cyst. JAMA 239:135, 1978.
16. Neer CS, Grantham SA, Foster RR: Femoral shaft fracture with sciatic nerve palsy. JAMA 214:2307, 1970.
17. O'Connell JEA: Maternal obstetrical paralysis. Surg Gynecol Obstet 79:374, 1944.
18. Patterson FP: Neurological complications of fractures and dislocations of the pelvis. J Trauma 12:1013, 1972.
19. Seddon HJ: Surgical Disorders of Peripheral Nerves, 2nd ed. Edinburgh, Churchill Livingstone, 1975, pp 224.
20. Silverstein A: Neuropathy in hemophilia. JAMA 190:554, 1964.
21. Spiegel PG, Johnston MJ, Harvey JP: Complete sciatic nerve laceration in a closed femoral shaft fracture. J Trauma 14:617, 1974.
22. Sunderland S: Nerve and Nerve Injuries, 2nd ed. Edinburgh, Churchill Livingstone, 1978, pp 967.
23. Tillman AJB: Traumatic neuritis in the puerperium. Am J Obstet Gynecol 29:660, 1935.
24. Walton JN: Brain's Diseases of the Nervous System, 9th ed. Oxford, Oxford University Press, 1985, pp 509.
25. Whittaker WG: Injuries to the sacral plexus in obstetrics. Can Med Assoc J 79:622, 1958.
26. Williams PL, Warwick R: Functional Neuroanatomy of Man. Philadelphia, W.B. Saunders Co., 1975, pp 1056.

CHAPTER 18

Nerve Entrapment Syndromes of the Foot and Ankle: Part I

Roger A. Mann, M.D.
Paul F. Plattner, M.D.

Prior to reviewing specific entrapment syndromes in the lower extremity it would be helpful to define entrapment neuropathy. Kopell defines this as "a region of localized injury and inflammation in a peripheral nerve that is caused by mechanical irritation from some impinging anatomical neighbor."[19] It can be a result of direct axonal compression or vascular effects. In the experimental literature the debate centers on the relative importance of the ischemic versus the mechanical aspects of these lesions, but it seems that both factors are operative and most likely additive.

A common factor is a nerve passing through a narrow rigid compartment at a point where movement or stretching of that nerve occurs. Common sites of occurrence are points where a nerve passes through a fibrous or fibro-osseous tunnel or at an area where the nerve changes its direction over a fibrous or muscular band.

The role of trauma in the initiation of these neuropathies is not always discernible. A traumatic incident may set up a local inflammatory process at an area where the anatomic configuration is such as to maintain a neuropathy. In other cases a patient's awareness of the condition may follow an accumulation of repeated small trauma. Repetitive motions can cause an encroachment on a nerve as it passes through a narrow passageway. Peripheral nerves must be able to move with relation to neighboring structures, and an entrapment point may be a region of significant pressure and interference with passive motion of a nerve. This becomes more important when it is realized that nerve trunks are relatively inelastic.

Entrapment neuropathies of the foot and ankle are important not only because of the pain and impairment that may result but also because they must be distinguished from other clinical situations. This was recognized by Kopell and Thompson in 1960 when they identified those patients with continuing pain and impairment after a foot and ankle injury. "A concurrent neuropathy is often overlooked and all the complaints and dysfunctions are attributed to ligamentous or joint residuals."[18]

Pain is prominent in entrapment neuropathies. It is usually present at rest and can be worse at night. Activity can cause pain but close correlation between discomfort and activity, and ease at rest (prominent in tenosynovitis and arthritis), are absent. Retrograde pain often occurs and the nerve can be tender both above and below the compression point, the Valleix phenomenon. Sensory nerves give a clear distribution of pain which often is sharp or burning and can be associated with paresthesias in many forms, including hyperesthesia, hypesthesia or dysesthesia. The pain in motor nerve compression is less well localized and can range from a dull ache to severe pain. Atrophy of the innervated muscles can occur. When both sensory and motor nerves are involved, pain is usually more evident than motor loss, and in chronic lesions vasomotor changes can occur.

History of a radiating pain present at rest and often worse at night, with an inconsistent relationship to activity, is suggestive of entrapment. When the pain is burning in nature this likelihood is increased. Examination might reveal tenderness over the nerve or a positive nerve percussion sign (reproduction of pain by tapping over the nerve). Sometimes the application of a tourniquet will precipitate symptoms. Nerve conduction studies are most valuable if the sites are accessible. Axonal conduction velocities commonly are normal in the early stages. The conduction velocity might be slow in becoming abnormal but conduction delays and progressive fall-off in action potential amplitudes occur.

Plantar Nerves

The medial and lateral plantar nerves are the two major terminal branches of the tibial nerve. They arise beneath the flexor retinaculum behind the medial malleolus and run forward deep to the abductor hallucis muscle. These nerves continue distally to give off, in the foot, muscular and cutaneous branches. Recently reports have described a branch of the lateral plantar nerve that arises proximally and runs beneath the fascia of the abductor hallucis muscle and courses between the median portion of the quadratus plantae muscle and the plantar fascia to innervate the abductor digiti quinti muscle.[6,12]

The medial calcaneal nerve is another distal branch of the tibial nerve, although some authors have found this to be a branch of the lateral plantar nerve. The calcaneal nerve usually has two major branches which exit beneath the lancinate ligament dorsal to the abductor hallucis muscle to supply cutaneous sensation to the plantar and medial aspects of the heel. The anterior branch of the calcaneal nerve, as described by Henricson et al. and Tanz, may be the same branch of the lateral plantar nerve that innervates the abductor digiti quinti muscle described already.[10,15]

Although the painful heel syndrome is a commonly encountered problem in orthopaedic practice, the etiology of this disorder has never been clearly demonstrated. One cause of a painful heel syndrome is entrapment neuropathy. A variety of terms have been used to describe particular types of individuals in which heel pain is commonly seen. A few such terms include tennis heel, policeman's heel, jogger's heel, and stone bruise.

Painful conditions about the heel can be classified according to location. Posterior heel pain may be the result of a prominence of the posterolateral aspect of the calcaneus and the formation of a superficial adventitial bursa (pump bump), or be the result of inflammation of the deep subfascial retrocalcaneal bursa or peritendinous lining of the Achilles tendon. More typically plantar pain is classified into such entities as plantar fasciitis, painful calcaneal spurs and subcalcaneal bursitis or periostitis. Entrapment neuropathy of the plantar nerve or medial calcaneal nerve may also be a source of plantar or medial heel pain. Several recent articles have elucidated this potential source of heel pain quite well.[6,7,10,12,13]

The potential sites of entrapment are shown in Figures 18-1 through 18-4. As shown in Figures 18-1 and 18-2, the nerve to the abductor digiti quinti muscle, which arises from the lateral plantar nerve, may become entrapped by the inelastic and unyielding deep fascia of the abductor hallucis muscle as the nerve courses to the lateral border of the foot beneath the long plantar ligament and medial calcaneal tuberosity. More distally the medial plantar nerve may become entrapped behind the navicular tuberosity (Figs. 18-3 and 18-4). This has been reported in joggers who run long distances in a valgus posture.[13]

Clinical Presentation

Characteristically the patient with the painful heel syndrome complains of pain with weight bearing, often noting that the pain is worse in the morning, that it improves somewhat as the day progresses and again worsens later in the day. Onset is often gradual with only an occasional patient reporting a history of trauma prior to the onset of symptoms. Symptoms are often of weeks to months in duration before the patient seeks medical attention.

Examination reveals tenderness most often on the medial aspect of the heel. Lapidus found 91.8 percent of patients had medial heel pain, 7.4 percent central heel pad pain and 0.8 percent had pain both medially and laterally. The lateral heel pain is rare.[11]

Attempts have been made to subdivide the painful heel syndrome into a number of different entities on the basis of physical examination. Plantar fasciitis is characterized by pain along the medial one-third of the plantar fascia, with an area of maximal tenderness located distal to the medial calcaneal tuberosity. Passive dorsiflexion of the toes places increased tension on the origin of the plantar fascia and may aggravate the pain. The painful heel pad is characterized by tenderness in the center of the heel pad. Pain localized to the medial calcaneal tuberosity is attributed by some to be

Continued on page 277

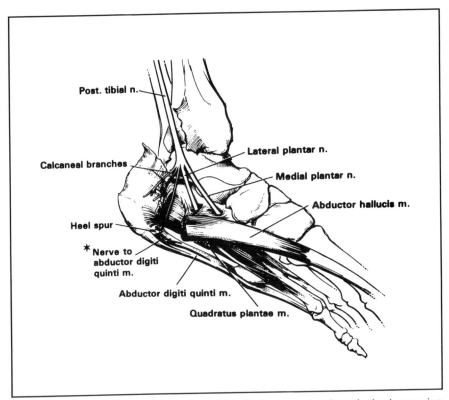

Figure 18-1. The deep fascia of the abductor hallucis muscle has been incised, exposing the nerve to the abductor digiti quinti muscle. (From Baxter DE, Thigpen CM: Heel pain: operative results, Foot & Ankle 5(1):16, 1984.)

Figure 18-2. Relation of nerves to anatomic structures: 1, long plantar ligament; 2, plantar fascia; 3, skin; 4, medial plantar nerve; 5, lateral plantar nerve; 6, nerve to abductor digiti quinti; 7, medial calcaneal nerve. (From Bordelon RL: Subcalcaneal pain: A method of evaluation and plan for treatment, Clin Orthop Rel Res 177:49, 1983.)

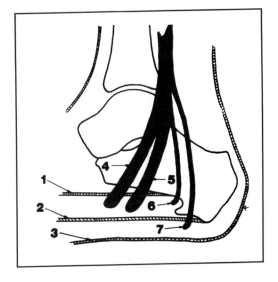

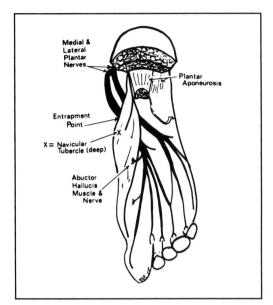

Figure 18-3. This schematic representation of the plantar aspect of the right foot shows the entrapment point just posterior to the navicular tuberosity. Instilling 2 percent lidocaine hydrochloride at this point should completely relieve the patient's burning heel pain. (From Rask MR: Medial plantar neuropraxia (jogger's foot): Report of three cases, Clin Orthop Rel Res 134:193, 1978.)

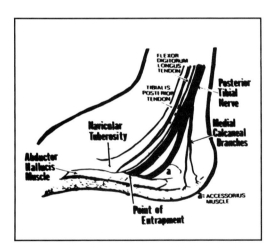

Figure 18-4. This schematic representation of the medial aspect of the right foot shows how the medial calcaneal branches share a common origin with the medial plantar nerve. The entrapment point of the medial plantar nerve comes from a valgus stretch of the nerve in its fibromuscular tunnel and longitudinal arch trauma of valgus running. (From Rask MR: Medial plantar neuropraxia (jogger's foot): Report of three cases, Clin Orthop Rel Res 134:193, 1978.)

calcaneal bursitis. Tenderness below and posterior to the tarsal tunnel over the origin of the abductor hallucis muscle may represent entrapment neuropathy of the medial calcaneal nerve or branch of the lateral plantar nerve to the abductor digiti quinti muscle.

Treatment

As has been indicated, there are multiple causes of heel pain, and treatment needs to be directed as specifically as possible at the cause. Most agree that nonoperative measures will be effective in the vast majority of patients. Conservative treatment usually consists of a program of anti-inflammatory medicine, local injections of steroids, or both, along with measures to reduce pressure on the tender areas. Orthotic devices which can be utilized include hard plastic heel cups, soft rubber waffle heel cups, felt arch supports, foam rubber or plastizote heel pads and UC-BL inserts.[8,9,14]

In the rare individual for whom nonoperative treatment fails to offer pain relief, surgical treatment may be indicated. Numerous surgical procedures have been described for treatment of the painful heel syndrome. These are divided into two major groups: those aimed at reducing the prominence of the calcaneal spur and those that strive to release compressed neural or fascial tissue. Baxter reviewed his experience with the operative results of 26 patients with recalcitrant heel pain who had failed a minimum of six months of conservative therapy.[6] His operative procedure involved isolated neurolysis of the nerve to the abductor digiti quinti muscle by release of the deep fascia of the abductor hallucis. Release of the tight plantar fascia or excision of the impinging heel spur was performed only if it caused entrapment of the nerve. Of the 34 operated heels, 32 were considered to have obtained good results. Isolated neurolysis appeared to give results similar to more extensive surgical procedures with less postoperative morbidity and recovery time.

Although entrapment neuropathy of the plantar nerves may be an etiologic factor in patients with medial and plantar heel pain, a nonoperative approach of treatment for a minimum of one year is highly recommended. The surgical release as described seems deceptively simple, but isolation of the nerve to the abductor digiti quinti muscle through a 4 cm incision under ankle block without tourniquet on an outpatient basis can be quite frustrating and potentially hazardous. The potential for inadvertent division of this nerve or one of the superficial medial calcaneal branches is a danger. A postoperative painful stump neuroma or annoying medial heel numbness may be more bothersome than the original entrapment neuropathy.

Sural Nerve

The sural nerve is a continuation of the tibial nerve formed by the medial sural cutaneous and peroneal communicating branch of the common peroneal nerve. The sural nerve accompanies the small saphenous vein behind the lateral malleolus and supplies the skin on the back of the leg, the lateral heel, lateral border of the foot, and lateral side of the little toe (Fig. 18-5). Sarrafian reviews the anatomic variations and innervation of the nerve in greater detail.[20]

There have not been many reports of entrapment neuropathy of the sural nerve. This may reflect unfamiliarity with the condition but more likely represents the fact that this is not a common problem. Pringle et al. reported the first four cases of sural nerve entrapment in 1974.[32] Since then several additional isolated case reports have appeared in the literature.[29,30,31]

For the most part, the sural nerve is well protected throughout its course, being surrounded by adequate subcutaneous tissue, and is not subjected

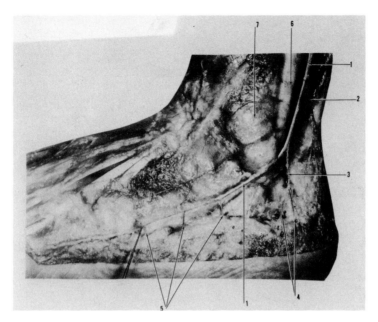

Figure 18-5. Sural nerve. 1. Sural nerve; 2, branch of sural nerve to posterolateral aspect of Achilles tendon area and calcaneal region; 3, lateral calcaneal branch of sural nerve with bifurcation branches [4]; 5, branches of sural nerve to lateral border of foot; 6, peronei tendons; 7, lateral malleolus [sural nerve passes 1 cm to 1.5 cm below tip of lateral malleolus]. (From Sarrafian SK: Anatomy of the foot and ankle: Descriptive, topographic, functional. Philadelphia, J.B. Lippincott Co, 316, 1983.)

to sharp fascial edges or tight constricting points. In the cases cited in the literature, the predisposing factors leading to entrapment were pressure from adjacent ganglia, direct contusion or crush of the foot or leg leading to subsequent fibrosis or adhesion about the nerve, or entrapment of the nerve secondary to a fracture fragment. Unless one of these well-defined conditions exists, diagnosis of sural nerve entrapment neuropathy should be viewed with suspicion.

Clinical Features

The most reliable feature in making the diagnosis would be a history of neurogenic pain in the distribution of the sural nerve. The other features of entrapment neuropathy as discussed earlier may also be present. These include pain at rest with inconstant relation to activity, night pain, reproduction of pain with direct pressure over the entrapment point, and distal paresthesias or retrograde pain.

Treatment

As with other entrapment neuropathies, treatment should initially be nonoperative. This would include avoidance of direct pressure over the trigger point, perhaps a trial of cast immobilization, anti-inflammatory medicine and injection of local anesthetic or steroid into the involved area. If the relief obtained is only transient, the entrapment may be mechanical in nature and subsequently require surgical decompression and neurolysis.

Superficial Peroneal Nerve

The superficial peroneal nerve is a branch of the common peroneal nerve that innervates the peroneus longus and brevis muscles in the lateral compartment. The nerve pierces the fascia in the distal anterolateral leg approximately 10 cm proximal to the lateral malleolus to become a cutaneous branch to the dorsum of the foot except the first webspace. The superficial peroneal nerve divides into two terminal sensory branches to form the medial dorsal cutaneous and intermediate dorsal cutaneous nerves (Fig. 18-6). Variations in the distribution of the cutaneous nerves on the dorsum of the foot are reviewed in greater detail by Sarrafian.[20]

The superficial branch of the peroneal nerve may become entrapped as it exits through the sharp fascial edges in the distal anterolateral leg. There is often a history of trauma such as repeated ankle sprains or exacerbation of symptoms with jogging or vigorous sports activity.[1,3,5] Exertional anterolateral compartment syndrome, fascial defect with muscle herniation tenting the superficial peroneal nerve, compression by lipoma, and entrapment in callus from a fibular shaft fracture have also been reported as causes of entrapment neuropathy.[1,2,4,5]

The pain distribution in superficial peroneal nerve entrapment may mimic a common peroneal neuropathy or L5 radiculopathy or be misdiagnosed as chronic ankle sprain. Electrodiagnostic studies can be helpful in differentiating a more proximal neurologic lesion. Table 18-1 summarizes some of the differentiating features.

Clinical Presentation

Patients usually report numbness and tingling over and ankle and foot dorsum, sparing the first webspace. There may be a swelling or fullness over the anterolateral leg with a positive nerve percussion sign over the soft tissue bulge. Resisted ankle dorsiflexion reveals normal motor strength and may increase the size of the soft tissue bulge. This usually implies a muscle herniation through a fascial defect, and symptoms may be exacerbated with prolonged vigorous activity.

Blocking the superficial peroneal nerve at its exit-point through the fascia or at the most tender trigger area will usually provide a sensation of numbness and temporary relief of pain.

Treatment

If the symptoms are unrelieved by steroid injection or other conservative measures, partial fasciectomy with decompression and neurolysis of the superficial peroneal nerve is indicated. Most patients make a significant recovery after surgical release.

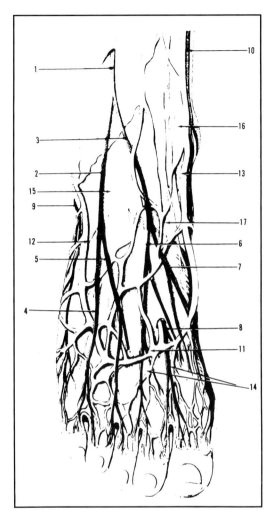

Figure 18-6. Superficial layer of the dorsum of the foot and ankle. 1, superficial peroneal nerve; 2, intermediate dorsal cutaneous nerve; 3, medial dorsal cutaneous nerve; 4, dorsal cutaneous nerve to fourth webspace; 5, dorsal cutaneous nerve to third webspace; 6, dorsal cutaneous nerve to second webspace with branch to dorsum of big toe; 7, dorsomedial cutaneous nerve to big toe; 8, nerve branch from deep peroneal nerve to first interspace; 9, sural nerve; 10, saphenous nerve; 11, dorsal venous arcade; 12, lesser saphenous vein; 13, greater saphenous vein; 14, dorsal metatarsal veins; 15, stem of inferior extensor retinaculum; 16, superomedial band of inferior extensor retinaculum; 17, inferomedial band of inferior extensor retinaculum. (From Sarrafian SK: Anatomy of the foot and ankle: Descriptive, topographic, functional. Philadelphia, J.B. Lippincott Co, 336, 1983.)

Deep Peroneal Nerve

The deep peroneal nerve (anterior tibial nerve) arises from the common peroneal nerve between the fibula and peroneus longus. It travels distally, passing through a fibro-osseous tunnel formed by the origin of the extensor digitorum longus muscle to the anterior surface of the interosseous membrane, where it is joined by the anterior tibial artery. Distally the deep peroneal nerve passes beneath the superior extensor retinaculum on the anterior surface of the tibia. It courses distally over the ankle joint beneath the inferior extensor retinaculum where it divides into a medial and lateral branch. The lateral branch innervates the extensor digitorum brevis muscle and nearby tarsal, tarsometatarsal and metatarsophalangeal joints. The medial branch accompanies the dorsalis pedis artery and divides into two dorsal digital branches that supply the skin between the first and second toes (Fig. 18-7).

A variation of the innervation of the extensor digitorum brevis by the accessory deep peroneal nerve, which arises from the superficial peroneal nerve, occurs in approximately 22 percent of legs.[23,25] The extensor digitorum brevis is usually innervated by the deep peroneal nerve, and its anomalous innervation may lead to errors in localization of deep and superficial peroneal nerve lesions.

The terminal branches of the deep peroneal nerve may become entrapped beneath the inferior extensor retinaculum. A compression neuropathy at this location has been designated anterior tarsal tunnel syndrome.[27] This entity must be distinguished from the posterior or medial tarsal tunnel syndrome caused by compression of the tibial or plantar nerves beneath the flexor retinaculum posterior to the medial malleolus.

The anterior tarsal tunnel syndrome may be partial or complete depending upon whether the motor or sensory branch of the deep peroneal nerve is involved. If the motor branch is involved, atrophy and diminished strength of the extensor digitorum brevis may be evident. Involvement of the sensory branch usually results in sensory deficits in the web between the first and second toes.

Deep peroneal nerve compression may be associated with previous trauma to the dorsum of the foot or ankle resulting from fractures, exostoses, or chronic edema. Compression by an osteophyte on the talus and by an os intermetatarsareum have also been reported.[28] The etiologic factor most often implicated is external compression from tight shoes or boots.[21,22,24,26] Cadaveric dissections have shown that the deep peroneal nerve is placed under maximal neural stretch with the foot plantar flexed and the toes dorsiflexed. This is the same position induced by high-heel (nonphysiologic) shoes.[21]

Deep peroneal entrapment neuropathy like that of the superficial peroneal nerve must be differentiated from other more proximal neurologic lesions. Electrodiagnostic studies resulting in an increased distal motor latency of the deep peroneal nerve (>5 msec) with normal conduction velocity proximal to the ankle and signs of chronic denervation in the extensor digitorum brevis are considered positive findings.[22,24]

Clinical Presentation

About three-quarters of the cases presented in the literature occur in females. The most common complaints are an ache or tightness over the ankle and dorsum of the foot with numbness and paresthesias in the first dorsal web. This may be exacerbated by tight shoes, but symptoms are often worse at night, with inactivity, or with certain positions.

Examination may reveal both sensory and motor changes. Decreased sensation to light touch or pin prick in the first dorsal web, a positive nerve percussion sign over the deep peroneal nerve, or atrophy and weakness of the extensor digitorum brevis may be present. The full-blown syndrome may mimic an L5 radiculopathy or neuropathy of the common or

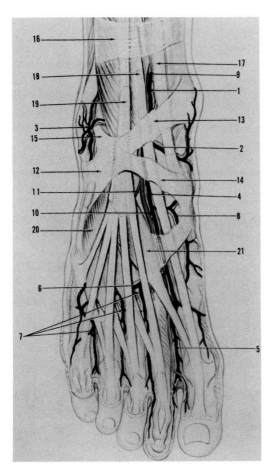

Figure 18-7. Second layer of the dorsum of the foot and ankle. 1. Anterior tibial artery; 2, anterior medial malleolar artery; 3, anterior lateral malleolar artery; 6, arcuate artery; 7, dorsal metatarsal arteries 2,3,4; 8, medial tarsal artery; 9,10, deep peroneal nerve; 11, motor nerve branch to extensor digitorum brevis; 12, inferior extensor retinaculum; 13, superomedial band of inferior extensor retinaculum; 14, inferomedial band of inferior extensor retinaculum; 15, superolateral band of inferior extensor retinaculum; 16, superior extensor retinaculum; 17, tibialis anterior tendon; 18, extensor hallucis longus tendon; 19, extensor digitorum longus tendon; 20, extensor digitorum brevis muscle to toes 2,3,4; 21, extensor hallucis brevis muscle. (From Sarrafian SK: Anatomy of the foot and ankle: Descriptive, topographic, functional. Philadelphia, J.B. Lippincott Co, 337, 1983.)

superficial peroneal nerve. Electrodiagnostic studies are helpful in differentiating the etiology of the lesion.

Treatment

Treatment should first be directed at avoiding tight footwear and positions which place the deep peroneal nerve on stretch. Nonsteroidal anti-inflammatory medicines and/or an infiltration of local anesthetic and steroid into the anterior tarsal tunnel may also alleviate symptoms. If nonoperative measures are unsuccessful after four to six months, surgical decompression of the anterior tarsal tunnel may be indicated.

Common Peroneal Nerve

The common peroneal nerve and the tibial nerve are the terminal divisions of the sciatic nerve. The common peroneal nerve separates from the sciatic nerve at the upper border of the popliteal fossa. It passes distally beneath the biceps femoris tendon and is separated from the lateral femoral condyle by the lateral head of the gastrocnemius and the plantaris muscle. The common peroneal nerve curves around the neck of the fibula and passes through a fibromuscular tunnel formed by the peroneus longus muscle and intermuscular septum. Kopell and Thompson[18] noted that the fibromuscular opening of the tunnel may have a J-shaped outline and the common peroneal nerve or its terminal divisions may be arched over the fascial band of the peroneus longus muscle (Fig. 18-8).

The common peroneal nerve's terminal branches, the superficial and deep peroneal nerves, supply the dorsiflexors of the ankle and evertors of the foot. The skin of the lateral leg and dorsum of the foot is also supplied by these terminal branches.

The common peroneal nerve is vulnerable to injury. It is exposed over the bony neck of the fibula, covered only by skin and subcutaneous tissue and susceptible to direct blows, lacerations, fractures of the tibia and fibula, dislocations of the knee, and external compression from casts or prolonged pressure following unconsciousness or abnormal posture.

Nobel[37] noted the limited longitudinal mobility of the nerve and observed that traction on the nerve could be produced with ankle inversion. After an inversion ankle sprain or distal torsional fibular fracture, the peroneal nerve is drawn distally and compressed against the J-shaped fibrous fascial band of the peroneus longus muscle. This may result in an immediate peroneal palsy. A delayed peroneal palsy may result from the formation of an intraneural hematoma within the nerve sheath.[34,37] Sidey[38] noted that mild evertor weakness may persist following an ankle sprain secondary to partial denervation from a peroneal neuropathy. The instability or "weak

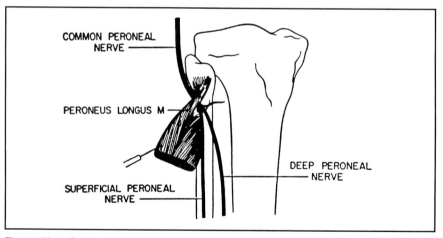

Figure 18-8. Common peroneal nerve—anatomical relationships at fibular neck. (From Kopell HP, Thompson WAL: Peripheral entrapment neuropathies of the lower extremity. N Engl J Med 262(2):56, 1960.)

ankle" that results is often blamed on ligamentous laxity rather than peroneal muscle weakness.

Compression of the common peroneal nerve can also be caused by ganglia or Baker's cysts.[33,35,36,39]

Clinical Presentation

Peroneal compression neuropathy results in pain over the lateral aspect of the legs, foot drop, and paresthesias in the lateral leg or dorsum of the foot. Muscle weakness affects the dorsiflexors and evertors of the foot and the extensors of the toes. Complete foot drop may result in a steppage gait. A positive nerve percussion sign may be present over the fibular neck.

An L5 radiculopathy may present similar features but would usually have associated low back pain, positive straight leg raising and also weakness in the tibialis posterior, hamstrings and gluteus medius muscles.

Electrodiagnostic studies can be helpful in differentiating a more proximal neurologic lesion. Table 18-1 summarizes some of the differentiating features between L5 radiculopathy and peroneal neuropathies.

Treatment

Management of peroneal nerve palsy depends upon the etiology. Compression neuropathies developing after diminished consciousness due to head injury, or anesthesia, or from external pressure by casts or braces usually recover within a few weeks.

Blunt injuries about the knee, dislocations of the knee or hip, and fractures of the femur, tibia, fibula, or ankle usually do not result in severance of the nerve. Incomplete lesions generally improve and can be followed by clinical observation. Complete lesions which are caused by a stretch or traction injury generally carry a poorer prognosis. Electrical testing and more careful followup are required. If there is no evidence of recovery by three to six months, surgical exploration of the nerve should be performed. Observations made at surgery as to the attenuation of the nerve and length of segment involved will help indicate the severity of the injury and the prognosis for recovery.

In cases of penetrating or lacerating injury, severance of the nerve should be suspected. If nerve conduction is absent, surgical exploration and repair is indicated.

Compression of the common peroneal nerve by a ganglion or cyst resulting in pain, paresis, or sensory changes is best treated by early exploration and excision of the cyst.

Incomplete injuries that are improving can be splinted or braced during the recovery period. Complete nerve injuries that are permanent need to be braced, or considered for a tendon transfer to restore lost muscle function.

Further discussion of peroneal nerve compression can be found in Chapter 20.

Table 18-1.

	L5 Radiculopathy	Common Peroneal Neuropathy (Fibular Neck)	Deep Peroneal Neuropathy (Anterior Tarsal) Tunnel Syndrome	Superficial Peroneal Neuropathy (Distal anterolateral Leg)	Ankle Sprain
Back Pain	Yes	No	No	No	No
Motor Weakness	L5 innervated muscles including tibialis posterior, gluteus medius.	Ankle dorsiflexors, foot evertors, toe extensors.	Extensor digitorum brevis.	No	No
Paresthesias	Lateral leg, Dorsum foot.	Lateral leg, Dorsum foot.	First toe web.	Dorsum of foot excluding first toe web.	No
EMG/NCV	Abnormal in L5 innervated muscles.	Abnormal motor conduction of peroneal nerve innervated muscles.	Prolonged distal latency of deep peroneal nerve. Denervation of extensor digitorum brevis.	Abnormal superficial peroneal nerve conduction.	Normal

Incisional Neuromas

Incisional neuromas should not be confused with entrapment neuropathies about the foot and ankle. Cutaneous innervation to the dorsum of the foot is supplied by branches of the sural nerve, superficial and deep peroneal nerves, and saphenous nerve, as depicted in Figure 18-9. As mentioned previously there is variation in the exact pattern of cutaneous innervation depending upon which nerve predominates.[16,17,20]

Entrapment of the dorsal cutaneous sensory nerves may arise from compression by ganglia, fascial bands, bony exostoses, marginal joint osteophytes, accessory ossicles, fractures, callus, or after crush injuries to the dorsum of the foot. Iatrogenic nerve injury can also occur after surgical incisions, causing symptomatic neuroma formation.

In 1984 an excellent review of symptomatic incisional neuromas on the dorsum of the foot was reported by Kenzora.[16] He reviewed 17 patients with 25 highly symptomatic neuromas over a two-year period after routine orthopaedic procedures on the dorsum of the foot. During this review of cases, he identified a region along the dorsomedial aspect of the foot where 76 percent of the highly symptomatic neuromas occurred. He termed this region the neuromatous or N-zone (Fig. 18-10).

Clinical Presentation

Patients with symptomatic incisional neuromas usually present with marked burning neurogenic pain with any pressure over or near the surgical scar. In addition to scar tenderness there are usually bothersome distal paresthesias. An exquisitely tender Tinel's sign with percussion accurately localizes the site of neuroma entrapment in underlying scar tissue. Occasionally the neuromatous thickening can be palpated within the subcutaneous tissue.

Treatment

Highly symptomatic neuromas are usually best treated with surgical excision allowing the nerve to retract proximally into soft tissue. Occasionally it may be necessary to bury the cut end of the nerve into bone if adequate soft tissue coverage is not available.

In Kenzora's series, 14 of the 17 patients underwent surgery with 12 highly satisfactory, two satisfactory, and two unsatisfactory results. His general recommendations were to avoid selective surgery within the neuromatous zone whenever possible and avoid deep subcutaneous closing stitches, which may entrap nearby cutaneous nerve branches.

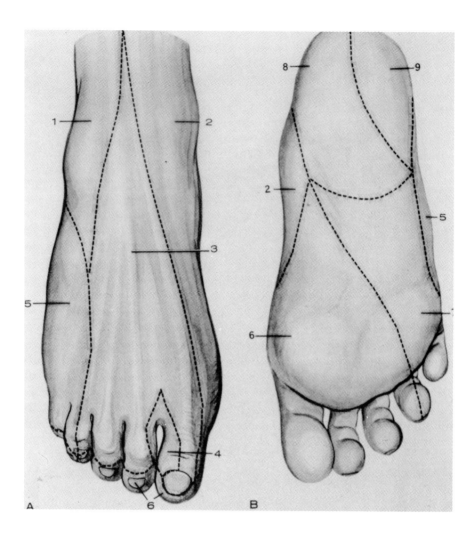

Figure 18-9. Cutaneous innervation of the foot. (A) Dorsum of the foot. (B) Sole of the foot. 1, peroneal cutaneous nerve; 2, saphenous nerve; 3, superficial peroneal nerve; 4, deep peroneal nerve; 5, sural nerve; 6, medial plantar nerve; 7, lateral plantar nerve; 8, medial calcaneal nerve; 9, lateral calcaneal nerve. (From Sarrafian SK: Anatomy of the foot and ankle: Descriptive topographic, functional. Philadelphia, J.B. Lippincott Co, 328, 1983.)

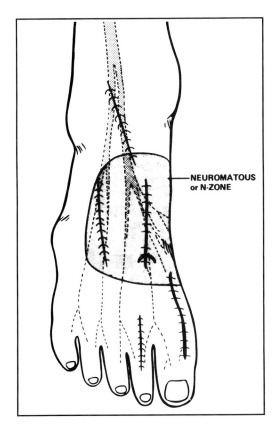

Figure 18-10. For unknown reasons, most of the highly symptomatic neuromas (19 of 25 or 76 percent) were located over the dorsomedial aspect of the midfoot. It appears that incisions placed within this neuromatous or N-zone are more likely to cause symptomatic neuromas than incisions elsewhere on the dorsum of the foot. (From Kenzora JE: Symptomatic incisional neuromas on the dorsum of the foot, Foot and Ankle 5(1):2, 1984.)

NEUROMATOUS or N-ZONE

Bibliography

Superficial Peroneal Nerve
1. Banerjee T, Koons DD: Superficial peroneal nerve entrapment: Report of two cases, J Neurosurg 55:991, 1981.
2. Garfin S, Mubarak SJ, Owen CA: Exertional anterolateral compartment syndrome: Case report with fascial defect, muscle herniation, and superficial peroneal nerve entrapment, J Bone Joint Surg 59A:404, 1977.
3. Mackey D, Colbert DS, Chater, EH: Musculocutaneous nerve entrapment, Irish J Med Sci 146:100, 1977.
4. Mino DE, Hughes EC: Bony entrapment of the superficial peroneal nerve, Clinic Orthop Rel Res, 185:203, 1984.
5. Sridhara CR, Izzo KL: Terminal sensory branches of the superficial peroneal nerve: An entrapment syndrome, Arch Phys Med Rehabil 66:789, 1985.

Plantar Nerve
6. Baxter DE, Thigpen CM: Heel pain: Operative results, Foot and Ankle 5(1):16, 1984.
7. Bordelon RL: Subcalcaneal pain: A method of evaluation and plan for treatment, Clin Orthop Rel Res 177:49, 1983.

8. Campbell JW, Inman VT: Treatment of plantar fasciitis and calcaneal spurs with the UC-BL shoe insert, Clin Orthop 103:57, 1974.

9. Eggers GWN: Shoe pad for treatment of calcaneal spur, J Bone Joint Surg 39(A):219, 1957.

10. Henricson AS, Westlin NE: Chronic calcaneal pain in athletes: Entrapment of the calcaneal nerve? Am J Sports Med 12(2):152, 1984.

11. Lapidus PW, Guidotti FP: Painful heel: Report of 323 patients with 364 painful heels, Clin Orthop 39:178, 1965.

12. Przylucki H, Jones CL: Entrapment neuropathy of muscle branch of lateral plantar nerve: A cause of heel pain, J Am Podiatry Assoc 71(3):119, 1981.

13. Rask MR: Medial plantar neurapraxia (jogger's foot): Report of three cases, Clin Orthop 134:193, 1978.

14. Snook GA, Chrisman DDO: The management of subcalcaneal pain, Clin Orthop 82:163, 1972.

15. Tranz SS: Heel pain, Clin Orthop 28:169, 1963.

Incisional Neuromas

16. Kenzora JE: Symptomatic incisional neuromas on the dorsum of the foot, Foot & Ankle 5(1):2, 1984.

17. Kozinski C: The course, mutual relations and distribution of the cutaneous nerves of the metazonal region of the leg and foot, J Anat 60:274, 1926.

General References

18. Kopell HP, Thompson WAL: Peripheral entrapment neuropathies of the lower extremity, N Engl J Med 262(2):56, 1960.

19. Kopell HP, Thompson WAL: Peripheral entrapment neuropathies. Malabar, FL. R. E. Krieger Publishing Co, 1976.

20. Sarrafian SK: Anatomy of the foot and ankle: Descriptive, topographic, functional. Philadelphia, J. B. Lippincott Co., 1983.

Deep Peroneal Nerve

21. Borges LF, Halle HM, Selkoe DJ, Welch K: The anterior tarsal tunnel syndrome: Report of two cases, J Neurosurg 54:89, 1981.

22. Gessini L, Jandolo B, Peitrangel A: The anterior tarsal tunnel syndrome: Report of four cases, J Bone Joint Surg 66A(5):786, 1984.

23. Gutmann L: Atypical deep peroneal neuropathy, J Neurol Neurosurg, Psychiat 33:453, 1970.

24. Krause KH, Witt T, Ross A: The anterior tarsal tunnel syndrome, J Neurol 217:67, 1977.

25. Lambert EH: The accessory deep peroneal nerve: A common variation in innervation of extensor digitorum brevis, Neurology 19:1169, 1969.

26. Lindenbaum BL: Ski boot compression syndrome, Clin Orthop 140:19, 1979.

27. Marinacci AA: Neurological syndrome of the tarsal tunnels. Bull LA Neurol Soc 33:98, 1968.

28. Murphy PC, Baxter DE: Nerve entrapment of the foot and ankle in runners, Clin Sports Med 4(4):753, 1985.

Sural Nerve

29. Colbert DS, Cunningham F, Mackey D: Sural nerve entrapment: Case Report, J Irish Med Assoc 68(21):544, 1975.

30. Docks GW, Salter MS: Sural nerve entrapment: An unusual case report, J Foot Surg 18(1):42, 1979.
31. Gould N, Trevina S: Sural nerve entrapment by avulsion fracture at the base of the fifth metatarsal bone, Foot & Ankle 2:153, 1981.
32. Pringle RM, Protheroe K, Mukherjee SK: Entrapment neuropathy of the sural nerve, J Bone Joint Surg 56B(3):465, 1974.

Common Peroneal Nerve

33. Firooznia H, Golimbu C, Rafii M, Chapnick J: Computerized tomography in diagnosis of compression of the common peroneal nerve by ganglion cysts, Comput Radiol 7(6):343, 1983.
34. Meals RA: Peroneal nerve palsy complicating ankle sprain: Report of two cases and review of the literature, J Bone Joint Surg 59A(7):966, 1977.
35. Muckart RD: Compression of the common peroneal nerve by intramuscular ganglion from the superior tibiofibular joint, J Bone Joint Surg 58B(2):241, 1976.
36. Nakano KK: Entrapment neuropathy from Baker's cyst, JAMA 239:135, 1978.
37. Nobel W: Peroneal palsy due to hematoma in the common peroneal nerve sheath after distal torsional fractures and ankle sprains: Report of two cases, J Bone Joint Surg 48(A):1484, 1966.
38. Sidey JD: Weak ankles: A study of common peroneal entrapment neuropathy, Brit Med J 3:623, 1969.
39. Stack RE, Bianco AJ, MacCarty CS: Compression of the common peroneal nerve by ganglion cysts: Report of nine cases, J Bone Joint Surg 47A(4):773, 1965.

CHAPTER 19

Nerve Entrapment Syndromes of the Foot and Ankle: Part II

Roger A. Mann, M.D.

Tarsal Tunnel Syndrome

The tarsal tunnel syndrome is the result of compression of the posterior tibial nerve within the tarsal canal or one of its terminal branches distal to the tarsal canal. The tarsal canal is created by the distal tibia behind the medial malleolus and becomes the tarsal tunnel when covered by the flexor retinaculum. Distal to the tarsal tunnel the terminal branches of the posterior tibial nerve, namely the medial plantar nerve, the lateral plantar nerve, and the medial calcaneal branches, are exposed to intrinsic compression, usually from a lesion that arises from a tendon sheath, such as a ganglion, or from the ankle or subtalar joint. Occasionally, enlarged varicose veins or a tumor such as a lipoma may be within the tarsal tunnel or distal to it, placing pressure upon the posterior tibial nerve or one of the terminal branches. The initial published reports pertaining to the tarsal tunnel syndrome were by Keck[1] and Lam[2] in 1962.

We believe the tarsal tunnel syndrome is a very distinct clinical entity, the diagnosis of which is made by the correlation of the patient's history, physical findings, and electrodiagnostic studies. It is imperative in properly diagnosing a tarsal tunnel syndrome, from our point of view, that all three clinical criteria are present to reduce the possibility of an incorrect diagnosis. The tarsal tunnel syndrome should not be equated to the carpal tunnel syndrome, since the diagnosis of a tarsal tunnel syndrome is much more difficult to make with assurity, and the results of surgical intervention do not approach those seen with the carpal tunnel syndrome.

Clinical Symptoms

The most frequent clinical complaint noted by the patient with a tarsal tunnel syndrome is that of burning, tingling, numb feeling on the plantar aspect of the foot which cannot be well localized.[3] The dysesthesias noted by the patient occasionally are distributed along one of the three terminal branches of the posterior tibial nerve; however, this usually occurs when one of the terminal branches is involved rather than when the compression is within the tarsal tunnel. The dysesthesias on the bottom of the foot are often aggravated by activities and relieved by rest, but conversely there is a group of patients whose main complaint is that of dysesthesias when in bed at night which are relieved by getting up, moving around, rubbing the foot, or at times by soaking the foot in hot or cold water.

There is a certain group of patients with tarsal tunnel syndrome who complain of the dysesthesias passing up along the medial aspect of the distal tibia, occasionally as high up as the knee. This, however, is not a frequent complaint.

The clinical complaints usually become progressively more severe until the patient is significantly affected by the pain and has to reduce his level of activity.

Etiology

In approximately 50 percent of cases of the tarsal tunnel syndrome a specific etiology can be identified. The etiology may be a space-occupying lesion-for example, a ganglion, synovial cyst, lipoma or other soft tissue tumor, or venous varicosities—tenosynovitis; severe pronation or valgus hind foot deformity; trauma such as fracture of the distal tibia or calcaneus; or following a severe ankle sprain.

Physical Examination

A careful physical examination is important in evaluating patients with a tarsal tunnel syndrome. The patient should be examined initially standing, in order to evaluate the posture of the foot, significant swelling of the extremity, venous varicosities, or the presence of swelling with the tarsal tunnel area.

With the patient seated, the range of motion of the ankle and subtalar joint, as well as the function of the tendons along the medial aspect of the ankle, should be carefully noted. Percussion along the course of the posterior tibial nerve is carried out, starting well above the tarsal tunnel and proceeding along the tarsal tunnel and then distally along the terminal branches of the posterior tibial nerve. This careful percussion is carried out in order to identify areas of irritability of the posterior tibial nerve or one of its terminal branches. It is only in this manner that the precise area of the compression can be identified. As this is carried out, careful note is made as to where the dysesthesias radiate to help identify which branch or branches of the posterior tibial nerve might be involved. If sensitivity of the nerve is noted proximal to the tarsal tunnel, is should be pursued because in cases in which there is a positive nerve percussion sign proximally the etiology probably does not involve the tarsal tunnel.

Careful evaluation of the medial aspect of the ankle joint, looking for any type of a small lump beneath the skin, which could represent a ganglion, or some type of synovial cyst emanating from a tendon sheath that would put pressure against the posterior tibial nerve or one of its terminal branches is carried out. At times the lesion might be extremely subtle, so caution and patience must be utilized when palpating these structures.

A careful neurologic study is carried out to determine which part of the posterior tibial nerve or its terminal branches is involved, but also to try to determine whether a more generalized type of neuropathy is present. It has been our experience that the sensory examination can be confusing at times, in that in less than 50 percent of patients can the clinician demonstrate reproducible numbness, loss of two-point discrimination, or vibratory sense. Weakness in the intrinsic muscles has been an infrequent finding, although it should be carefully sought by attempting to assess muscle strength and by comparing the muscle bulk of the two feet, looking for atrophy.

Electrodiagnostic Studies

The final criterion for establishing a diagnosis of tarsal tunnel syndrome is a positive electrodiagnostic study. This should include the conduction velocity of the posterior tibial nerve in order to rule out the possibility of a peripheral neuropathy. The conduction velocity of the posterior tibial nerve through the tarsal canal, which measures the terminal latency of the medial plantar nerve to the abductor hallucis, and of the lateral plantar nerve to the abductor digiti quinti are determined. The terminal latency of the medial plantar nerve to the abductor hallucis should be less than 6.2 msec, and that of the lateral plantar nerve to the abductor digiti quinti should be less than 7.0 msec. There is some variation noted between different electromyographers, and this needs to be taken into account when evaluating nerve conduction velocities.

The abductor hallucis and abductor digiti quinti should be sampled, looking for fibrillation potentials which would indicate dysfunction of the posterior tibial nerve or one of its terminal branches. Some electromyographers favor sensory testing of the posterior tibial nerve to diagnose a tarsal tunnel syndrome, but there seem to be conflicting reports as to the reliability of these studies.

Differential Diagnoses

As mentioned previously, the diagnosis of tarsal tunnel syndrome should be based upon the history, the physical findings and the electrodiagnostic studies. If all three of these do not point strongly to the diagnosis of a tarsal tunnel syndrome, then one has to consider carefully an alternative diagnosis. The differential diagnosis of the tarsal tunnel syndrome is outlined in Table 19-1.

**Table 19-1 Differential Diagnosis of Tarsal
Tunnel Syndrome**

Remote causes
    Interdigital neuroma
    Intervertebral disc lesion
    Plantar fasciitis
    Plantar fibromatosis

Intraneural causes
    Peripheral neuritis
    Peripheral vascular disease
    Diabetic neuropathy
    Leprosy
    Neurolemmoma
    Neuroma

Extraneural causes
    Ganglion
    Nerve tethering
    Fracture (callous, mal-union, non-union, displaced fragment)
    Blunt Trauma
    Valgus hindfoot
    Rheumatoid arthritis
    Venous varicosities
    Tenosynovitis
    Ligament constriction
    Abductor hallucis origin constriction
    Metatarsal arch strain
    Longitudinal arch strain
    Lipoma

(Wilemon W.K.: Tarsal tunnel syndrome: A 50-year survey of the world literature and a report of 2 new cases. Orthop. Rev., *8*(11):111, 1979.)

Conservative Treatment

Once the diagnosis of tarsal tunnel syndrome has been established, there are various types of conservative management that might be of benefit. If the etiology is felt to be postural, then some type of an orthotic device may provide the patient with relief. If there is significant edema of the lower extremity, it should be controlled. Oral nonsteroidal anti-inflammatory medications, or occasionally a steroid injection into the area of the tarsal tunnel, are of benefit. On a few occasions use of a short-leg walking cast to immobilize the area in order to assess the patient's response might be of benefit. If indeed immobilization does significantly relieve the symptom complex, then possibly the use of a polypropylene ankle-foot orthosis would be more desirable than surgical intervention.

Once conservative management has been exhausted, then surgical release of the tarsal tunnel or one of the terminal branches of the posterior tibial nerve may be of benefit. If a specific etiology is known to be present, such as a ganglion, a synovial cyst, or some mechanical pressure in the area of the tarsal canal or distally, then the prognosis following surgery is extremely good. If, however, the etiology is not secondary to mechanical pressure and the diagnosis is based upon the criteria presented already, it has been our experience that approximately 75 percent of patients who undergo surgical release of the tarsal tunnel syndrome have a satisfactory clinical response with a significant improvement. This, however, leaves about 25 percent of patients who are not improved following surgery, and the patient should be counseled about this prior to surgery. The success noted with release of the carpal tunnel should not be equated with release of the tarsal tunnel.

As a general rule, if the irritability of the posterior tibial nerve, as noted by percussing it, extends more than approximately 10 to 15 cm proximal to the tip of the medial malleolus, it has been our experience that there is some type of neuritis of the posterior tibial nerve that usually does not respond to release of the tarsal tunnel.

Surgical Treatment

The surgical treatment of the tarsal tunnel syndrome consists of releasing the constriction of the posterior tibial nerve and/or its terminal branches. If a specific diagnosis is known prior to the surgery, such as a ganglion distal to the tarsal tunnel area, then a complete release does not need to be carried out. Conversely, if there is no specific area of irritability, then a complete release of the posterior tibial nerve and its terminal branches must be carried out. A thigh tourniquet is used for hemostasis. The skin incision is made approximately 1 to 2 cm posterior to the posterior border of the tibia and ends approximately 8 to 10 cm proximal to the tip of the malleolus, and is then brought distally behind the malleolus and along a course between the medial and lateral plantar nerves, ending at about the level of the talonavicular joint. The incision is deepened through the subcutaneous tissue and fat in order to expose the deep fascial layer. By blunt dissection the fascial layer is adequately exposed and the blood vessels that are encountered are cauterized. In the proximal portion of the wound the fascia is opened posterior to the sheath of the posterior tibial tendon in order to expose the posterior tibial nerve and vessels before they enter the tarsal canal. The advantage of exposing the nerve in this area is that the nerve is still surrounded by soft fatty tissue and is readily mobilized (Figs. 19-1 and 19-2). The deep fascia is opened distally down toward the tip of the medial malleolus and then beyond, and the posterior tibial nerve traced distally by blunt dissection. The dissection at times is difficult if there are many large venous varicosities present around the nerve. Occasionally these may need to be ligated in order to expose the nerve adequately. As the posterior tibial nerve is traced distally, it branches within the tarsal canal, giving off the medial plantar nerve, the lateral plantar nerve, and medial calcaneal branches, which arise off of the posterior aspect of the lateral plantar nerve. The posterior tibial nerve at the level of its bifurcation is frequently surrounded by a vascular leash, so that it is easier at times to trace the medial plantar nerve down to the level of vascular

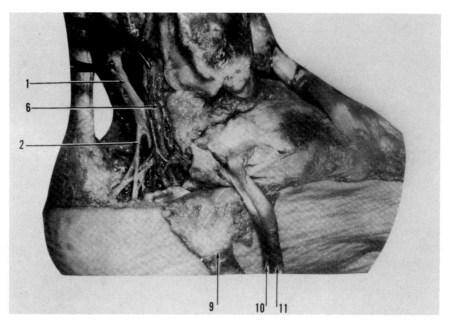

Figure 19-1. *A* and *B*. Neurovascular bundle in the tibiotalocalcaneal canal. (1. posterior tibial nerve; 2. posteromedial calcaneal nerve; 3. medial plantar nerve; 4. lateral plantar nerve; 5. medial calcaneal nerve; 6. posterior tibial artery and veins covering posterior tibial nerve in *A* and reflected downward in *B*; 7. upper calcaneal chamber; 8. interfascicular septum; 9. reflected flexor retinaculum; 10. reflected flexor digitorum longus tendon; 11. reflected posterior tibial tendon; 12. flexor hallucis longus tendon.) (From Serrafian, S. K.: Functional Anatomy of the Foot and Ankle, J. B. Lippincott Co., Philadelphia 1983.) Note in *A* the way the vascular leash (#6) obscures the division of the posterior tibial nerve into its two main terminal branches. In *B* note the relationship of the tendon sheaths of the tibialis posterior, the flexor digitorum longus, and the flexor hallucis longus tendons to the tarsal tunnel and the medial and lateral plantar nerves.

leash and then proceed distally beyond the vascular leash in order to identify the medial plantar nerve just along the superior border of the abductor hallucis. The nerve, once identified, is then traced proximally behind the vascular leash. In this manner one is able to fully expose the nerve without having to become too involved with the vascular leash. The medial plantar nerve is then traced distally until it passes through an opening in the abductor hallucis muscle, where it crosses into the plantar aspect of the foot. If a specific area of constriction or scarring is noted, a careful dissection of the area needs to be carried out in order to identify the etiology, for example, a possible ganglion or cyst arising from one of the adjacent tendon sheaths.

The surgeon now returns to a more proximal level in order to identify the lateral plantar nerve and trace this distally to the area where it passes deep to the abductor hallucis origin. As this is carried out, it should be kept in mind that the medial calcaneal branches arise from the posterior aspect of the lateral plantar nerve, and therefore the dissection should be

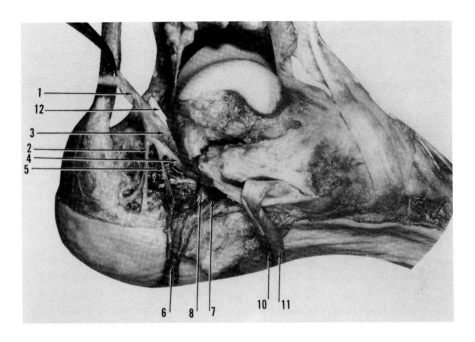

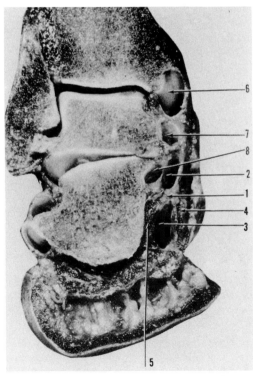

Figure 19-2. The compartments of the tarsal tunnel as seen in a frontal cross section of the ankle and hind foot. (1. interfascicular septum; 2. upper chamber; 3. lower chamber; 4. abductor hallucis muscle with its investing fascia forming the medial wall of the lower chamber; 5. quadratus plantae muscle forming lateral wall of the lower chamber; 6. posterior tibial tunnel; 7. flexor digitorum longus tunnel; 8. flexor hallucis longus tunnel.) (From Serrafian, S. K.: Functional Anatomy of the Foot and Ankle, J. B. Lippincott Co., Philadelphia 1983.) Note the relationship of the tendon sheaths to the upper and lower chambers of the tarsal tunnel. Through the upper chamber (2) passes the medial plantar nerve and its vessels, and through the lower chamber (3) passes the lateral plantar nerve and its vessels. Note that the interfascicular septum (1) passes between the two nerves and at times should be divided when releasing the tarsal tunnel.

carried out along the anterior aspect to avoid damage to these fine structures. An effort is made, however, to identify the medial calcaneal branches, which may be one or more, and they should be carefully traced distally in order to be sure that they are in soft fatty tissue and are not entrapped by a heavy fascial band. The origin of the abductor hallucis should be carefully released in order to adequately identify the lateral plantar nerve as it passes behind it toward the plantar aspect of the foot. Depending upon the patient's main area of clinical symptoms, the degree of dissection behind the abductor hallucis varies. If the majority of the symptom complex involves the lateral plantar nerve, then the entire origin of the abductor hallucis must be carefully released and the nerve traced beneath it over the edge of the plantar aponeurosis and then to the plantar aspect of the foot. Needless to say, this may be a difficult and time-consuming dissection.

Once the posterior tibial nerve and its branches have been carefully dissected, the nerve needs to be carefully explored, looking for any changes along its course, such as alterations in color, the presence or absence of the fine capillary tree, and the presence or absence of fat. Whenever a specific constriction is identified, or some type of a growth such as a ganglion or synovial cyst, it needs to be traced to its origin in order to be sure that it does not recur. Once the dissection has been carried out, the tourniquet is released and careful hemostasis is obtained. The wound is then closed in a routine manner and a compression dressing is applied. The patient is treated postoperatively in a nonweight-bearing compressive dressing for three weeks, following which they are gradually encouraged to ambulate with the use of adequate support hose. It is very important to control the edema in the postoperative period.

Clinical Results

As a general rule, patients who immediately after surgery state that their pain has been relieved tend to have the best prognosis for a successful tarsal tunnel release. If immediately following surgery the patient does not feel that the symptom complex has been relieved, the prognosis is not as favorable.

At times there is a great deal of scarring around the posterior tibial nerve sheath or one of its terminal branches, which necessitates a neurolysis or stripping away of the enclosed neural sheath as well as freeing of the individual fascicles from the adherent tissue. Not infrequently following this type of dissection, the patient experiences varying degrees of numbness on the plantar aspect to the foot, since the posterior tibial nerve seems to be very sensitive to surgical trauma. In these cases, after a latent period of approximately four to six weeks, a progressive Tinel's sign may be noted along the course of the posterior tibial nerve and its terminal branches. It may be well over a year until the final result is known in cases such as this. Not infrequently, even following a successful tarsal tunnel release, there is still a positive nerve percussion sign along the course of the posterior tibial nerve.

As mentioned previously, approximately 75 percent of patients who undergo release of the tarsal tunnel have relief of symptoms. Not infrequently the patient still notes some dysesthesias, but generally speaking most are quite satisfied with the surgical outcome. There is a group of about 25 percent of patients who still demonstrate little or no improvement following the surgical procedure.

The question often arises after a failed tarsal tunnel release whether or not one should consider reexploration of the tarsal canal, and as a general rule, in our limited experience with this group of patients, the results are not satisfactory. We have rarely seen a patient who, following a second release of the tarsal tunnel, has a satisfactory clinical result.

Conclusion

Diagnosis of tarsal tunnel syndrome is based upon three criteria—the history, the physical findings, and the electrodiagnostic studies. If all three criteria are not present, then the diagnosis of the tarsal tunnel syndrome is in doubt. Initially conservative management of the condition is warranted, but if after an adequate clinical trial has failed to relieve symptoms, then surgical release of the tarsal canal would be indicated. Following the release of the tarsal tunnel approximately 75 percent of patients experience significant improvement; however, this leaves 25 percent with minimal or no improvement as a result of the surgical procedure. It is important to forewarn the patient that release of the tarsal tunnel may not bring about a satisfactory clinical response. Re-exploration of the tarsal canal in our experience has not yielded very satisfactory results.

Interdigital Neuroma

An interdigital neuroma is a frequent cause of metatarsalgia. The condition has had a rather interesting history since it was first described by Louis Durlacher[6] in 1845. Following a report by Thomas G. Morton[15] in 1876 the eponym "Morton's neuroma" was applied to the clinical condition. In 1892 a Thomas S. K. Morton[15] confirmed the findings of Thomas G. Morton. An unrelated form of metatarsalgia was described in 1935 by Dudley J. Morton.[14] I personally prefer to use the term "interdigital neuroma" since it is somewhat more descriptive of the patient's problem, although the condition is not a neuroma per se. The etiology of an interdigital neuroma is somewhat controversial and therefore, the various etiologies will be discussed in detail.

Etiology

The etiology of an interdigital neuroma includes trauma, mechanical pressure against the transverse metatarsal ligament, enlargement of the intermetatarsal bursa, the anatomic arrangement of the nerve supply to the third interspace, the mobility of the fourth metatarsal head in relation to the third metatarsal head, impingement by a synovial cyst, and vascular changes within the nerve.

Trauma to the plantar aspect of the foot can produce a contusion of the common digital nerve and result in neuritic symptoms. This is not thought to be a frequent cause of a neuroma, but it occurs at times when people fall from a height or step on a sharp object.

The possibility that an interdigital neuroma is the result of mechanical pressure against the transverse metatarsal ligament was advanced by Graham et al.,[8,9] who demonstrated changes secondary to pressure in the common digital nerve, particularly as it crosses beneath the proximal portion of the transverse metatarsal ligament. He and his colleagues demonstrated that the common digital nerve was narrowed at the proximal end of the transverse metatarsal ligament and demonstrated degenerative changes within the nerve fascicles as well as venous congestion. The fact that the ratio of females to males with this condition is approximately 10 to one lends further credence to this theory, since the metatarsophalangeal joints of women are often held in a chronically dorsiflexed position by the use of high-heeled shoes.

Enlargement of the intermetatarsal bursa at times can give rise to a sufficiently large mass so that pressure is exerted against the common digital nerve, which could give rise to symptoms of an interdigital neuroma.

The anatomic alignment of the nerve to the third interspace is such that the common digital nerve to the third interspace receives a communicating branch from the lateral plantar nerve. Jones and Klenerman,[10] as well as Graham,[9] noted a consistent communicating branch between the medial and lateral plantar nerves and hypothesized that this might result in a tethering effect that could lead to the development of an interdigital neuroma.

The anatomic alignment of the foot is such that the medial three rays are rather rigid whereas the two lateral rays are not. This permits motion to occur between the third and fourth metatarsal heads, which could result in irritation of the digital nerve to the third interspace, according to T. G. Morton[14] and DuVries.[7] The constant motion between these metatarsal heads may lead to thickening of the tissues surrounding the nerve.

At times a synovial cyst may arise from the joint space and result in compression of the nerve as it passes beneath the transverse metatarsal ligament.

The possibility that an interdigital neuroma is the result of degeneration of the nerve has been advocated by McElvenny[12] in 1943, and by Baker and Kuhn[4] in 1944. The possibility that this represents a vascular type of degeneration has been advocated by Nissen[17] in 1948 and by Lassmann[11] in 1979.

Clinical Evaluation

Patients with an interdigital neuroma complain of pain which is well localized to the plantar aspect of the foot. As a general rule patients note that the onset of symptoms was gradual in nature and cannot remember any specific trauma. Occasionally they have the feeling that they are walking on a "lump" on the plantar aspect of their foot. Not infrequently the pain radiates out toward the tip of the toe on either side of the involved interspace. The patient, when asked, can usually place his or her finger exactly on the area on the bottom of the foot where the pain occurs. This is in contradistinction to the patient with a tarsal tunnel syndrome, who cannot localize the pain to any specific area. The pain itself is usually characterized as a tingling, burning, very uncomfortable type of feeling, which not infrequently radiates toward the toes. Occasionally the patient notes that the pain radiates proximally within the foot. Some patients complain of a cramping feeling within the foot.

As a general rule the pain is aggravated by activities and wearing shoes. Women in particular state that the symptoms are made worse by wearing a high-heeled shoe and men by tight loafers. The symptoms are relieved by removing the shoe and massaging the foot. Frequently patients remove their shoes when they return home from work and walk around barefooted on carpet, which usually brings about complete relief. Persistent use of a high-heeled, fashionable, pointed-toe women's shoe almost invariably significantly aggravates the condition. As a general rule, once the weight-bearing stress is removed from the foot little or no pain occurs.

The third interspace is involved about 55 percent of the time and the second interspace about 45 percent. Neuromas involving the first or fourth interspace rareley, if ever, occur. Occasionally two neuromas occurring in adjacent interspaces have been noted, but this is very uncommon. As a general rule, although a neuroma can occur at almost any age, it is most frequent in the fourth to sixth decades. A neuroma may occur bilaterally, in about 5 to 10 percent of cases.

Physical Findings

The physical examination of a patient with a neuroma is extremely important, since it is on this basis that the diagnosis is made. First of all the patient should be asked be stand so that the overall alignment of the feet can be analyzed. Occasionally a neuroma or at least symptoms similar to a neuroma are noted in patients who have deviation of the toes as a result of a degenerative change within the capsule of the metatarsophalangeal joint. When the toes deviate the metatarsal heads are forced closer together, and this may be the etiology of the persistent discomfort, rather than an interdigital neuroma per se. When the patient stands, the dorsal aspect of each interspace should be carefully palpated, looking for any fullness that might represent a ganglion or a synovial cyst within the plantar aspect of the foot.

The examination of the forefoot is then systematically carried out. Initially each metatarsophalangeal joint is grasped between the examiner's fingers and gently squeezed in order to ascertain whether or not there is any pathology present within the joint, since this not infrequently mimics the symptoms of a neuroma. Following this, each interspace is grasped in a dorsiplantar direction in order to evaluate any fullness. As the interspace is grasped, the patient's foot is squeezed together in a medial-lateral direction so as to apply pressure across the interspace. Not infrequently patients with a significant neuroma that has been forced up into the interspace by palpation of the plantar aspect of the foot experience a snap and rather acute pain that reproduces their clinical symptoms. This should strongly suggest the possibility of a neuroma. A sensory deficit can be looked for in patients with a neuroma, although one is rarely found.

Not infrequently a patient with a suspected neuroma needs to be examined on two or three occasions in order to assess carefully, the patient's foot pain and to be sure which interspace is involved. If more than one interspace appears to be involved, which is rarely the case, it is important to attempt to evaluate which interspace is the more sensitive on three or four visits. Whem more than one interspace is suspected, the patient is also re-examined on several occasions until the most sensitive interspace is identified.

A weight-bearing radiograph of the foot is obtained, just for completeness, to rule out the possibility of bone or joint pathology.

Differential Diagnoses

There are many conditions that can mimic an interdigital neuroma and as such these should be carefully considered before the diagnosis of an interdigital neuroma is made. These include the following:

1. Pain of neuritic origin other then interdigital neuroma:
    a. Degenerative disc disease.
    b. Tarsal tunnel syndrome.
    c. Lesion of the medial or lateral plantar nerve.
    d. Peripheral neuritis.
2. Metatarsophalangeal joint pathology:
    a. Synovitis of the metatarsophalangeal joint secondary to rheumatoid arthritis, nonspecific synovitis, gout, trauma, etc.
    b. Impending subluxation or dislocation of the metatarsophalangeal joint.
    c. Freiberg's infraction.
    d. Degenerative lesion of the plantar capsule.

3. Lesions of the plantar aspect of the foot:
    a. Synovial cyst.
    b. Lesions not involving the metatarsophalangeal joint, such as a ganglion, a lipoma, or other soft tissue tumor.
    c. Tumor involving a metatarsal bone.

Treatment

The initial treatment of an interdigital neuroma should be conservative in nature. This consists of relieving pressure on the involved interspace. This is most easily accomplished by placing the patient into a low-heeled shoe with a broad toe box and soft sole material. A soft metatarsal support is placed in the shoe proximal to the metatarsal heads of the involved interspace. It has been our experience that a soft metatarsal support within the shoe is more effective than the use of a metatarsal bar or plastic orthosis. On occasion an anti-inflammatory medication, or even judicious use of local steroids, may be of benefit, although in my experience the success rate with these has been low.

Caution must be taken when injecting steroids into the interspace because if the joint capsule is injected it may result in degeneration of the joint capsule, and deviation of the toe may follow, or possibly atrophy of the plantar fat pad.

Approximately one-third of patients treated conservatively are satisfied with this method of treatment and their symptoms subside. The majority of patients, however, require surgical intervention.

Surgical Treatment

An interdigital neuroma should be excised through a dorsal approach made in the involved web space. The incision is made in the midline so as to avoid the small superficial dorsal cutaneous nerve that are present on either side of the web space. The incision is deepened directly in the midline, following which a Weitlaner is expanded, the transverse metatarsal ligament is placed under tension and is cut. This exposes the tissues beneath, which consist of the neurovascular bundle and the plantar fat. Working cautiously in a longitudinal manner, utilizing a neurologic freer, the surgeon readily identifies the nerve just proximal to the transverse metatarsal ligament and traces it distally just beyond the bifurcation of the nerve. The common digital nerve is now traced proximally to the level of the neck of the metatarsal, where it is cut sharply and allowed to retract. If it is noted that the common digital nerve makes a very oblique angle beneath the metatarsal head, so that when it is cut it will retract to lie beneath the metatarsal head, then an effort is made to cut the nerve more distal and then to suture the nerve to the side of the metatarsal just proximal to the metatarsal head. This is done in order to prevent a stump neuroma from forming underneath a metatarsal head when this anatomic alignment is present.

If some other type of pathology is present within the interspace, such as a synovial cyst, this too can be excised through the same dorsal approach. When carrying out any type of a dissection looking for a synovial cyst or a ganglion within the plantar fat pad, care should be taken to preserve as much of the plantar fat pad as possible to prevent unnecessary scarring within this tissue that might result in metatarsalgia. Following the excision of the neuroma, which is carried out under tourniquet control, the wound is closed in a single layer and a compression dressing applied. The patient is ambulated postoperatively in a wooden shoe for approximately three weeks, following which the patient is permitted to resume activities as tolerated. Preferably the patient should not return to narrow, high-heeled shoes or high impact activities such as running for at least two months from the time of surgery.

Complications

As mentioned, we prefer to excise the neuroma through a dorsal approach. Although some surgeons use a plantar approach to remove a neuroma, at times a painful plantar scar occurs, which unfortunately is in a weight-bearing area. If a scar becomes hyperkeratotic, the fat pad atrophic, or by chance the cut end of the nerve becomes adherent within the scar tissue, this may result in a significant problem. Not only does the patient have a painful scar, but the treatment of such a condition is very difficult. Unfortunately, not infrequently following the excision of a neuroma through a plantar approach, there is some atrophy of the plantar fat pad, which may cause metatarsalgia.

Results

In a review of excisions of interdigital neuromas carried out in my private practice,[13] it was noted that 80 percent of patients believed that they were substantially improved by the surgery; six percent felt that they were improved but still had some tenderness on the plantar aspect of the foot; and 14 percent believed that the surgery did not significantly change their preoperative symptom complex.

This group of patients was carefully studied, and no specific etiology could be determined for their continued postoperative complaints. None of these patients went on to develop any type of other condition in the metatarsophalangeal joint which had been misdiagnosed prior to the excision of the neuroma. It is for this reason that patients with a neuroma should be treated conservatively and should be informed that there is possibility that excision of the neuroma may not necessarily represent a panacea but that indeed there is a failure rate of about 15 percent. A small percentage of patients noted numbness in the web space and some had numbness on the plantar aspect of the foot in an area of about 2 cm adjacent to the web space. Some patients interpret this numbness as walking on a lump on the bottom of the foot.

Recurrent Neuromas

At times following excision of a neuroma the patient initially experiences relief, only to have the symptoms recur anywhere from six months to several years later. This is often called "recurrent neuroma," although in reality it is the only true neuroma that the patient has experienced. It is well known that following transection of a nerve a traumatic neuroma will form over the free end of the nerve, and this is what has occurred in these patients with a recurrent neuroma. This can be an extremely frustrating problem for both the patient and the physician.

The diagnosis of the recurrent neuroma is based upon the history given by the patient of recurrent symptoms as well as on the physical findings. The physical examination usually demonstrates an area of rather exquisite tenderness which is localized to the plantar aspect of the foot, usually beneath a metatarsal head or adjacent to the interspace. Associated with this area of tenderness is a positive Tinel's sign, which I believe is the best evidence that a recurrent neuroma exists.

The conservative management of a recurrent neuroma is the same as that for a virgin neuroma, namely adequate padding to relieve weight bearing, and proper shoe wear. If the symptoms persist, the re-exploration of the interspace is indicated.

The surgical technique that we prefer is, again, through a dorsal approach, but through a slightly longer incision. A Weitlaner is used to spread the metatarsal heads apart and place the transverse metatarsal ligament on stretch. Even if the transverse metatarsal ligament has been cut previously, it reforms postoperatively. Once the transverse metatarsal ligament has been cut, it is easier to search for the common digital nerve as proximally as possible, so that hopefully one is working within virgin fat, which makes the identification of the common digital nerve much simpler. The nerve is then traced distally, again utilizing a neurologic freer to carefully free the nerve from its surrounding tissue, following which it is transected at a more proximal level. Other authors have discussed the possibility of going in through a plantar approach and burying the nerve within bone or muscle, but again we prefer not to place a scar on the plantar aspect of the foot if possible.

Postoperatively the patient is treated the same as for a virgin neuroma, as already discussed.

The results following excision of a recurrent neuroma demonstrate that approximately 70 percent of patients have a satisfactory result, but 30 percent persist in having pain of varying degrees on the plantar aspect of the foot. The reason this occurs remains an enigma.

Based upon our own series of patients who had a neuroma excised, it is was noted that in approximately 60 percent of the patients numbness occurred in the web space as well as in a small localized area on the plantar aspect of the foot adjacent to the web space. This area of numbness is occasionally bothersome to the patient, particularly in the immediate postoperative period, but as a general rule it fades away and becomes minimally symptomatic. Patients also at times following surgery complain of the feeling that they are walking on a lump on the plantar aspect of the foot, but again this feeling usually diminishes in time.

References

1. Keck C: The tarsal tunnel syndrome. J.B.J.S. 44A:180, 1962.
2. Lam SJS: Tarsal tunnel syndrome. J.B.J.S. 49B:87, 1967.
3. Mann RA: The tarsal tunnel syndrome. Orthop Clin North Am 5:109, 1974.
4. Wilemon WK: Tarsal tunnel syndrome. Orthop Rev 8(11):111, 1979.
5. Baker LD, Kuhn HH: Morton's metatarsalgia. South Med J 37:123, 1944.
6. Durlacher L: A treatise on Corns, Bunions, the Disease of Nails and the General Management of the Feet. Simpkin, Marshall, London, 1845, p 52.
7. DuVries, HL: Surgery of the Foot, 2nd. Ed. St. Louis, The C.V. Mosby Co., 1965.

8. Graham CE, Graham DM: Morton's neuroma: A microscopic evaluation. Foot Ankle 5(2):150, 1984.
9. Graham CE, Johnson KA, Ilstrup DM: The intermetatarsal nerve: A microscopic evaluation. Foot Ankle 2:150, 1981.
10. Jones JR, Klenerman L: A study of the communicating branch between the medial and lateral plantar nerves. Foot Ankle 4(6):313, 1984.
11. Lassmann G: Morton's toe: Clinical, light, and electron microscopic investigations in 133 cases. Clin Orthop 142:73, 1979.
12. McElvenny RT: Etiology and surgical treatment of intractable pain about the fourth metatarsophalangeal joint (Morton's toe) J Bone Joint Surg 25:675, 1943.
13. Mann RA, Reynolds JC: Interdigital neuroma: A critical clinical analysis. Foot Ankle 3:238, 1983.
14. Morton DJ: The Human Foot: Its Evolution, Physiology and Functional Disorders. New York, Columbia University Press, 1935, pp 184 and 211.
15. Morton TG: A peculiar and painful affection of the fourth metatarsophalangeal articulation, Am J Med Sci 71:37, 1876.
16. Morton TSK: Metatarsalgia (Morton's painful affection of the foot). Tr Phila Acad Surg 1893.
17. Nissen KI: Plantar digital neuritis J Bone Joint Surg 30B:84, 1948.

CHAPTER 20

Pudendal and Peroneal Nerve Compression

Timothy J. Bray, M.D.,
and Ross K. Leighton, M.D.

Pudendal Nerve Compression

Anatomy

Lindenbaum, Fleming and Smith have elegantly described the pudendal nerve anatomy, and this discussion reflects their most recent work.[1] The pudendal nerve complex arises from the second, third, and fourth sacral nerves. Once these nerve roots exit the pelvis, the pudendal nerve regains its intrapelvic course by passing under the sacrotuberous ligament. With a rich vascular supply, the nerve passes anteriorly near the intrapelvic wall in dense fascia called the obturator fascia or Alcock's Canal (Fig. 20-1 and 20-2). The inferior rectal nerve, which is responsible for sphincter tone and perianal sensation, is one of the first branches. Where the urogenital diaphragm and levator ani muscles meet, the pudendal nerve divides into the perineal nerve and dorsal nerve of the penis (Fig. 20-3). The perineal nerve supplies scrotal sensation, and the muscular branches of the pudendal nerve supply the transversis perinei superficialis, the bulbocavernosus, the ischiocavernosus, transversus perinei profundus and sphincter urethrae. The dorsal nerve of the penis gives off terminal branches to the corpus cavernosum.

The functional deficits associated with pudendal nerve palsies are great. The complex neurologic interactions for erection and ejaculation involve both distal sensory impulses and major motor nerve reflex arcs. In the 1950s and early 1960s unilateral or bilateral pudendal neurectomies were reported to result in a 50 to 60 percent rate of impotence. In addition to the problem of impotence was the loss of perianal and perivaginal sensation. From this

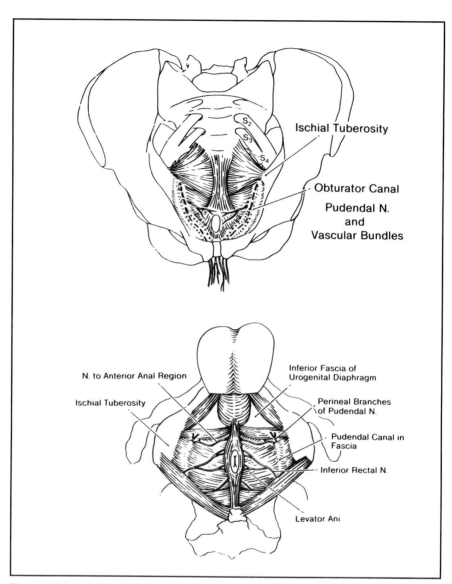

Figures 20-1 and 20-2. With approval, Lindenbaum, Fleming and Smith. Journal of Bone and Joint Surgery, Vol. 64-A, Number 6, July, 1982. p. 934-938.

experience we now know the critical importance of preserving function of the pudendal nerve.

Due to the close proximity of the pudendal nerve and its terminal branches to the pelvis, the pelvic and hip surgeon unfortunately must negotiate these critical complexes and painstakingly protect them from injury during surgical procedures.

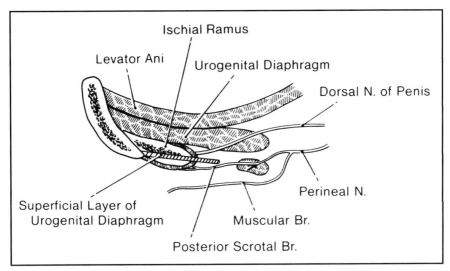

Ischial Ramus

Levator Ani   Urogenital Diaphragm

Dorsal N. of Penis

Superficial Layer of
Urogenital Diaphragm

Perineal N.

Muscular Br.

Posterior Scrotal Br.

Figure 20-3. Division of inferior rectal nerve to perineal nerve and dorsal nerves of the penis. (With approval, Lindenbaum, Fleming and Smith. Journal of Bone and Joint Surgery, Vol. 64-A, Number 6, July, 1982. p. 934-938.)

The Problem

Operative management of hip, femur, and pelvic fractures has demonstrated predictably good results during the past decade. Smith Peterson[3] initiated the operative management of hip fractures, which significantly reduced patient mortality and returned patients to ambulatory status with high rates of success. Professor Gerhardt Kuntscher[4] described intramedullary nailing of the femur which today is the method of choice for treating femoral shaft fractures, and Professor Emile LeTournel[5] has described excellent results in the operative treatment of acetabular and pelvic fractures, which is now an accepted alternative to long term traction. However, the great interest in the operative management of fractures has its drawbacks.

In order to manipulate bones of the pelvis and femur, which are surrounded by strong muscle masses, the fracture table has become the mainstay of intra-operative reduction. By stabilizing the pelvis on a perineal post attached to the fracture table and applying distal counter-traction, forces can be generated to assist reduction. There are disadvantages to the use of the fracture table, including skin complications, fixed patient positions, and potential compression neuropathies around the pelvis. Specifically, the proximity of the pudendal nerve to the ischial tuberosity (Fig. 20-2) creates the potential for iatrogenic injury during reduction maneuvers utilizing the perineal post. Although pudendal nerve palsies are found infrequently associated with pelvic surgery, they should be considered in any of the following procedures;

1. Pelvic Fracture Fixation
2. Acetabular Fracture Fixation
3. Hip Fracture Fixation

4. Tumor Resection
5. Children's Pelvic Osteotomy

Pelvic and Acetabular Fractures

LeTournel,[5] Mears[6] and others have demonstrated excellent results with the operative treatment of pelvic fractures. Use of the fracture table and the perineal post are an integral part of fracture reduction at the time of surgery and, therefore, pose a potential problem of compression to the pudendal nerve complex. The fracture table and perineal post are used for temporary reduction of pelvic fractures in the supine, prone, and lateral decubitus positions. Currently, the main indication for open reduction and internal fixation of pelvic fractures is the unstable Malgaigne fracture, frequently referred to as the vertical shear injury. The sacroiliac joint and the pubic symphysis have both been disrupted, leaving the entire hemipelvis unstable.

After obtaining temporary reduction using skeletal traction in the hopsital, the patient is brought to the operating room and placed on the fracture table in the prone position. Using distal femoral skeletal pins, a significant distracting force can be applied that aids the surgeon in reducing the proximally migrated hemipelvis. To reduce the amount of traction force necessary to obtain a reduction intra-operatively, it is imperative that the

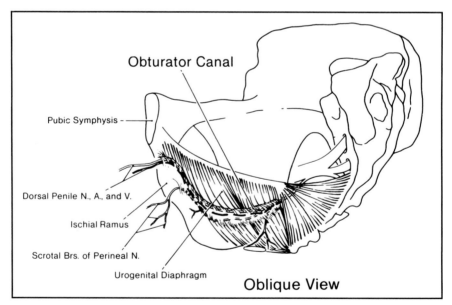

Figure 20-4A. Anatomic relationships of the scrotal branches to the perineal nerve. (With approval, Lindenbaum, Fleming and Smith. Journal of Bone and Joint Surgery, Vol. 64-A, Number 6, July, 1982. p. 934-938.)

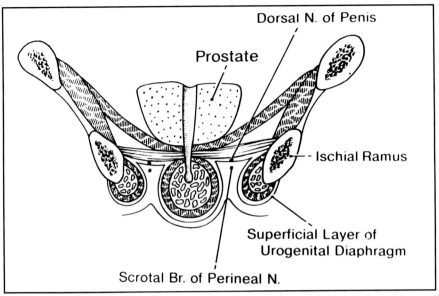

Figure 20-4B. Table I—Perineal pressure significantly reduced by increasing size of perineal post. (With approval, Lindenbaum, Fleming and Smith. Journal of Bone and Joint Surgery, Vol. 64-A, Number 6, July, 1982. p. 934-938.)

fracture be reduced preoperatively in skeletal traction. This will assist the surgeon and protect the pudendal nerve and the distal sensory branches intra-operatively.

After this reduction maneuver, the sacroiliac joint can be stabilized. With the aid of fluoroscopy, the sacroiliac joint is fixed with two large cancellous screws placed from the outer ilium across the sacroiliac joint to the sacral ala. The pubic symphysis can then be stabilized using plate fixation with the patient supine. The pudendal nerve and distal branches are usually protected during this fixation as the approach is directly over the pubic symphysis and too superficial to cause injury.

Acetabular fractures are frequently operated on the fracture table and therefore the same care and protection of the pudendal nerve should be exercised as described in the operative management of pelvic fractures. Certain complex fracture patterns involve the pelvic bones close to the pudendal nerve in Alcock's canal. Due to the thick fascial coverage, the nerve is frequently spared from injury. However, internal fixation of these complex fractures is a potential source of iatrogenic injury. Uncontrolled or misguided drill bits, inappropriately applied reduction clamps, and long screws may damage the pudendal nerve at or near its course under the sacrotuberous ligament, or near the obturator canal. The dorsal nerve of the penis and perineal nerve must also be protected from the perineal post during reduction maneuvers as described for pelvic fractures.

Hip Fractures

Hip fractures have routinely been operated in the supine position on the fracture table with the perineal post placed between the legs and pressing against the pubic symphysis for pelvic stability. In all of these cases there are compressive forces to the pudendal nerve in its anatomic position against the pelvis. Schulak, Bear, and Summers discuss transient impotence resulting from pudendal nerve injury due to excessive perineal pressure during surgery. They conclude that traction should be the minimum necessary for reduction and should be released as soon as possible after stabilization of the fracture.

The true incidence of iatrogenically caused impotence in hip fracture patients may be greater than suspected. As opposed to fractures of the pelvis and femur found frequently in young sexually active males, fractures of the hip are found in the elderly, less sexually active population. Therefore, impotence secondary to overzealous pull on the perineal post during hip fracture fixation may go unreported.

Tumors

Complete or incomplete resections of the pubic symphysis, superior ramus, and inferior ramus may be indicated for the treatment of pelvic neoplasia, granulomatous infections, or other hematogenous bacterial infections. Many surgical approaches have been described; however, during any operative approach to the anterior pelvis, there is potential injury to the pudendal nerve complex.

Milch[7] described an approach using a large perineal incision from the anterior pelvis near the pubic symphysis and extending to the ischial tuberosity. This provides access to the pubic symphysis and body of the pubis. After the abductors, pectineus, and rectus abdominus muscles have been removed from bone, the pudendal vessels and nerves that emerge from the pelvis through the greater sciatic foramen must be protected. If the dissection is subperiosteal in this area, the pudendal neurovascular bundles can be easily protected. However, with overzealous soft tissue retraction, a compression or stretch neuropathy can occur. It is essential that all retractors be placed carefully near the bone so that no soft tissue interposition occurs.

Children

Many pelvic osteotomies have been described for the treatment of congenital hip dysplasia. Pelvic osteotomy can injure the pudendal nerve complex along its course from the central nerve to the dorsal penile sensory nerves. Sutherland and Greenfield[8] have described a double innominate osteotomy which is at particular risk. They have emphasized the importance of a subperiosteal dissection around the pubic symphysis, taking care to avoid damage to the internal pudendal artery which runs along the margin of the inferior pubic ramus. After the osteotomy of the pubic symphysis, a second osteotomy through the iliac wing is performed, thus allowing a free segment of pelvis to be rotated over the femoral head and increase femoral head coverage.

Hind quarter amputations or hemi-pelvectomies must also be performed with special care taken to protect the pudendal nerve complex. Retraction during large exposures to the acetabulum and pelvis are also dangerous, and careful soft tissue techniques should always be utilized.

Clinical Studies Investigating Pressure on the Pudendal Nerve

Lindenbaum, Fleming, and Smith measured the pressure exerted in the perineal region during actual and simulated closed femoral reaming using a semi-conductor transducer connected to a computer. Volunteers as patients were placed on a fracture table in the lateral position. Three sizes of perineal posts were studied—a normal 3 cm diameter post, a 3 cm diameter post with 1.5 cm diameter thick rolled cotton used as padding, and a 9 cm diameter post without an outer layer of padding. The amount of pressure exerted against the perineal post was compared to the number of turns of the traction crank on the fracture table.

The results of this study, summarized in Table I, clearly demonstrate that the large diameter post and the smaller post with padding produced far less perineal pressure than the smaller diameter post without padding. This demonstratres that a well designed perineal post can decrease pressure in the perineum, thereby decreasing the likelihood of compression neuropathy.

Table 20-1. Perineal Pressure Readings on Twenty Volunteers

No. of Turns of Traction Crank	Perineal Pressure* (kg/cm²)		
	Post I	Post II	Post III
0	0	0	0
10	1.4	0.7	0.7
20	3.5	1.2	1.2
25	6.3	1.4	1.4
30	9.1	2.1	1.4
40	—	2.8	1.9
45	—	2.8	1.9
50	—	3.5	2.1
60	—	4.2	2.6
70	—	4.9	2.6

*Post I — three-centimeter diameter without padding; Post II — three-centimeter diameter with 1.5 centimeters of padding; and Post III — nine-centimeter diameter without padding.

Perineal pressure significantly reduced by increasing size of perineal post. (With approval, Lindenbaum, Fleming and Smith. Journal of Bone and Joint Surgery, Vol. 64-A, Number 6, July, 1982, p. 934-938).

Schuleck, Bear, and Summers[9] suggested that iatrogenic nerve injuries can occur when a large traction force is required to distract fractures for more than three hours, which would likely result in sufficient perineal compression to cause impotence.

These clinical studies indicate that traction force and duration of applied traction are variables which can be controlled by the surgeon to reduce the risk of pudendal nerve injury.

Recommendations for Prevention of Pudendal Nerve Injury

Pre-operative Planning

To decrease the amount of axial pull required to reduce femoral shaft or hip fractures, patients should be kept in skeletal traction preoperatively. By keeping the fragments out to length and in their appropriate anatomic position preoperatively, a very minimal amount of distal axial pull is required intraoperatively. The fracture table can then be used simply as a positioning tool rather than as a distracting tool for fracture reduction.

In the management of acetabular and pelvic fractures the fracture table is not necessarily required. Frequently, intraoperative distraction can be achieved with the AO/ASIF femoral distractor, (Fig. 20-5). The lateral decubitus position on the fracture table is potentially the most dangerous patient position for iatrogenic pudendal nerve compression. If the lower part of the patient's torso is partially supported by the fracture table, the resulting force vector in the perineum will be in a safer, vertically oriented direction. If a lower part of the torso is allowed to hang free so that all of the force is carried by the perineal post, the force will then be directed toward the branches of the pudendal nerve as they cross the ischial ramus, causing excessive compression against this bony prominence. For intramedullary nailing of the femur and certain approaches to the sacroiliac joint, the appropriate patient position laterally on the fracture table is demonstrated in Figure 20-6A and B.

Surgical Approaches

During surgical approaches to the superior ramus, pubic symphysis, inferior ramus, and the ischium, the pudendal nerve and its distal branches are at risk for injury. Patients should be informed of this risk preoperatively and all efforts should be made to prevent iatrogenic injury.

Pressure applied intraoperatively from an assistant's hand or the overzealous use of retractors can compress these nerves, especially during approaches that are in close anatomic proximity during superior pubic and inferior pubic ramus resections, as well as pelvic osteotomies. Care should be taken not to use towel clips or skin staples around the penis or vagina for fear of injury to these delicate sensory nerves. The surgeon should also drape enough room for pelvic surgery so that retraction is kept at a minimum. The surgical team should never try to make up for the

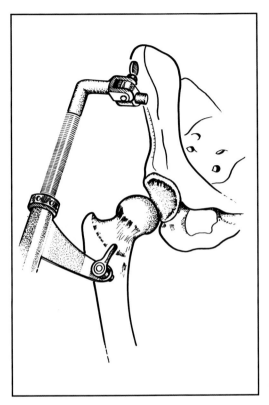

Figure 20-5. AO/ASIF femoral distractor can be used to sublux the hip for acetabular articular visualization and intra-operative reduction for certain acetabular and pelvic fractures.

lack of space from an inadequate drape by overzealous retraction on the soft tissues. Finally, review of the anatomy preoperatively is mandatory when operating in the floor of the pelvis. It is of great benefit to dissect a cadaver pelvis preoperatively or to ask for the assistance of a surgeon familiar with pelvic anatomy prior to undertaking these often difficult orthopaedic approaches.

Perineal Post:

The perineal posts most commonly available are 3, 5, or 8 centimeters in diameter. It is clear from the data on Lindenbaum, Fleming, and Smith[1] that the larger diameter post exerts less pressure. Since pressure as low as 1.4 kg per square centimater for 90 minutes can produce severe nerve conduction deficiencies, a large well-padded perineal post is preferred. Distraction techniques using the perineal post for fracture reduction should be used for the shortest intra-operative time possible. When the skeletal fixation is complete, the reduction pressure from the fracture table should be released as soon as possible.

Anesthetic Assistance:

Large muscle forces are required to maintain the upright position across the hips, knees, and ankles. Most of the large muscle forces can be

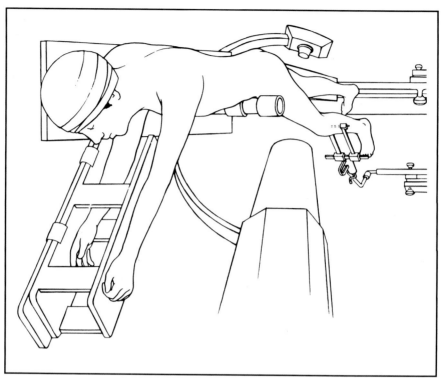

Figure 20-6A. The lateral patient position for intramedullary nailing of the femur as seen from the head of the table. Set-up represents position for left femoral nailing. Upper body and torso stabilized with stacked armboard, contralateral leg adducted to allow fluoroscopy unit to swing free and fractured leg slightly flexed and pulled into upright bar of perineal post for countertraction. All peripheral nerves are well-padded and protected. (With approval, Chapman, M., Upjohn: Strategies in Orthopaedic Surgery, Volume 4, Number 1, January, 1985.)

completely neutralized intraoperatively by the use of anesthetic agents for total muscle paralysis. By relaxing these large muscles, the amount of traction necessary to obtain anatomic reduction during operative fixation is greatly decreased. In the case of pelvic surgery where temporary over-distraction is necessary for bony reduction or hip joint inspection, muscle relaxation is mandatory. It is the responsibility of the operating surgeon to request the assistance of his anesthesiologist in these difficult reductions.

Peroneal Nerve Compression

Anatomy

The common peroneal nerve, a branch of the sciatic nerve, has its origins from the L4, L5, S1, and S2 plexes.[10] It may be differentiated from the tibial branch of the sciatic nerve as far proximal as the sciatic notch, but does not become a separate branch until the level of adductor canal. It

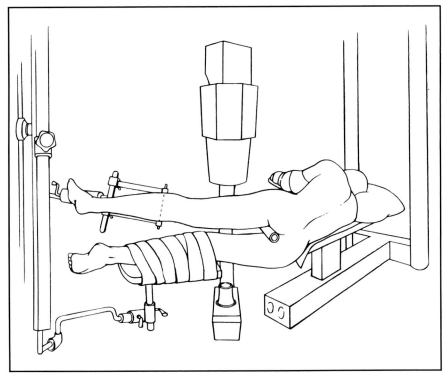

Figure 20-6B. Lateral patient positioning for closed intramedullary nailing of the left femur as seen from surgical viewpoint. Note adducted right leg to allow easy fluoroscopic access to fracture visualization.

then separates, posterior and medial, at the head of the biceps femoris. It lies between the tendon of the biceps femoris and the lateral head of the gastrocnemius (Fig. 20-7). It becomes superficial at the biceps femoral insertion and passes around the neck of the fibula. It then passes anteriorly through a foramen near the attachment of the long peroneal muscle group, where it divides into two branches—the superficial peroneal and deep peroneal nerve.

There are three articular branches at this level; one accompanies the superior, another the inferior lateral geniculate, and the third branch is the recurrent articular nerve which arises near the point of decussation of the common peroneal nerve and ascends with the anterior recurrent tibial artery (Fig. 20-8). The cutaneous branches frequently arise from a common trunk, the lateral cutaneous nerves of the calf, or the sural communicating branches.

The deep peroneal nerve begins at the bifurcation of the common peroneal nerve, between the fibula and the proximal part of the peroneus longus. It passes obliquely forward deep to the extensor digitorum longus. It then descends with the anterior tibial artery to the front of the ankle joint where it divides into lateral and medial terminal branches. In the

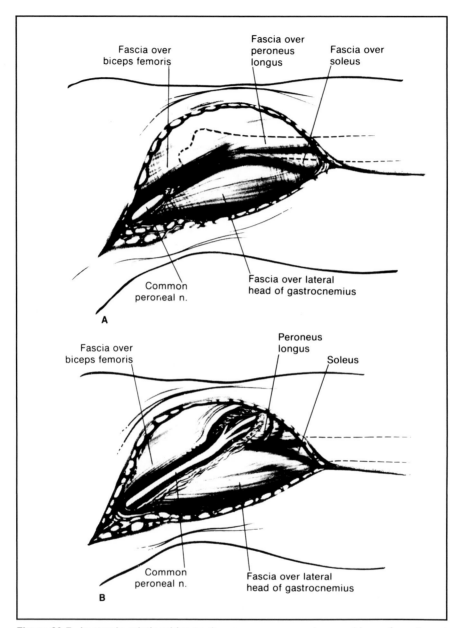

Figure 20-7. Anatomic relationships to the common peroneal nerve, biceps femoris and lateral head of the gastrocnemius. (With approval, Hoppenfield: Surgical Approaches in Orthopaedics. Lippincott, 1984, p. 454.)

leg the deep peroneal nerve supplies branches to the tibialis anterior, extensor digitorum longus, extensor hallucis longus, and the peroneous tertius.

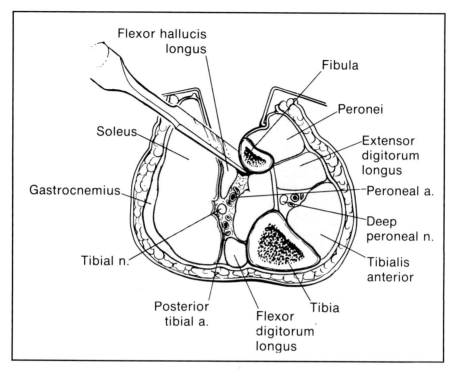

Figure 20-8. Anatomic relationships of the deep peroneal nerve and artery. (With approval, Hoppenfield: Surgical Approaches in Orthopaedics. Lippincott, 1984, p. 454, figure 10-17.)

Classification of Peroneal Injuries

1. Trauma
2. Compression
3. Ischemia & Surgical Insult
4. Skeletal Pins
5. Peripheral Neuropathy

Trauma

Hip Trauma

The peroneal nerve is frequently injured in high energy trauma to the lower extremity. The two most important prognostic variables are the level and type of injury.

Fracture dislocation of the hip or simple dislocations frequently traumatize the peroneal component of the sciatic nerve due to the lateral position of the peroneal nerve fibers in the sciatic sheath. Hip dislocation is a true orthopaedic emergency, and immediate reduction is indicated. Frequently, the palsy will spontaneously resolve. However, with posterior wall or posterior column acetabular fractures, the nerve may become entrapped in fracture fragments necessitating careful exploration at the time of open reduction and internal fixation.

Complete transection of the peroneal nerve at high levels may cause additional loss of part or all of the biceps femoris function of the hamstrings. The prognosis for functional return of the foot is generally poor with those injuries that require surgical repair or nerve grafting. With peroneal nerve lesions above midthigh, the axons usually do not regenerate rapidly enough to reverse the effects of prolonged distal denervation.

Knee

Injury to the peroneal nerve can be caused, at this level, by open fracture dislocations of the proximal tibia or by closed high energy injuries. Because of its superficial anatomic position, the peroneal nerve is particularly susceptible as it passes around the head of the fibula. Contusion, stretch, and compression have been implicated in these complete neuropathies of the peroneal nerve.

Peroneal palsy resulting from varus stress on the knee usually involves a lateral collateral ligament injury and sometimes is associated with rotational instability and/or anterior cruciate ligament injury. This neuropathy is usually caused by a stretching type of injury which is seen in high velocity motor vehicle injuries, falls from heights, and certain athletic injuries. The nerve is stretched in situ, and has an excellent chance of spontaneous recovery. Early exploration is generally contraindicated.[11]

A medial tibial plateau fracture can be seen in association with the ligamentous injuries to the knee mentioned above. If the palsy is identified pre-operatively and an open reduction is indicated, the nerve can then be explored. However, the great majority of the nerves are found intact, with the palsy caused by contusion or stretching. Therefore, early exploration is of limited benefit.

The lateral tibial plateau fracture is a more serious injury, especially with an associated fibular head fracture. In these associated fractures, a nerve palsy is more likely to be secondary to a laceration, and if open reduction is elected, nerve exploration is then indicated. If the fracture does not require operative treatment, immediate exploration of the nerve is seldom indicated.

A direct peroneal nerve contusion is frequently seen with associated soft tissue injuries and isolated proximal fibular head fractures.[12] The lateral knee area is usually swollen, ecchymotic, and frequently has associated ligamentous injuries.

It should always be remembered that injuries of the lower extremity can be associated with compartment syndromes. The index of suspicion should be high in any patient with a neurologic deficit associated with a fracture or major soft tissue injury of the leg. Compartment pressures and fasciotomy should be considered when swelling, pain with passive motion and distal sensory changes are present (see Chapter 3).

For most peroneal nerve injuries at the knee, a watch-and-wait treatment is the norm. The only absolute indications for exploration are lacerations with sharp objects such as knives, cuts, or industrial injuries. Severe lateral plateau fractures associated with fibular head fractures and a complete, preoperatively identified peroneal nerve palsy should be explored when open reduction is considered. Because the peroneal nerve sheath is attached to the periosteum of the fibula, stretch is a frequent component of nerve injury in this region, and therefore surgical correction is seldom possible.

The motor deficit accompanying peroneal nerve palsy involves the foot everters and dorsiflexion of the ankle and toes. This deficit is the so-called foot drop from the loss of the anterior tibial muscle. The extensor hallucis longus is always the first to lose function and usually the last to recover. In the interim period a polypropylene ankle-foot orthosis (AFO) will improve gait, and nerve recovery can be assessed with electromyographic studies beginning at six weeks after the injury.

Compression Injury

The peroneal nerve, as it crosses the fibular head and neck area, enters the lateral and anterior compartments of the leg in an area very susceptible to compression injury. One should be acutely aware of this susceptibility when applying dressings around the proximal tibia. Circular dressings and casts frequently end at this level. Their edges may compress the peroneal nerve. This can be avoided by applying long leg bulky dressings to the acutely injured lower extremity, especially when a patient is at bedrest. Short leg dressing and casts are frequently the cause of peroneal palsy in bedridden patients, as these patients tend to externally rotate the leg while lying in bed, thus pressing the edge of the cast or dressings into the nerve.

Peroneal nerve compression neuropathy can occur intraoperatively because of failure to pad the peroneal nerve appropriately during unusual patient positioning. It is the surgeon's responsibility to care for peripheral nerves during patient positioning.

The treatment of external compression-related peroneal nerve palsies is usually conservative and observational.[13] The great majority of these patients regain functional foot dorsiflexion strength by eight months, but frequently have a permanent extensor hallucis longus extension lag. There is no support for early exploration or decompression as improving the final functional outcome.

Ischemia and Related Orthopaedic Procedures

Ischemic peroneal nerve palsy accounts for a large group of patients with peroneal neuropathy and, possibly, is an explanation for some of the compression neuropathies as well.[14] Many authors have suggested that the superficial and unprotected portions of the nutrient artery to the nerve leave the nerve particularly susceptible to a pressure-induced ischemia. Roberts, in 1948 alluded to a patient with bacterial endocarditis who developed a popliteal nerve palsy and whose postmortem examination revealed thrombosis of the vasa vasorum in the center of the affected nerve.

Significant dissection around the posterior capsule of the hip has always carried a risk of sciatic nerve injury. Although an ischemic etiology is hard to scientifically prove, it has been suggested that surgical stripping of the perineurium during sciatic nerve exploration may result in focal ischemia and a functional neuropathy. Procedures that have been reported to occasionally result in sciatic nerve injury are total or hemi-arthroplasty of the hip, acetabular reconstruction, acetabular osteotomy, and open reduction of posterior hip dislocations.

Dissections around the fibular head and neck area are always dangerous due to the adherence of the peroneal nerve sheath to the fibular periosteum.[15] Related orthopaedic procedures that have been reported to cause peroneal nerve injuries in this area include reconstruction of the lateral tibial plateau, high tibial osteotomy, knee ligament replacement, knee arthroplasty, vascularized and nonvascularized fibular grafts, and tumor excisions.

All of these procedures carry an inherent risk of peroneal nerve palsy. Most, including tumor surgery, have an incidence of less than one percent. However, some authors have reported an incidence of up to five percent, especially with high tibial osteotomy when utilizing external pins and clamps.[16] The incidence of peroneal nerve injury in total knee replacement is approximately one percent, and is most likely related to direct traction on the nerve, traction on the syndesmosis causing a vascular compromise, or direct pressure dressings.[17] Once the palsy is discovered, loosening the dressing and flexing the knee is the treatment of choice. There is no indication for immediate exploration in these cases.

Skeletal Pins

Injury of the peroneal nerve can be caused by pins placed either for skeletal traction or for external skeletal fixation. Loose dressings are mandatory after pin placement for skeletal traction; the pin is frequently used to tether tight dressings around the fibular neck with resultant peroneal nerve injury. Good technique for skeletal pin placement is extremely important. The pins should be started laterally in the proximal tibia. As the pin passes from lateral to medial, the risk to the nerve is decreased as the pin exits medially. If the pin is placed from the medial portal, the pin can directly injure the nerve during uncontrolled or misguided lateral exit.

Care must be taken when placing external fixation pins in the proximal tibia as well. Peroneal nerve injury is more frequently encountered when transfixing pins are used with the quadralateral tibial external fixation frames. Recommendations currently include anterior or anteromedial half-pin frames rather than the transfixing pins. This places the pins anatomically medial to the proximal peroneal nerve and therefore decreases the chance of iatrogenic injury. If the nerve is injured with skeletal pin placement, exploration is indicated prior to removing or replacing the pin. The nerve or nerve sheath may be wrapped up in the pin threads and to remove it blindly may compound the injury.

Peripheral Neuropathies

The clinical diagnostic aspects of polyneuropathy is beyond the scope of this chapter but it is important to remember that a few genetic, metabolic and inflammatory conditions of peripheral nerves or roots may present as isolated mononeuropathies. These mononeuropathies may be misdiagnosed as entrapment neuropathies and therefore may lead to unnecessary peroneal nerve exploration.

Diagnostic Aids

The best method of detecting the level of nerve entrapment in the lower extremity continues to be the clinical exam. If the L5 nerve root is involved as opposed to an isolated peroneal nerve injury, there will usually be an associated weakness of the hamstrings or gluteus muscles. Electrophysiologic methods are less commonly used, but can be helpful in localizing lesions of the peroneal nerve.[19] Behse, et al. determined sensory and motor conduction along a 10 centimeter length of the peroneal nerve across the fibular head and compared it with the nerve velocity in the segment distal to the fibular head.[20] This procedure permits a lesion at the fibular head to be localized with great precision. The diagnostic yield can be increased by examining the motor and sensory fibers separately. This procedure has been used to localize lesions of the ulnar nerve and the cubital sulcus and of the radial nerve proximal to the elbow. The indication to perform this type of study is the patient in whom the clinical signs and symptoms leave doubt as to whether the peroneal palsy is due to involvement of the lumbar root or of the peripheral nerve.

Treatment

General Principles

The patient should be informed of the injury to the nerve and a plan should be outlined as to its treatment and followup. The acute management depends on the type of injury, but a common factor is the necessity of applying a dorsiflexion cast or splint to hold the foot in a neutral position during the recovery phase. The equinus deformity or fixed plantar flexion contracture is an avoidable complication. A very functional type of orthosis is the inexpensive polypropylene ankle-foot orthosis with removable velcro straps. This type of removable orthosis is more comfortable for the patient, is cosmetically acceptable, and can easily be removed for hygenic care.

When assessing recovery after an injury, muscle activity can be noted for the first time at the distal aspect of the fibula. The peroneal muscles that evert the foot are the first to return, followed by the anterior tibial muscle group. The extensor digitorum communis and the extensor hallucis longus are the last to return.

Open Injuries with Peroneal Palsies

The most common area for open peroneal nerve injury is the proximal fibula. With associated open fractures of the fibula and/or tibia, the wounds should be taken immediately to the operating room for formal irrigation, debridement and stabilization. If the nerve is felt by the surgeon to be at risk during methods of fixation and debridement, the nerve should be exposed and protected. With high energy trauma and open fractures, these nerves may be lacerated in association with the bony injuries. This can be suggested by the physical examination and x-ray characteristics of the fracture. If the nerve is explored and found to be clean and not associated with gross contamination, then microsurgical technique can be employed to repair these nerves acutely. However, in the face of severe crush, gross contamination requiring multiple debridements, or segmental nerve loss, then a delayed reconstruction of the nerve is advised. If physical examination of fracture characteristics do not suggest nerve injury, as is usually the case, exploration is not indicated.

Closed Injuries

Most closed injuries of the fibular head or proximal tibia associated with peroneal nerve palsies are direct contusions to the nerve. These injuries usually result in a neurapraxia and the treatment in this situation is conservative. These nerves should not be explored unless the elective incision to operate the closed fracture in that area passes directly in the anatomic position of the peroneal nerve. The patient is followed both clinically and electromyographically. The EMG's will detect nerve regeneration long before the patient is clinically able to dorsiflex his foot. The first electromyographic study should be obtained at six weeks; with progressive clinical evidence of return, no further EMG studies are indicated.

If there is no EMG of clinical recovery by three months, then it is recommended to consider exploration. It appears that the best time for exploration is between the third and fifth month, when the extent of intraneural fibrosis is easily assessed. In this fashion the neurapraxic lesion is less likely to be explored unnecessarily. Although up to ten centimeters of nerve have been reported resected and primarily repaired, it has become well-accepted that tension on any nerve repair is deleterious to function return. Nerve grafting using intrafascicular technique is the method of choice when reconstructing large segmental injuries. Despite the technical advances in microsurgery, the functional return of the peroneal nerve following nerve repair has been less than optimal. Therefore, with an injury at a low level, serious consideration should be given to transferring the posterior tibial muscle through the interosseous membrane at the dorsum of the foot to assist in foot dorsiflexion.[21] The patient will, therefore, have an active foot dorsiflexor during the recovery phase and his or her rehabilitation will not be prolonged should peroneal nerve return be delayed.

NOTE: The authors wish to thank Ms. Stephanie Griffith for her technical assistance in the preparation of this manuscript.

References

1. Lindenbaum SB, Fleming LL, Smith DW: Pudendal-nerve palsies associated with closed intramedullary femoral fixation. J Bone Joint Surg 64A:934, 1982.
2. Weiss HD: The physiology of human penile erection. Ann Intern Med 76:793, 1972.
3. Smith-Peterson MN, et al: Intracapsular fractures of the neck of the femur-treatment by internal fixation. Arch Surg 23:715, 1931.
4. Kuntscher G: Die Marknagelung von Knochenbruchen. Arch F Klin Chir 200:443, 1940.
5. LeTournel E, Judet R: Fractures of the acetabulum. New York, Springer-Verlag, 1981.
6. Mears DC, Rubash HE: Pelvic and acetabular fractures. Thorofare, NJ, Slack Inc, 1986.
7. Milch H: in Campbell's Operative Orthopaedics, St. Louis, C.V. Mosby, 1980, Vol. II, p. 1289.
8. Sutherland DH, Greenfield R: J Bone Joint Surg 59A:1082, 1977.
9. Schulak DJ, Bear TF, Summers JL: Transient impotence from positioning on the fracture table. J Trauma 20:420, 1980.
10. Gray's Anatomy, 28th Edition, Philadelphia, Lea & Febiger, 1969.
11. White J: The results of traction injuries to the common peroneal nerve. J Bone Joint Surg 50B:346, 1968.
12. Bateman SE: Trauma to nerves in limbs. Philadelphia. W.B. Saunders, 1962.
13. Waltman H: Crossing the legs as a factor in the production of peroneal palsy. J Am Med Assoc 93:670, 1929.
14. Ferguson FJ, Liversedge LA: Ischemic lateral popliteal nerve palsy. British Medical Journal. August 1934. p. 333.
15. Kettlekamp DB, Brueckman FR: Proximal tibial osteotomy. Orthop Clin North Am 21:3, 1982.
16. Kettlekamp DB, Leach RE, Wasca R: Pitfalls of proximal tibial osteotomy. Clin Orthop 106:232, 1975.
17. Rose HA, Hood RN, Otis JC, Ranawat CS, Insall, JN: Peroneal nerve palsy following total knee replacement. J Bone Joint Surg 64A:347, 1982.
18. Berry H, Richardson P: Common peroneal nerve palsy: a clinical and electrophysiological review. J Neurol Neurosurg Psychiatry 30:1162, 1976.
19. Singh N, Behse F, Buchthal F: Electrophysiological Study of Peroneal Palsy. J Neurol Neurosurg Psychiatry 30:1202, 1976.
20. Behse F, Buchthal F: Normal Sensory Conduction for the Nerves of the Leg in Man. J Neurol Neurosurg Psychiatry 34:404, 1971.
21. Hudson A, Waddell JP: Peroneal Nerve Injuries. Personal Communication, 1986.

Index